A Promise Kept:
One Son's Quest for the *Cause* and *Cure* of Dis-ease

by

James Chappell, D.C., N.D., Ph.D., M.H.

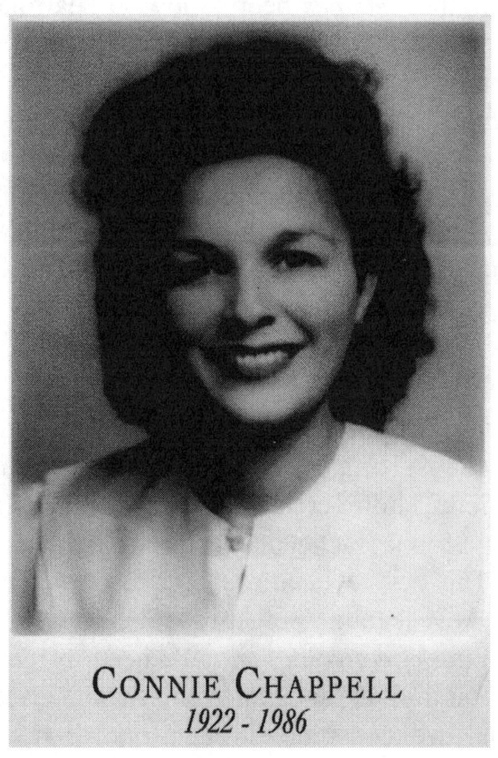

CONNIE CHAPPELL
1922 - 1986

This book is dedicated to the first person who loved me unconditionally, my mother, Constance Marie Chappell. I will *never* forget her kindness, guidance and devotion.

A Promise Kept:
One Son's Quest for the *Cause* and *Cure* of Dis-ease

by

James Chappell, D.C., N.D., Ph.D., M.H.

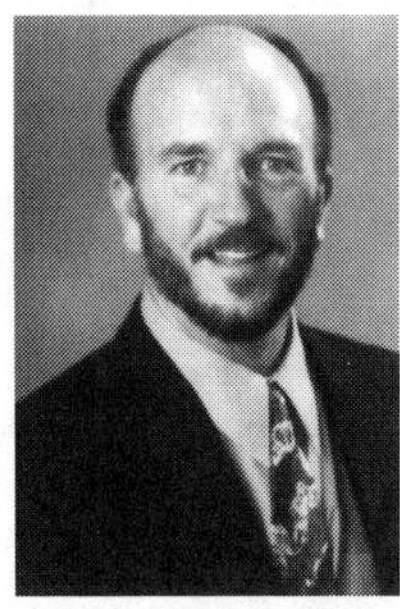

James Chappell is a chiropractic (D.C.) and naturopathic (N.D.) physician, clinical nutritionist (Ph.D.) and medical herbalist (M.H.). Since 1971, he has been a health *researcher* and *educator* specializing in chronic, severe and so-called "terminal" illnesses. He does not *treat* "disease," but rather *teaches* people how to heal themselves using classical, aboriginal, advanced quantum energy and natural healing protocols from around the world.

He is the president of Chappell Consulting Services, founder and formulator of QCI Products®, vice president of Heart to Heart Media/Publishing and former producer/co-host of The Shoong & Chappell Show aired on KTMS radio Santa Barbara, California. Dr. Chappell is a noted author, internationally recognized medical consultant and a leading authority on natural healing. In addition to having helped over 10,000 people, he worked ten years as a lot doctor at Universal, MGM, Paramount and Burbank studios in Hollywood, California providing healthcare to actors, producers and directors.

Whether consulting, participating in seminars, radio or television interviews, infomercials, writing articles, newsletters or books, Dr. Chappell is a teacher's teacher and a whole-food nutrition purist, stating, "The key to health is *not* treatment, be it natural or orthodox. The key is and has always been *love* and *attention*, *education* and taking *effective action*. We need to remember that we are what we eat, assimilate and don't eliminate. Caution should be taken as to what we consume through our food, air, water and especially our *minds*. I have devoted my entire adult life to sharing the wisdom contained in nature and what befalls us when we ignore Her. Ignorance is definitely *not* bliss and hence we continue to suffer because of it. Nothing is more important than our health. Nothing. The laws of nature are without negotiation. The key is in understanding and adapting to them. Those who fail to take the time to be healthy will ultimately have to take the time to be sick."

Dis-ease is defined as lack of ease or harmony, it is NOT the same as "disease," a medical term for illness treated by medicine. *NEVER* attempt to stop or reduce your medication without the supervision of your medical doctor.

Congratulations!

During my 34 years specializing in chronic, severe and so-called "terminal" illnesses, I spent the last 20 years researching the true *cause* and *effect* of dis-ease. You are about to learn the results of this valuable data reflecting my life's work.

This book is *not* a quick-fix approach to eating all the sugar, junk food, pasta, bread and animal flesh you want; without worry - because you are taking just *one magic pill.*

This book is *not* about taking pills, even vitamins or herbs, to be used as another *drug* to live a life in violation of the natural laws of good nutrition. I will teach you how to *prevent* and *cure* dis-ease, not *treat* it. You will learn how to truly nourish and heal the body, thereby achieving optimum health and longevity. This book is also about giving the body what it requires for only the body knows what it needs and when it needs it. If you are sick and tired of being sick and tired and you want to experience the healing benefits of *effective* natural healing, this book is for you.

Please Note: If you understand The H.O.N.S.T.E.C. Syndrome (see Chapter Two) and follow the four step protocol outlined in Chapter Six, most of all the condition specific nutraceuticals and botanicals recommended by well meaning healthfood store representatives and practicing natural healers, will NOT be necessary. Give your body foundational elements first and see what happens. You can always do more, if needed.

Government Ordered Disclaimer

[This book does *not* intend to diagnose, treat, cure or prevent any "*disease*," even if it does. The information herein is presented for educational purposes only and is *best* used in cooperation with your natural healing doctor. In the event the reader uses the within information to solve their own health problems, they are treating themselves, which is still (hopefully) their constitutional right. The author and publisher assume no responsibility or liability.]

Dis-ease is defined as lack of ease or harmony, it is NOT the same as "disease," a medical term for illness treated by medicine. *NEVER* attempt to stop or reduce your medication without the supervision of your medical doctor.

A Promise Kept:
One Son's Quest for the *Cause* and *Cure* of Dis-ease

© Copyright 2005 by Dr. James Chappell

1st Edition

October 19, 2005

Copyright © 2005 by Dr, James Chappell. All rights reserved. No part of this book may be reproduced or transmitted by any means, electronic or mechanical, without written permission from the publisher:

BL Publications, Detroit Lakes, MN

USA Distribution: Health Resources
Placenta, CA
1-714-223-1199
1-800-924-1907
www.naturalhealingnetwork.com

Library of Congress Cataloging-in-Publication Data
James Chappell
A Promise Kept: One Son's Quest for the Cause and Cure of Dis-ease / James Chappell
p. cm. --First Edition
Includes bibliographical references and index.
ISBN 1-890766-3563995

Cover Design by Frank Boross; Graphic artist: Olga Singer;
Edited by Connie Anderson; Nicole Shoong and Rose D. Sigman

NOTICE

This book is entirely *my* opinion based on 34 years of research, education and clinical experience. It does not represent any other individual, company, organization or association. To the contrary, I know no one save *G. Edward Griffin*, who are willing to say what you are about to read other than a few *natural healers* several of whom are currently serving prison terms for telling the truth. As long as we have a United States Constitution guaranteeing our *Freedom of Speech*, I will continue to voice *my* opinion.

Yours for health freedom, Dr. James Chappell

Dis-ease is defined as lack of ease or harmony, it is NOT the same as "disease," a medical term for illness treated by medicine. *NEVER* attempt to stop or reduce your medication without the supervision of your medical doctor.

FOREWORD
by
NICOLE SHOONG

What you are about to read will change your views on what you previously thought orthodox medicine was all about. If you already know these facts, it will offer further insight to help you stay healthy, feel better and look younger. No one can pull the wool over your eyes after reading this book. Remember, "The truth shall set you free."

Dr. Chappell's intuitive gifts are so varied and profound, and for sake of space, I will only mention one.

Throughout his career Dr. Jim, as he is affectionately called, has sought out and studied with some of the finest doctors and healers of our day, traveling to their clinics in the United States and Mexico. He's lived with shaman on their native lands, acquiring their herbal remedies and taught their mystic ways. You will learn about many of these amazing healers and their techniques in this priceless book.

In addition to Dr. Jim's academic accomplishments, his keen insight into the nature of dis-ease far exceeds even the gifts of the renowned medical intuit, Edgar Cayce.

One day while out about town, Dr. Jim and I ran into Carolyn McCabe, an old friend of the doctor's. "Jimmy," she said, grabbing his arm, "I've gone to three specialists for a terrible ear problem and tomorrow I'm scheduled for surgery. They think I have a brain tumor. What should I do?"

Dr. Jim asked her to explain her symptoms. She began with details of excruciating pain with a deafening non-stop ringing noise in her left ear. Suddenly, Dr. Jim said, "Stop, you don't have to say any more." Carolyn looked startled while the doctor told her not to have surgery for it could damage her inner ear, causing hearing loss. He also said, "You don't have a tumor." He told her to make up a certain herbal and oil mixture, and before bed, place three drops in her ear, then cover with cotton. He assured her, she would be fine in the morning.

Dis-ease is defined as lack of ease or harmony, it is NOT the same as "disease," a medical term for illness treated by medicine. *NEVER* attempt to stop or reduce your medication without the supervision of your medical doctor.

That little encounter took less than five minutes. Carolyn and I were literally speechless, to say the least. As Dr. Jim and I continued to walk, I asked how he knew what was wrong with her ear? He replied matter-of-factly, “I just saw her inner ear in my mind and the ossicles were dry and hot. She has lost her lubrication. Kind of simple, really.”

The next morning Carolyn called Dr. Jim, excited and relieved, almost shouting, “Jimmy, the pain is completely gone, my ear is totally better. I canceled the surgery! Thank-you, thank-you, thank-you!”

Throughout the six years I have worked with Dr. Chappell, I could easily fill two-hundred pages of these amazing stories, but what is even more remarkable is who he is as a man, a father, a friend, a doctor, a true healer and a man of God. Even his Navajo friends call him “See the Fire” for his great ability of seeing into the matrix of all life.

All who know him, each person he makes contact with, will admit to having their life transformed into a higher, more sensitive state of awareness.

Although no longer consulting with patients, he will continue to teach through his books, seminars and other media. In that way, we will continue to benefit from this most talented and gifted healer.

It was truly a privilege for me to contribute my skills in bringing this soon-to-be-classic book, *A Promise Kept: One Son's Quest for the Cause and Cure of Dis-ease*, to you. Read with an open mind and “The Promise” will be revealed.

Nicole Shoong
Investigative Journalist
Former Publisher of the
California Sun

TESTIMONIAL
From Consulting Editor
ROSE D. SIGMAN

I am thrilled that Dr. Chappell has asked me to share my healing experience.

Four years ago, I was diagnosed with cancer with no hope of survival. Today, thanks to Dr. Chappell, I am cancer-free.

After I was diagnosed, as most of us will do, I immediately ran to see an oncologist. This proved to be one of the *worst* mistakes I have ever made. However, I simply didn't know any better.

After one year and thirty-one fatiguing radiation treatments, the cancer came back. In addition, I became severely allergic to the medication prescribed, especially the chemotherapy cocktail.

My experience in the hospital, seeing other patients wearing only nightclothes, too sick to care, crammed into a waiting room in various stages of treatment and decline, made me feel I was part of a surrealistic nightmare.

I knew I didn't want to feel like them, vomiting and taking horrible drugs. Even though my odds of survival the second time around were dismal at best, I left the hospital vowing I would never see an oncologist again.

Although I didn't know what to do next, for reasons that are part of what Dr. Chappell calls the "Great Mystery," my son's fellow band member, Ms. Terri Nunn, the singer and co-founder of the rock group Berlin, urged me to call Dr. Chappell. Terri's advice saved my life. For that, I will be forever in her debt.

My first consultation with Dr. Chappell was a remarkable experience. He gave me hope, when I had none. He told me exactly what to do to turn around this thing called cancer and destroy it. He also promised his protocol would not make me sick or cause any more hair loss. Most importantly he gave me confidence that I could beat this terrible dis-ease. All of his promises came true.

Dis-ease is defined as lack of ease or harmony, it is NOT the same as "disease," a medical term for illness treated by medicine. *NEVER* attempt to stop or reduce your medication without the supervision of your medical doctor.

Dr. Jim, as I now call him, told me about healthy food that would energize my body. I went from being overweight to my normal weight without going hungry. He taught me how to listen to my body and how to take care of myself. He gave me the knowledge to heal my body and mind and return the confidence that false promises took from me. Dr. Jim does not guess on what needs to be done. He speaks from experience and knowledge.

Fortunately, cancer is just one of the many dis-eases Dr. Jim knows how to cure. He is blessed with the ability to intuit the function of the body and how to heal it.

Whether you have cancer, diabetes or any other chronic dis-ease, Dr. Jim's advice can help you.

I am living proof that you can believe every word Dr. Jim has written in this book. After you read it, you will believe too. His promise made, ***Is*** a Promise Kept.

I wish you good health.

Rose D. Sigman
Patient and Consulting Editor

Dis-ease is defined as lack of ease or harmony, it is NOT the same as "disease," a medical term for illness treated by medicine. *NEVER* attempt to stop or reduce your medication without the supervision of your medical doctor.

A Special Thank You

To:

Dorris 'Spike' Tenpenny for introducing me to the benefits of natural healing, when I was just eighteen years old. From that moment to this, I have always strived to be worthy of his kindness and time. His devotion to the ways of nature set a course for me to humbly follow. I will forever be grateful to my friend 'Spike'.

Thomas Cheng, my publisher and friend, without your enthusiastic confidence and support, this book would never have been written. Booklets are one thing. A book of this magnitude is something else. I thank you, Thomas, for the part you played in making everything come together.

Frank Boross, who designed the cover, using a picture that reminded him of my mom's best friend and his second mother, never knowing they knew each other. Great job!

Olga Singer, for her graphic design and expertise. Once I admitted my incompetent computer and design skills, Olga came and saved me. She is my cyberspace angel. Thank you.

Connie Anderson, Rose D. Sigman and Nicole Shoong, for their editing and patience. I apologize for my reluctance to graciously accept criticism. Your suggestions always proved best.

Patty Larkin (Running Angels), Beth Nielsen Chapman (You Hold The Key, Sand & Water) and to Merle Haggard (Unforgettable), the only music I listened to for the 900 hours it took me to write this book. I love where your music takes me. Thank you for the journey, my friends.

- James Chappell, D.C., N.D., Ph.D., M.H.

February 7, 2005

Dis-ease is defined as lack of ease or harmony, it is NOT the same as "disease," a medical term for illness treated by medicine. *NEVER* attempt to stop or reduce your medication without the supervision of your medical doctor.

A Promise Made, A Promise Kept:
One Son's Quest for the *Cause* and *Cure* of Diabetes

TABLE OF CONTENTS

Dis-ease is defined as lack of ease or harmony, it is NOT the same as "disease," a medical term for illness treated by medicine.
NEVER attempt to stop or reduce your medication without the supervision of your medical doctor.

ACKNOWLEDGEMENTS

It has been said, "You learn *more* about a person from their library than from their diploma". In that light, I would like to thank some of my mentors and masters without whom I would have only limited knowledge relative to the truth about natural healing. They include, but are not limited to:

Dale Alexander
Napoleon Hill
Eric Butterworth
Jack LaLanne
Rene Caisse
David Morsey
George Clason
Herman Aihara
Nicholas Culpeper
Jamie Sams
Mary Baker Eddy
Ken Wilber
Louise Hay
Eric Sloan

Christopher Hobbs
Richard Bach
Jethro Kloss
Henry Box
Neil Z. Miller
Mildred Carter
Paul Pitchford
Edgar Cayce
J.I. Rodale
Benjamin Disraeli
Neale Walsch
Joel Goldsmith
Gypsie Boots
Chief Seattle

George Anderson
V.E. Irons
Sam Biser
Ed McCabe
Joseph Campbell
John R. Price
James Redfield
Yogi Ramacharaka
Adelle Davis
W. Clement Stone
Epicteus
Gary Zukav
Richard Thomas
G. Edward Griffin

And to Doctors:

Henry Bieler
Robert Mendelsohn
Marlo Morgan
John Christopher
Linus Pauling
Norman V. Peale
Arnold Pike
Paul Eck
Royal Rife
Carlton Fredericks
Forrest Shaklee
Ernest Holmes
Jack Tips
D.C. Jarvis
Stuwart Wheelright

Paavo Airola
D.D. Palmer
Paul Bragg
Richard Passwater
Carolyn Myss
William Crook
Paul Dorosh
Carey Reams
Rocco Errico
Hans Selye
Max Gerson
Wilfrid Shute
Harry Hoxsey
Lowell Ward
William D. Kelly

Bennett Lust
Allen E. Banik
John N. Ott
Giraud Campbell
Carl S. Cleveland
Ray Peat
Weston Price
William Ellis
Otto Warburg
W.H. Graves
Edward Shook
Edward Howell
N. W. Walker
Bernard Jensen
Ann Wigmore

Dis-ease is defined as lack of ease or harmony, it is NOT the same as "disease," a medical term for illness treated by medicine. *NEVER* attempt to stop or reduce your medication without the supervision of your medical doctor.

George Lamsa	H. Curtis Wood	Royal Lee
James Murray	Charles A. Brusch	George Mienig
Hulda R. Clark	Col. Dinshah	Harold Manner
Joanna Budwig	Russell Blaylock	Masaru Emoto

The above-named gifted and talented people, many of whom earned doctorates, are *all* healers. There is a difference between a doctor and a healer. These healers helped me forge my mind in the fire of my will. They helped me to realize that *ability* is what one is capable of doing, while *motivation* determines what one does and *attitude* determines how well one succeeds. Thank you, my friends, for sharing your wisdom and knowledge. I will always be in your debt.

Although I have included some of those responsible for my education, inspiration and enthusiasm, I would be remiss if I didn't mention my deep-seated faith in God, Nature or the Great Mystery. You see, my faith extends far beyond mere belief. It includes a state of *knowingness*. I am fortunate because, I *know* who I am, where I came from, where I am going and what I was born to do. I have heard the quiet voice within direct me to and through my journey. From Abraham, Mohammed, Jesus, Buddha, Krisha, Mother Teresa, Chief Seattle to Eric Sloan as well as the other inspired aforementioned healers, I have been a devoted student, learning, sharing and then teaching others to be a blessing as they are blessed.

Is there any better way than to teach by example? I think not, for to teach by example, we must first learn what is being taught. What you are about to learn may save your life. I think it is well worth the effort to find a comfortable place to relax, take notes and be ready to acquire the information you will need to find the health and happiness you seek.

To learn more about the above authors and their contributions, turn to Index C - *Suggested Readings and References* at the back of this book. Having read all of these fine works, I can tell you, natural healing has worked since the beginning of time and will continue to work until time ceases to exist.

Dis-ease is defined as lack of ease or harmony, it is NOT the same as "disease," a medical term for illness treated by medicine. *NEVER* attempt to stop or reduce your medication without the supervision of your medical doctor.

WHY NOW?

In 1971, I was asked by Dr. Forrest Shaklee of the Shaklee Corporation - and then again in 1973 by Dr. Paul Dorosh two respected doctor-mentors - to *not* write a book for 25 to 30 years. They told me there were far too many so-called "natural healers" writing books before they were properly educated. Some write a 2,000 page all-you-need-to-know book about medicine or natural healing within days of graduation. How can anyone write from experience, if they have none? Drs. Shaklee and Dorosh said it takes at least 25 years of blood, sweat and tears to really know what you are writing about. After 34 years and *personally* seeing over 10,000 people, I now know what they meant. I am now ready to write.

If you study most medical or naturopathic writers, they are fresh out of school. They don't know the difference between isolated verses whole-food nutrition, what constituents the key to health or how to really communicate with a patient. After all, how could they? Even after ten years, they are just "getting their feet wet." But write they must for their ego or pocket book demands it.

Anyone can put on a white clinic coat and drape themselves with the symbol of arrogance and intelligence: the all-knowing stethoscope. But that doesn't mean you really have any experience in healing or medicine. It is just part of the costume the public has become acquainted with and now demands as the mark of a real "doctor." Look on the covers of most of the so-called "healing" books and you will see what I mean. Young smiling or serious faces, dressed in costume giving advice to the sick and infirmed without ever really having the experience to know what they are talking about. Worse yet, are medics (medical doctors) who after a lifetime career dispensing drugs and are now retired, writing about natural healing. What qualifies them to even pretend?

I am not one of those youngsters or impostors. Although I can't blame my hair loss on anything but genetics, one look at my face and you will see the signs of sleepless nights thinking about those who have asked me to save their lives. My eyes have even grown weak from the tens of thousands of hours reading, researching and writing, in spite of my own advice concerning good nutrition.

My voice has aged from the hundreds of thousands of hours of talking to anyone who will listen, be it one-on-one, in seminars, conference calls or through radio and television appearances. I am not a newcomer to this thing called natural healing. Unfortunately, I am one of the last of the breed of *real* naturopathic doctors who grew up on Jethro Kloss' *Garden of Eden,* the bible on healing.

Over the years I have learned about the infinite possibilities of 'being' human and divine simultaneously. With this knowledge, comes the ability to claim our spirituality in this and all moments, thus exemplifying 'being' the physical manifestation of the essence of truth or that which is God also known as the Great Mystery.

In the interim of attaining this realization, please remember this: *The most serious potential danger associated with experimental orthodox medicine is that a patient may avoid or delay receipt of safe, natural healing care in a timely fashion, leading to irreversible damage caused by toxic drugs, mutilating surgeries and medieval carcinogenic radiation.*

Although there may be a need for emergency medical care, I say, "Caveat Emptor; Let the consumer beware!" With this book, I wish you well on your journey to find the true meaning of love, health, peace and joy.

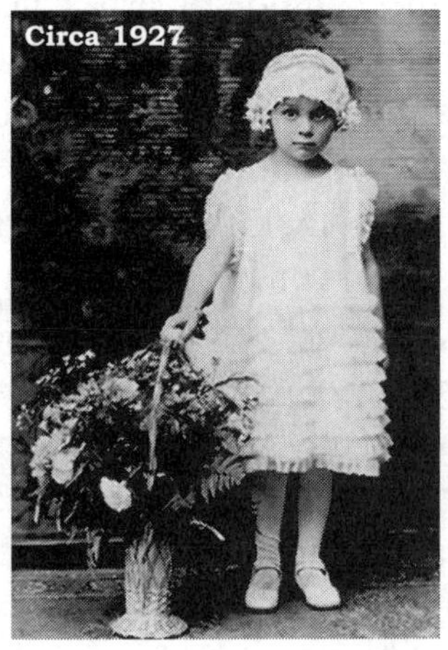
Circa 1927

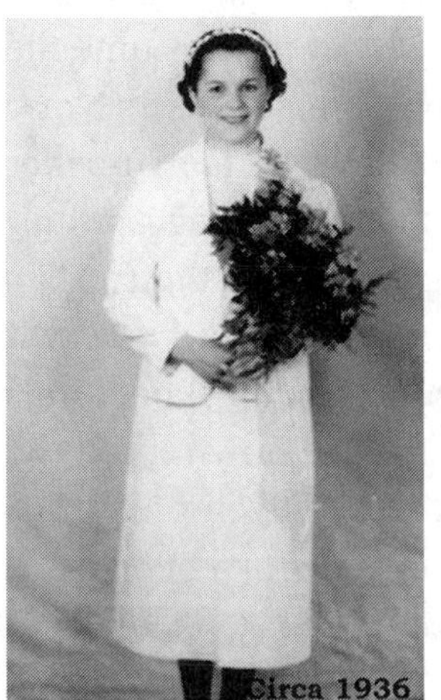
Circa 1936

"Roses are so colorful, so fragrant they take my mind to a place I long to be. If only I could live there." - Connie Chappell

Dis-ease is defined as lack of ease or harmony, it is NOT the same as "disease," a medical term for illness treated by medicine. *NEVER* attempt to stop or reduce your medication without the supervision of your medical doctor.

[Below is one of my mother's favorite poems by her favorite poet. She always told me it was her *choice* to live the way she did. I wonder if it was her *choice* to die that way as well? I suppose so.]

Choice

by
Eric C Wyndham

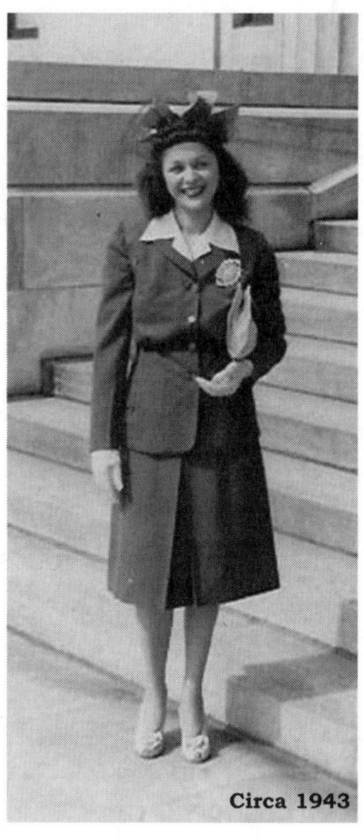
Circa 1943

My life so graciously received, I know is a *gift* as intended to be. In honor of the Giver, I respectfully endure every challenge set before me and even more.

Free to dream, free to learn, free to grow and free to yearn. From my beginning to the end, my life has been my friend.

I have *choice* in what I eat and what I wear on the street, in the books that I read and the plays I want to see. If I chose to give up this pride, releasing my spirit from inside, it is mine as I see fit and not a dictating government's.

If by religion you tempt me to change, I suggest further study in your god's name. For *Love* has no beginning or an end; we simply travel back home again.

Our essence can *never* die, unless you believe in the lie: that this life is all there is and God, which is Love, has been amiss.

By *choice* I have come and by same I may leave, but the *choice* is mine, forever to be. For no one may withhold the sun from the tree, and no man shall keep me from my eternity.

Dis-ease is defined as lack of ease or harmony, it is NOT the same as "disease," a medical term for illness treated by medicine. *NEVER* attempt to stop or reduce your medication without the supervision of your medical doctor.

The *New* American Death Ceremony

The *New* American death ceremony began as a crude ritual, back in the days when *experimental* orthodox medicine first started. Death came quickly as drug physicians gave out their toxic elixirs. In recent years, it has been developed into a deceitful, so-called "science." It now usually takes from ten to fifteen years to slowly poison and kill, however, modern advancements in "medicine" are ever shortening this period of time.

It starts with one simple aspirin for a simple headache. When the one aspirin will no longer cover up the headache, people then take two. After a few months, when two aspirin will no longer cover up the headache (a sign of an underlining problem), you can take one of the stronger compounds found either over-the-counter or by prescription, however, it will become necessary to take something for the ulcers that have been caused by the aspirin. Now that you are taking two or more drugs, you have a good start on your journey to the grave.

After a few months, your drug treatment will begin to disrupt your liver function. (It's easy to see your liver enzymes elevate through a blood test when under drug therapy). Of course, if an infection develops your "doctor" will prescribe antibiotics assuming all infections are caused by bacteria. These drugs lead to anemia and yeast infections. Both will require *additional* drugs, one being Nystatin, a known liver toxin.

Since all of these drugs filter through your kidneys it won't be long before they become affected. When the kidneys start to fail, they will be "treated" with their own "medication" and additional medical procedures.

By now your diet of drug therapy will have your body total confused, toxic and failing, but it doesn't really matter. If you have followed every step as directed, you can make an appointment with your local mortician.

American *experimental* orthodox medicine kills over 800,000 people every year. We not only suffer a terrible death, we spend all our savings paying for it! This game is played by practically all Americans, except for the few ignorant souls who follow nature. Unfortunately, my mother died believing her drug doctors knew what they were doing. Perhaps they did?

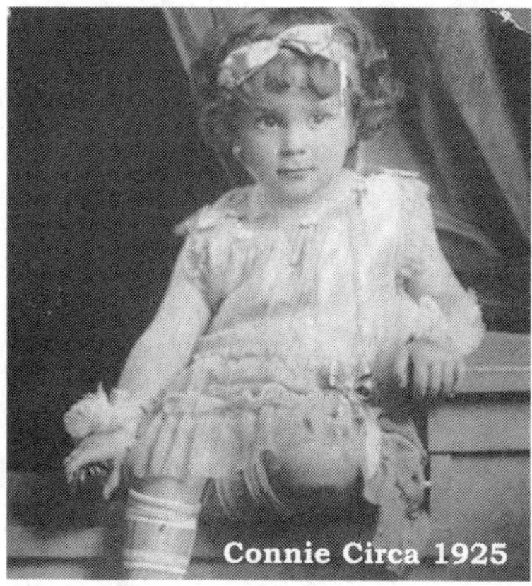
Connie Circa 1925

PREFACE

Children need not only the basics; nourishing food and water, proper clothes and shelter, they need *love* and *attention*. All are prerequisites for optimum health. When provided, both children and adults enjoy an excellent opportunity to flourish and prosper.

During my thirty-four years of clinical experience, I discovered the key to health is not medical treatment. In addition to the basics, the master key to health and longevity will always be *love* and *attention, education* and taking *effective action.*

Love is a meaningful and caring concern for ourselves and others in an *attentive* way. *Education* has to do with learning how to take care of yourself such as reading books like this, an excellent start to achieving optimum health and longevity. Unless the *action* you take is *effective*, it will have no benefit. Weight loss exercise is not *effective* unless you lose weight.

Once we take responsibility for our own health, we will depend less on doctors to "fix" us. With few exceptions, by learning the basic principles of health and healing and, more importantly, *practicing* them, we may expect a life full and rewarding. Good health is not a pipe dream or theory. Good health is a reality being experienced by millions of people all over the world.

Dis-ease is defined as lack of ease or harmony, it is NOT the
same as "disease," a medical term for illness treated by medicine.
NEVER attempt to stop or reduce your medication without the supervision of your medical doctor.

My mother, Connie Chappell, was a young, vivacious, energetic, fun-loving, beautiful Italian woman. She had hopes of one day having a life that she had dreamed of. She tried desperately to *forget* her haunting past, but could never *forgive*. Her inability to forgive proved a major stumbling block, for without *forgiveness,* we never truly *forget*. Without letting go of our painful memories that cause our fear, insecurity and lack of trust, we live and re-live them forever.

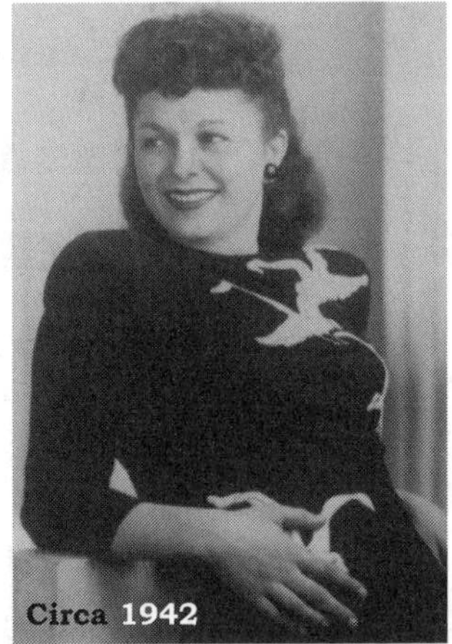
Circa 1942

Regardless of what we eat and how much we exercise, good thoughts or bad, we become what we *think* about all day long. We really do manifest our *fears*. My mother used to say she'd never live to sixty-five. She was right.

As far back as I remember, 'Mama' was always struggling with her weight and health. From one tragedy to the next, she suffered for many years, but during the last 10 years of her life, she endured horrific pain and torment. I watched helplessly as she became overweight, sickly, stubborn and angry. Behind her photogenic smile and heart of gold was a little girl still hurting, still angry at God and at the world for her "lot in life."

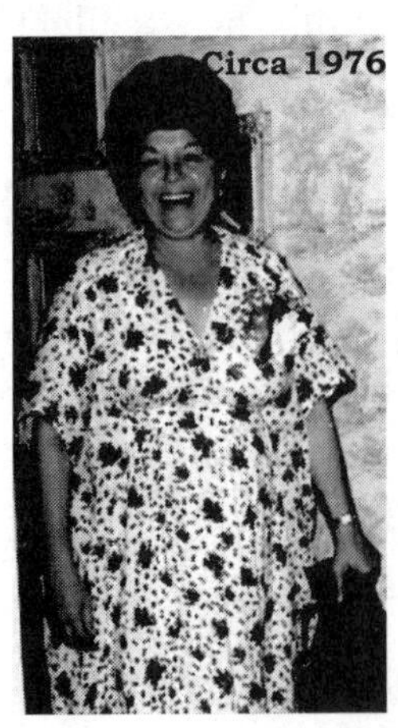
Circa 1976

Lack of forgiveness has devastating, deep and long-lasting consequences, some of them non-recoverable. The good news is if you *practice* what you learn in this book, you can prevent those lack of forgiveness experiences and most dreadful pending consequences.

Although being overweight and having diabetes was challenging enough, it wasn't until the next phase of her degenerative process that my mother took her health, or lack of it, seriously.

Dis-ease is defined as lack of ease or harmony, it is NOT the same as "disease," a medical term for illness treated by medicine. NEVER attempt to stop or reduce your medication without the supervision of your medical doctor.

After being diagnosed with cancer, my mother was literally overcome with fear of dying. As expected, self-pity, anger and denial consumed her. Now the final sentence hung over her head and she knew it.

Her modern medical cancer treatment consisted of drugs and surgery. After having part of her colon removed and being assured they "got it all," the cancer soon metastasized to her liver. During an exploratory surgery needed to "really know what is going on," her doctors said nothing more could be done. They gave her six months to live. Her death took longer than that, while she dwindled from approximately 300 pounds down to 88. On February 14, 1986, she quietly withered and died.

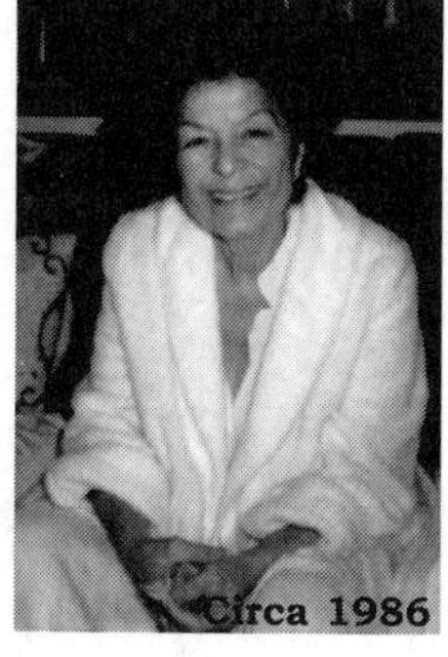
Circa 1986

I not only lost my best friend, my confidant, my supporter and admirer, but I lost my "Mama Lucia," as I lovingly nicknamed her.

From obesity, diabetes to cancer, my mother *never* gave up hope and neither did I. At her deathbed, I promised I would find the *cause* and eventual *cure* to her lingering illness. Now, after almost 20 years of research, trial and error, *I have found the answer to her core dilemma mistakenly called diabetes.* I want to share these answers with you.

In this book, I explain the *causes* of what we call dis-eases and what *cures* them. From obesity, diabetes, cancer and everything between, I discovered the *cause* of all dis-ease stems from the same thing: I call it The H.O.N.S.T.E.C. Syndrome, as thoroughly explained in Chapter Two.

What I discovered may shock you as it did me. But the answer is clear: There are NO incurable dis-eases, only our preconceived ideas about them. Again, the key is the basics; *love, attention, education* and taking *effective action.* It is *not* treatment be it orthodox or natural. Medicines may have a precise calculated effect, but unless they are used in harmony with respect to the body, they can have terrible side-effects, death being one.

What about you? Are you ready to change your life? Are you willing to let go of hatred, jealousy, resentment, anger and lack of forgiveness? Are you committed to eating healthy, wholesome, pure nurturing food and water? Will you dedicate a few minutes everyday to move your body in an *effective* way so as to prevent illness and dis-ease? Are you willing to stop all those things known to *cause* sickness, like smoking and over indulging in food and alcohol?

If you answered "yes" to all of the above, you can achieve optimum health. You can live a life free of sickness and dis-ease. But if you are one of the millions of people who simply do whatever anyone in perceived authority dictates to you, this book is NOT for you. Just keep trusting your doctors and take your drugs as needed...and needed they will be, for one drug will always lead to another. After all, that's the nature of drug therapy. And no drug has ever cured anything. Let me repeat: **NO DRUG HAS EVER CURED ANYTHING!** It may have postponed the inevitable, but only God or nature heals. We simply must go back to trusting God and nature for there isn't anything mankind can offer that God or nature hasn't already provided. As my late mother would say, "The proof is in the pudding."

Everyday, we lose plants and animals as they become extinct. Humans may be proliferating, but they have more sickness and dis-ease than ever before. Because we have violated natural laws and principles, our planet is dying. Most of our waterways, lakes, rivers and oceans are polluted. Our air is contaminated. Our "civilized" food is processed, de-vitalized, genetically engineered, fumigated, irradiated and saturated with toxic pesticides, synthetic growth hormones and fertilizers.

We live in an ocean of electromagnetic radio waves penetrating and mutating cell after cell in our body. And yet, this glorious, wonderful body continues to struggle, heal and repair, but at what cost? *Sickness and dis-ease is the result of the struggle. We have caused our own dilemma.* Through our ignorance of nature and Her natural laws and principles, we have created and live in a decaying world. Are you really surprised when everyone around you is getting sick? I mean really surprised? Of course not, for in your heart you know the truth.

Unfortunately, many of you reading this will struggle to understand what I have said. It falls outside of your paradigm or comfort zone, not your intelligence, just your acceptance. You may be a non-believer in God or nature and so those words have triggered a disconnection. That's okay. I wrote this book for those with "eyes to see" and "ears to hear." Be *open* to the infinite possibilities of life and learning and you will find what you seek.

If you step outside of your preconceived ideas of what you have been told about health, sickness and dis-ease, I promise you, you will learn how to *cure* yourself from almost every acquired illness. It won't be easy, but you *can* do it. There are exceptions like congenital deformities and post-traumatic physical damage, but barring those exclusions, I *know* all other so-called "diseases" can be eradicated. Notice, I did not say, I believe. I said I *know*. There is a difference. Belief connotes faith with the possibility of doubt or uncertainty. Knowing comes from knowledge, which we acquire from learning or experience. After years of helping almost every imaginable human ailment and observing thousands of people recover from their health challenges naturally, I *know* there are no incurable conditions.

Ask yourself this: Why would he say these things if they were not true? Just to sell a book? I have written other books and hundreds of newsletters, health reports and articles where I just gave statistical information. Why risk my credibility making statements such as "There are no incurable dis-eases," when I can play it safe? The answer is simple; we are running out of time. We are not being told the truth. In fact, we are being purposefully misled and it's all about money. If you read at the same pace I do, in the time it took you to get this far, six people just died from cancer in the United States. That's right. One dies from cancer every minute in this country alone, more than 500,000 people every year. Add all the other premature and totally unnecessary deaths from obesity, diabetes, heart dis-ease, stroke and so-called "natural causes," and we suffer millions of deaths yearly, many preventable if we would just go back to trusting God and nature.

Have you wondered why no one dies from "natural causes" unless they are over eighty years old? That's because our government has declared eighty to eighty-two years old as the upper limit of the average American's life expectancy. What is a "natural cause" anyway, wearing out, wearing down? Shouldn't we live like a lit candle brightly reflecting until the last flicker goes out? Most of us die with half of our life remaining. Worse yet, we burn the candle at both ends with our constant "doingness," forgetting what it is to just 'Be.'

Shakespeare said, "To be or not to be, that is the question." Ask yourself. Are you always striving to 'do' something in order to 'be' someone? Cars, boats and planes mean nothing, while relationships, love and peace bring true joy and happiness.

I know what you are thinking. "How can we live without money? It takes money to buy food, clothes and shelter." I will answer that *later* and you will *not* like the answer. But if you are a truth seeker, my answer shouldn't surprise you. You should already know about the medium of exchange we call money.

DEDICATION

This book is not dedicated only to my mother Connie, but to all those seeking optimum health. Although it is too late for her, it may not be too late for you. I hope and pray the inspired wisdom herein blesses you as it has so many others. If you or anyone you know suffer from *any* dis-ease, you owe it to yourself and your family to learn what you can about overcoming your health challenge and then take *effective action.* Remember the key to health is not only having the basic nutrients, but you must have *love*, *attention* and health *education*, and you must take *effective action.* If you learn and do not act, there will be no appreciable benefit. Reading this book is an excellent start.

INTRODUCTION

In the sixties I read a book entitled, *Anything Can Cause Everything and Everything Can Cause Anything*. It didn't take me long to realize lack of hydration, oxygen deprivation, nutritional excesses or deficiencies, spinal-structural-neurological aberrations, toxic waste accumulation, emotional stress, electromagnetic, environmental and chemical contamination, all contribute to what we call dis-ease. There are many reasons why people get sick, and it isn't for the reasons you have been told.

Basically the above named book focused on bacteria, viruses, parasites and other pathogens that are attracted to nutrient-deficient, dehydrated, stressed-out, toxic bodies. The end result is what we commonly call "disease." Yes, there are exceptions to this fact. Some genetic disorders can be traced to the womb and its blood-nutrient supply. However, the core message is, we become our mental, physical and emotional environment.

When we compound one contributing factor with another, our "disease" risk factors increase dramatically. Just smoking a few cigarettes daily will not automatically *cause* cancer. As damaging as they may be, not everyone who smokes gets sick. Logic says there must be other factors involved. Emotions like fear, anger, anxiety, resentment, hatred, lack of forgiveness and jealously all contribute to suppressing the immune system. Add a poor diet, lack of exercise and environmental toxins found in our food, air and water, and you have the perfect recipe for a litany of so-called "diseases." But as you will read, "disease" is not dis-ease. Dis-ease is defined as lack of ease, lack of harmony demonstrated by *signs* and *signals*. "Disease" is a medical term used to classify conditions or groups of *symptoms*, mostly created and necessary for insurance reimbursement, competitive protectionism and drug treatment.

From my mother's birth, losses, life challenges and sickness to The H.O.N.S.T.E.C. Syndrome, this book will take you on a journey ultimately giving you all the information you need to overcome so-called "diabetes," "obesity," "cancer" and other ailments.

Dis-ease is defined as lack of ease or harmony, it is NOT the same as "disease," a medical term for illness treated by medicine. *NEVER* attempt to stop or reduce your medication without the supervision of your medical doctor.

From the *experimental,* ineffective, drug-based, orthodox medical approach to the time-tested and true natural healing approach, you will learn about the seven key elements that are historically and scientifically proven to regulate, normalize and lower glucose, thus *reversing* diabetes! Finally, you will be taught how to initiate a proper food and exercise program and how to eliminate known contributors to illness. With plenty of statistical data, scientific evidence, references and resources, nothing has been left out.

Twenty years of research have gone into this work inspired by my mother Connie and her mother before her. Although my mother was kind and loving, her loss, fear, hatred, insecurity, ignorance, UN-forgiveness and profound stubbornness, plus her lack of exercise and a poor, excessive diet, she eventually developed obesity, diabetes and cancer. This ultimately led to her premature death at age sixty-four.

To a teenager, she was a senior citizen and perhaps was old enough. But when you consider the Hunza Kats from the mountains of Northern Pakistan living to one hundred and twenty years and doing so virtually dis-ease free, my mother definitely died prematurely.

It is possible for those of us living in this-less-than perfect modern civilization to double our life expectancy? Yes!

My intention is to provide you with accurate information. When coupled with your willingness to take *effective* action, it should lead you to the prevention of sickness and dis-ease. If you have young children, reading this book may not only save yourself from a future of pain and suffering, you will save them, as well. Remember, nothing is more important than your health. Nothing.

To understand the ill-fated web we weave, I start with my grandmother, Rose.

(In order to protect the innocent, I have changed my mother's maiden name to 'Smith.' As you continue to read, you will know why.)

Dis-ease is defined as lack of ease or harmony, it is NOT the same as "disease," a medical term for illness treated by medicine. *NEVER* attempt to stop or reduce your medication without the supervision of your medical doctor.

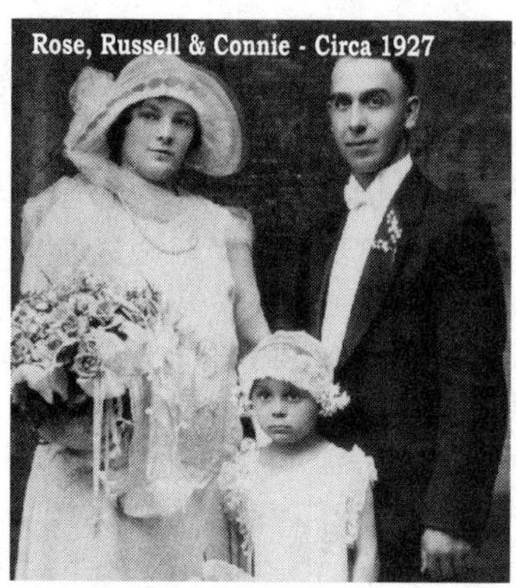
Rose, Russell & Connie - Circa 1927

CHAPTER 1 - IT STARTED WITH A ROSE

"*There is no love like that of a mother for her child. Surely she gives life and truly would willingly die for it.*" **- EC Wyndham**

Rose was just fourteen years old, her husband seventeen when Connie was conceived. Born Constance Marie 'Smith,' February 7, 1922 in Buffalo, New York, Connie lived no ordinary childhood. From her mother's parents of the DeSalvo and Amato families in Sicily and Rome, to her parents, Rose and Russell 'Smith' of New York, Connie was born into the old-world Italian tradition where children married very young.

For the first six years of her life, Connie knew only love and attention. She enjoyed two loving parents, a home in a good neighborhood, relatives all around her and plenty of excellent home-cooked Italian food to grow up on. She played outside with her friends in the fresh air and sunshine in the days when pollution in her town was a word few ever spoke. Her mother was always there to comfort her and her father couldn't wait to come home from work to play games with his little brown-eyed princess. Her life was exactly what dreams are made of, but this dream soon became a nightmare without reprieve.

Some of us live a lifetime sheltered from the possibilities of reality, either protected from the "dark side" by others or by refusing to acknowledge its existence. For whatever reason, like children in the holocaust, my mother's reality came early.

My mother's nightmare began one morning just before the sun cleared the asphalt gray rooftops on a cold New York day in May of 1927. There was a knock on the front door. In fact, it was more of a pounding. Six-year-old Connie woke up, startled and ran for the security and comfort of her mother's arms. Half way across the upstairs landing overlooking the front door, little Connie met her mother, who instinctively knew her child would be frighten and was on her way toward her.

As Connie wrapped her arms around her mother's legs and Rose embraced her by her side, they watched as a young father and husband cautiously approached the front door. "Who is it?" Russell whispered. "It's your brother. Let me in." Uncle 'Tony' was always welcome and often ate dinners with Connie and her parents. The sound of her uncle's voice lessened her fear, but there was still something in the air that didn't feel right.

As Russell and Anthony stood in the doorway, their conversation purposefully muted for no known reason, mother and daughter witnessed Anthony give her father the sinister cheek-to-cheek Italian "kiss of death." As if time stopped, Connie and Rose watched in horror as Uncle Anthony pulled out a handgun and shot little Connie's father. One shot to the head and the love of her life was gone. Anthony immediately dropped the gun and ran to a waiting car. Screaming, Rose grabbed her baby and ran down the stairs to her husband's lifeless body.

The knock on the door, and the high-pitch sound of tires screeching down the street taking the murderer away, couldn't have taken five minutes. But because of that five minutes, Connie's life would never be the same.

Losing a loved one is never easy, but watching in horror as your father is murdered, forever leaves an imprint that is difficult if not impossible to overcome.

Loss

Why would Russell's own brother kill him? They had their differences as any two "hot-headed" Italian brothers might, but nothing could justify Anthony killing his own flesh and blood. Nothing, unless, of course, you were part of the *Family*.

Called by many names and originating in Sicily as far back as the ninth Century, the *Family, Costra Nostra* or *Mafia* started as a secret society organized specifically for self-preservation and for protection against Arab and Norman invaders. Legend has it, upon being invaded, the Sicilians escaped into the hillsides. Forming a bond under one cause, the *Family* took the name *Mafia* from the Arabic word 'refugee' and, one by one, fought the invaders forcing them to leave Sicily in defeat. Now, with a sense of unity and strength, the *Mafia* became a force unto itself. By the 1700s their symbolic code of honor, the notorious *Black Hand,* was a sign that instilled fear and intimidation in those not in the clan.

If one was not accepted by the clan, one wanted to be. Otherwise one paid and paid dearly. This system was really nothing new. Governments have been using it for centuries; pay the tax or go to jail. Give us money or we punish you.

Business was easy. By sending letters to the rich demanding they pay the *Mafia* for protection, those who did not heed the warning found themselves victims of their so-called "protectors." By the late 1800s the *Mafia* found its foothold in America, first in New Orleans and then in New York City.

Being young, strong and Italian, Russell and Anthony were easily accepted into the American *Costa Nostra*. Not being "wise, tough guy or hit man" material they became runners or gophers, until my grandfather, Russell, wanted out. Therein was the answer: my grandfather was in the *Mafia* and he no longer wanted to be. Unfortunately, once in the *Mafia*, you are in until "Death do us part." Anthony, wanting to rise in the ranks, took the contract and killed his brother. Case closed? Well, not really.

Barely two days after the funeral, attended only by my grandmother and my mother, two detectives appeared at the house. Rose thought they wanted more information. Although she was an eyewitness and already explained, in detail, what happened, it wasn't clearly "cut and dried." The police had the gun, the killer's fingerprints, a credible witness and even a little girl's testimony saying, "My uncle killed my papa," but there was one thing missing: Justice.

Say what you will, the Italian *Mafia* is not naive. Power and money can buy anything you want, including most of the whores masquerading as politicians. *Covering up a killing for hire is no exception.*

Loneliness

The detectives shackled my grandmother and threw her into the infamous "patty wagon" while six-year-old Connie was pulled away, screaming. Rose was arrested, tried and convicted for killing her husband. Now the case was closed. She was sentenced to twenty-five years to life in prison and if she did not "confess" to the murder, her daughter, my mother, would be next.

If you are part of the *Family* you are in the in-crowd. If you are not, you are simply an outsider. But if you are in and you want out, you are a traitor, a mutineer, one "*disprezzato*," and so is everyone in your family. It made no difference if you were six-years-old or eighty. My mother was treated by her Italian relatives as if she had leprosy. She was a non-person, an outcast. Someone to be seen and not heard.

With her father dead and her mother in prison, little Connie lived in the attics and basements from family to family, treated like Cinderella without a magic slipper. Weeks led to months and months led to years, never a kind word, never a feeling of belonging, never a loving moment. Connie was alone. She was given scraps to eat and skim milk watered down with old coffee. During her formative years her diet was dismal. In later years this would play a major role in her sickness and premature death.

Although they wrote to each other often, for twelve long years, with no one to take her, Connie never saw her mother. Finally, at age 18, she could sign herself in at the prison as a visitor and travel the over 60 miles from Buffalo to the state penitentiary in Albion.

Nothing could prepare her for what she was about to see.

The once radiantly glowing, youthful olive-skinned, sparkling brown-eyed, confident Rose, now shamefully hung her head and looked twice her age. There was a slight graying of her hair and harshness about her that dimmed the old glitter in her eyes. Her smooth beautiful olive skin turned blotchy, dry and rough. Most frightening were Rose's sunken eyes hidden in deep, dark circles as if to further show her unyielding confinement and hopelessness.

After a few months of weekly visits, while waitressing during the swing shift, my mother got a call from a monotone voice simply saying, "Connie Smith? Your mother is being released from prison. She's dying."

Apparently, the state wanted one incarcerated for as long as possible, guilty or not, unless, of course, one required expensive medical treatment. Then, regardless of the sentence, you were paroled. And so it was for my grandmother Rose.

Now at the age of thirty-three and after twelve years in prison for a crime she did not commit, Rose contracted infectious peritonitis, a life-threatening illness. Whether it was the infection or just someone thinking she suffered enough, rather than the state spending any money on medical treatment, in 1939 Rose was paroled and sent to live with her daughter.

From a daughter's love or simply just being away from prison life, Rose's health slowly improved. Rose married a non-*Mafia* Italian gentleman named Joseph in 1940. For the first time since she was six years old, Connie had her mom and a new papa.

Within a year, Rose gave birth to a little baby girl named Joannie. That birth came with consequences. For some unexplainable reason her peritonitis came back and this time it killed her. It was 1942, and Rose was only thirty-six.

Seeing her father murdered, her mother taken away and sent to prison was painful enough. Being left to the whim of dictating relatives for over twelve years only added to Connie's suffering. Reuniting with her mother, only to see her die prematurely, left Connie emotionally, mentally, physically and spiritually damaged. My mother's early life was truly the epitome of the "dark side."

This proved later to be another factor in her future illness.

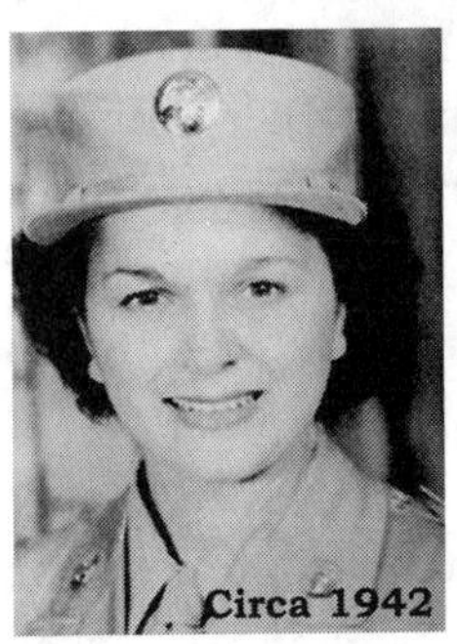
Circa 1942

Lost, confused, lonely and scared, Connie joined the Army. It was 1942 and America was at war. This was a time when Carole Lombard was selling war bonds and movie stars John Wayne, Jimmy Stewart, Bob Hope and Bing Crosby were making *Uncle Sam Wants You* films.

Connie changed her last name to Branton, and spent the next two years in Europe where no one knew who she was or where she came from.

With thick black hair, deep excitable brown eyes, perfect olive skin and an hourglass figure that could "stop a clock," Connie was beautiful. She was also smart and gutsy. During her tour in the Army, she learned how to relax, party, drink and smoke. Connie was the "bell of the ball," but there was one thing she did not do. She did not date Italians. She wanted nothing to do with anyone from Italy.

Betrayal

Upon her Army discharge in 1943, she returned to Buffalo where her stepfather Joseph and stepsister Joannie still lived. In a whirlwind of emotion, she married a non-Italian named Douglas Hughes. Within one year she gave birth to a beautiful girl, Deirdre. For the first time in her life, she was happy. However, this also was too good to be true.

Apparently Douglas felt Connie was spending too much time and attention with their daughter and not enough with him. Before long, he had an affair.

From one loss to another, first her father, then her childhood, then her mother and now her husband, Connie was desperately disillusioned. So much so, she lost her faith in God and discovered food and alcohol to escape her misery.

Begging her husband to come back home fell on deaf ears. She was losing him and she knew it. In spite of her hatred for what had happened to her mother and father, she felt the only solution was to ask the 'Don' of the *Family* for help. ('Dons' are the leaders of a *Mafia* clan). Everyone goes to the 'Don' if they have a problem. She was given an audience where she pleaded her case. "Please ask my husband to come home. I love and miss him," she said. After a promise to "look into it," Connie left, praying for a miracle from a God she didn't know. The miracle never came. Three days after her visit, her husband and his girlfriend were found dead, the victims of a single car accident. Case closed.

Upon hearing the news and without a second thought, Connie packed her bags and with her daughter in tow moved as far away as she could from New York: San Luis Obispo, California.

Abandonment

It didn't take long to find an apartment, a job and a line of young, available suitors. She may have had a young daughter, but she was still an Italian "bomb shell." For the most part, being a single mom is a great qualifier. You quickly find out if a man really cares about you. When a man comes on strong, bringing flowers and wine, and you tell them you have a child, most will run. One didn't.

They met at the restaurant where Connie worked. Jim was a graduate student at 'Cal Poly' majoring in horticulture. He wasn't very good looking, funny or even intelligent and of course he didn't have much money, but he was ambitious and she thought he was kind and considerate. Above all, he was *not* Italian.

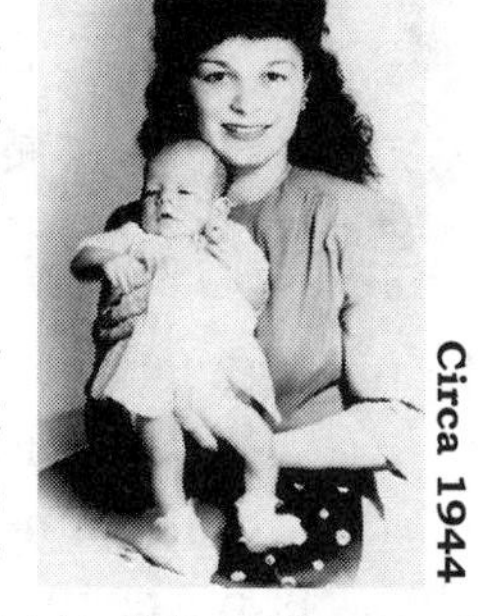
Circa 1944

Whether for love or security, within a year they married and life couldn't be better, at least until my mother announced she was pregnant with me. It seemed the "curse" followed her to California or at least she thought it did. (She used to say she felt it was God's way of punishing her for being a "bad" person).

When my father demanded she have an abortion, she refused and lost whatever respect and love she thought she had for him. Being a Roman Catholic she was not at liberty to divorce for idle cause. And being a survivor, she was not about to be thrown out on the street pregnant and with a young daughter.

Eventually she convinced my father having a child would be okay. She would stay home to mother, cook, clean and perform her wifely "duties" if only he would provide for their family and *not* leave or have an affair. (Up to this point, she had not told him about her *Mafia* past. Sometimes I wish she had).

Their relationship was more a mutual arrangement. My father fell in love with his work and my mother fell in love with her children. Her children were the only love she never lost and she was the first love I ever knew.

On the surface we appeared to be a normal family. My parents both loved to drink, smoke, eat out, party, laugh and dance. Really, my mother danced while my father drunk and philosophized with anyone who would listen. Still everyone thought the Chappells were one big happy family.

And so it was until my mother became pregnant again. This time there was no demand for an abortion. My father knew he was just the provider, and he didn't really care. He worked more and drank more. Not having a loving husband was nothing new for my mother. The love she had for her children sustained her from my father's cruel, intentional, emotional abandonment. Abandonment is one emotional "straw" that can contribute to "breaking a camel's back." Connie's back was heavy and near breaking.

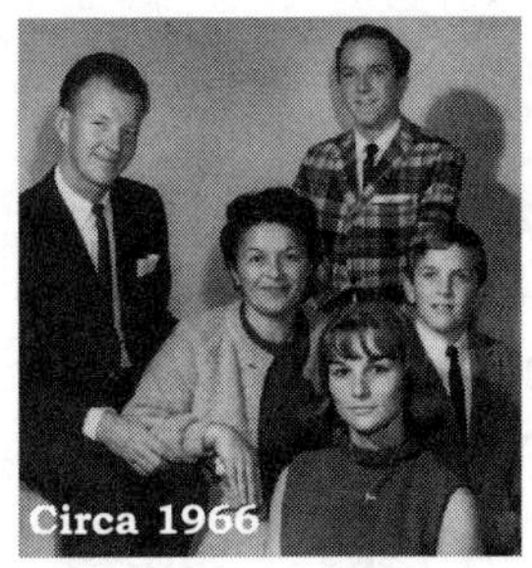
Circa 1966

Connie's First Warning Sign

By the time I was old enough to notice my mother's body, she was on her way to becoming overweight. Prior to that, she developed pyorrhea, an infectious gum and jaw bone "disease." Even dentistry refuses to seek the *cause* of dis-ease, when they, like the medics (medical doctors) only treat symptoms. After several rounds of the most powerful antibiotics known, the medical cure

Dis-ease is defined as lack of ease or harmony, it is NOT the same as "disease," a medical term for illness treated by medicine. <u>*NEVER*</u> attempt to stop or reduce your medication without the supervision of your medical doctor.

for her pyorrhea was to extract her teeth. Sadly, before she was thirty-five years old, my mother wore dentures. Although embarrassed, she eventually learned to smile again.

Don't think this is something of the past. A dear friend who is currently a dentist in Maine, said he knows of several cases in Canada when after a child reached the age of sixteen, the parents had all their teeth removed and gave them dentures. It was literally their sixteenth "coming out party." The reasoning is simple; by removing one's teeth at this age, they will save a lifetime of money, inconvenience and dental pain. I guess they have never heard of the dental meridian pathway to illness?

Every tooth is connected neurologically to the entire body, therefore teeth are much more important than for chewing food. My mother made an unrecoverable error by allowing the removal of her teeth, as you will discover in *Chapter 2 - The H.O.N.S.T.E.C. Syndrome.*

The next physical sign of my mother's illness was her increasing weight. Instead of realizing our body is trying to tell us something, we write off weight gain as settling into a relationship or part of growing older, when, in reality, obesity is a sign of nutritional deficiencies, imbalances, stress and a laundry list of other dysfunctionalities.

Remember when being fat was just an observation? Today, it is called obesity and has become a "disease." Interesting.

Another contributing factor to illness is stress and how we handle it. When it came to a stressful, dysfunctional family, the Chappells were it, personified. As you can imagine, my mother and father did not get along. Without love, how could they? From prescription drugs, alcohol, coffee and cigarettes, my parents were both constantly self-medicating. Food became mother's aphrodisiac and especially anything sweet. When she was happy she ate. When she was depressed, she ate more. Because of *what* she ate, she became increasingly unhealthy and overweight.

I was one major factor in my parent's daily and nightly stressful arguments. I became the most decisive contributor to my parents' warring relationship. By the time I was five years old, I became my father's punching bag and the focus of his anger and escalating frustrations. It was simple: six days a week my father would work all day, come home at night, get drunk, have something to eat, beat me and then watch TV until he fell asleep. On Sunday's he didn't work so he got drunk earlier. My mother was helpless to protect me. She was dependent on her husband with three children and no education, so she drank herself into denial.

I was *not* an innocent victim. My father had no idea what it meant to be genetically linked to my Sicilian heritage. Even as a young boy, I was extremely protective of my mother both physically and emotionally. I was willing to go into battle with my father for the slightest reason.

One night, when I was about eleven he was yelling at my mother while trying to force her into a room. I chased him down the hallway with a baseball bat, screaming at him to get out of the house. He did.

I learned from my mother early that my father never wanted me to be born. So, every chance I got, I tried to make his life miserable. By all accounts, I was doing a good job. Getting beaten was the trade-off. To this day, I still have the 'protector' trait, although I now choose peace over aggression.

When I turned fifteen, my mother sent me to martial arts class after school three days a week. I had one goal: to learn how to defend myself enough to fight my father and win. That day came when I turned sixteen. During dinner, my father got so drunk, he threw his chair and knocked me to the ground. Grabbing me by the neck, he dragged me outside to teach me a lesson.

I glanced at my mother while being dragged through the dining room doorway to the back yard. Her eyes told me "take him if you can." That's all I needed. I put him on the ground in ten seconds. He never saw it coming. And he never hit me again. When I graduated from high school, he kicked me out of the house. I was seventeen years old.

The Sum of Connie's Life

From a lifetime of smoking, eating processed devitalized junk food, refined carbohydrates, sweets and more sweets, drinking alcohol daily, having no effective exercise program and living without the love of her spouse, my mother grew obese, developed pre and then Type II diabetes. Finally, she acquired cancer and died.

What really killed my mother? Was it not having enough love and attention when she was a little girl or watching the murder of her father, or living in basements and attics after her mother was sent to prison? Was it malnutrition from lack of healthy food during her formative years? Perhaps it was her stressful, dysfunctional relationship with my father or smoking cigarettes and over-indulging in alcohol? Maybe it was because she *mistakenly* thought God punishes those He or She doesn't like, or to teach them a lesson?

I believe it was all that and more.

Unless we consider the entire body, mind and spirit of a person as did Deepak Chopra when bringing 5,000-year-old Ayervedic medicine from India to the west, we will *never* get to the *cause* of illness, a *cause* I call The H.O.N.S.T.E.C. Syndrome.

No matter what you have been told, it is *never* too late to learn something new, unless you refuse to accept or consider the infinite possibilities found in this life.

My mother used to say, "ignorance is bliss." She was wrong. Ignorance is directly related to suffering. If you don't know how dangerous a snake is and you pick it up, one bite, and now you know. However, it may be the last thing you will ever know. Her snake was a cigarette, junk food, alcohol, lack of exercise and forgiveness. It kills almost the same. It just takes a little longer.

Perhaps it's your time to find what you have been looking for? This book just maybe a portal into your new world. I pray it is.

Dis-ease is defined as lack of ease or harmony, it is NOT the
same as "disease," a medical term for illness treated by medicine.
NEVER attempt to stop or reduce your medication without the supervision of your medical doctor.

[My mother loved being outside in her garden. She loved the flowers and plants. This is another one of her favorite poems.]

Bliss

by

Eric C Wyndham

Oh, how I love my time worn trail of polished earth, hardened by shuffled step, from garden wall to the sweet water spring, a daily ritual that pleases the soul.

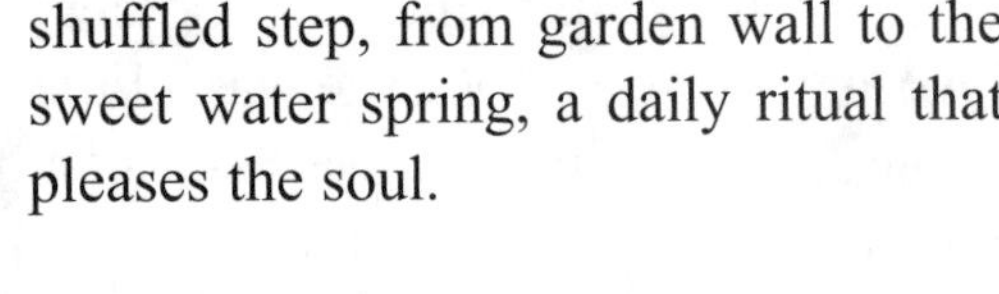

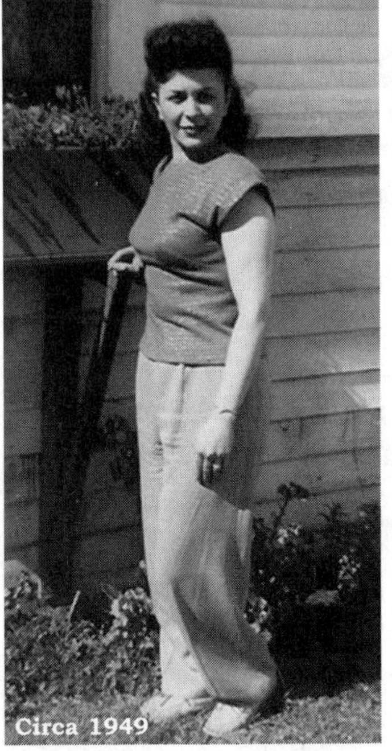

Circa 1949

On the bench I made, no sturdier found, I sit for hours smelling wild flowers and watching sparrows, wing on wind, fly to and home again.

Oh, how I love my mind to soar in my secret place. To take the time to commune with Him that sent me for purpose I long ago achieved. My just reward lies here with nature, in peace and harmony.

Let the world spin at full speed, throwing those not one with it to the universe. I will spend my days here in my beloved meadow, never regretting a day in the life of this thing called me.

With no regret of life in total, I am all that was, is and will be. I am the sum total. And only the Grand Architect knows why I've come this way.

Find your meadow, wear your trail and regret not your life. A moment in time. A chance to be. For this is *Bliss*, you see...

[I found this in *A Collection of Writings* by EC Wyndham. It seemed he was describing my life. For all of you having similar circumstances, there is hope and its called forgiveness.]

Forgiveness

by

Eric C Wyndham

My mouth runs dry as I feel my heart pounding in my throat,
the approaching footsteps becoming louder.

The front door opens, I run to hide; my home once secure and
warm is now piercing cold by contrast, the air heavy with fear.
The ritualistic ceremony has begun, it's only a matter of time.

Regardless of what I say or do, I am doomed.
There is no place of safety, for I will be found,
rest assured, I will be found.

I scream, cry and plead to no avail;
my pain only nourishes my attacker.
The more I beg, the more torment befalls me.
How can one do such things?
I am so young, so vulnerable, so innocent.

After years of horrific punishment,
I learn to stare aimlessly in the distance
as I am struck time and again.
The tears long ago dried, leaving nothing left to give.

I now live with a lifetime of unwanted memories,
my only hope is releasing them to what was, so I can now "Be.'
For without *forgetting* there is no *forgiveness,*
without *forgiveness* there is no *Love*,
without *Love* .....what's the purpose?

Notes

Dis-ease is defined as lack of ease or harmony, it is NOT the
same as "disease," a medical term for illness treated by medicine.
NEVER attempt to stop or reduce your medication without the supervision of your medical doctor.

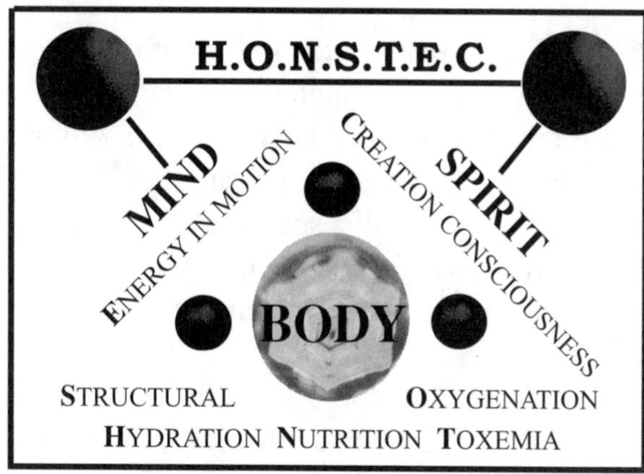

CHAPTER 2 - THE H.O.N.S.T.E.C. SYNDROME: THE ONLY *CAUSE* OF DIS-EASE.

"Balance is the key to health and longevity, and nothing is more important than your health. Nothing." **- Dr. James Chappell**

My mother clearly demonstrated what happens to someone when they don't eat properly, exercise or have a system in place to deal with stress and forgiveness. Her losses were unavoidable, her reactions her own. She willingly surrendered to *experimental* orthodox medicine, a mistake with *irreversible* consequences. The lesson here is clear: We can not concede to blindly trying drugs and other medical procedures as our parents and ancestors have. We *must* use common sense and logic before we accept any protocol allegedly promoting health, including that which I outline in this book. If what I have said does not feel right to you, perhaps you should take pause and re-evaluate what you are reading.

We go now from Chapter 1, the colorful, yet painful history of why I wrote this book, to the more clinical, but critically important end result of my research. In Chapter 2, I will take you through The H.O.N.S.T.E.C. Syndrome (known as the *cause* of all dis-ease). In Chapter 3, I will discuss the top twelve dis-eases, including obesity, diabetes and cancer. Chapter 4 is a basic food, supplement, exercise and emotional release program to cure dis-ease. Chapter 5 covers the politics of medicine and drug therapy.

Chapter 6 is an *intensive* protocol I developed for my patients during my clinical service. Chapter 7 announces the six herbal and one mineral element that have been *scientifically* proven to *cure* diabetes. In Chapter 8, I include a comprehensive health questionnaire allowing you to actually see your current health status. In Chapter 9, you will learn about the current health status in America. We have a lot to cover, so let's start with The H.O.N.S.T.E.C. Syndrome.

Most of the time people look for one isolated event that caused their health challenge and one magic pill to cure it. If it isn't a bug, germ or some other alien invasion, it's our parents, siblings, relatives, friends or strangers. Some how we feel we "catch" dis-eases, never accepting responsibility for *causing* them ourselves.

Haven't you heard we *catch* a "cold" or *get* the "flu"? It seems easier to blame someone or something for our health circumstances rather than looking inward. Of course the medical profession tells us it isn't our fault we are sick and in some cases, it isn't. But the vast majority of us have acquired our illnesses through our lifestyle, poor diet, lack of exercise and the way we think, or more often, the way we *don't*.

With this understanding, I discovered at least seven common denominators found in *all* dis-eases which I coined The Chappell H.O.N.S.T.E.C. Syndrome or simply The H.O.N.S.T.E.C. Syndrome, which is an acronym for the following:

The H.O.N.S.T.E.C. Syndrome:

H - Hydration or the lack thereof

O - Oxygen/Tissue deprivation

N - Nutritional deficiencies and/or excesses

S - Spinal/Structural/Neurological aberrations

T - Toxic waste accumulation

E - Emotional/Energetic blocks or release

C - Creation Consciousness

Dis-ease is defined as lack of ease or harmony, it is NOT the same as "disease," a medical term for illness treated by medicine. *NEVER* attempt to stop or reduce your medication without the supervision of your medical doctor.

The H.O.N.S.T.E.C. concept is fairly easy to understand, as long as you keep an open mind. As you will see, any one or more of the above H.O.N.S.T.E.C. components can *cause* anything or everything, from a common "cold" to cancer. All components of the syndrome can directly or indirectly *cause* malnutrition, subtle dehydration, toxemia, tissue hypoxia (lack of oxygen), cellular fermentation and subsequent immune disorders. If we can't absorb sufficient amounts of nutrients from our food and/or oxygen from the air and proper breathing and water consumption, we will be malnourished and dehydrated. In addition, toxic waste accumulation and contamination keep us from functioning properly. Without proper nutritional absorption, hormonal, biochemical, musculo-skeletal and neurological systems, will be out of balance and problematic. This is what really *causes* dis-ease, not a defective gene, germ, bacteria or virus. These scapegoats are merely after the fact, not before. By the time you finish this book, you will know the truth and the difference.

Have you ever considered what causes a cancer cell to multiply uncontrollably? If a virus causes the cell to become infected and then divide uncontrollably, what causes the virus to behave in this manner? If genetics cause the immune system to be programmed to be susceptible to viral infections, what causes that? The medical profession has simply been looking at the *after* affect of "disease" rather than the *cause* and *effect* of dis-ease.

Any one or more of the components of The H.O.N.S.T.E.C. Syndrome may cause genetic mutations and viral, bacterial, fungal or parasitic infections, all leading to uncontrollable cellular proliferation, i.e., cancer. The same pathway leads to obesity, diabetes, heart dis-ease, Parkinson's, Alzheimer's, muscular dystrophy, lupus, multiple sclerosis, arthritis and Attention Deficit Disorder to name a few. These so-called "diseases" are simply physical manifestations of The H.O.N.S.T.E.C. Syndrome. The key to understanding the dis-ease process will be discussed in *Chapter 3 - Top Twelve Dis-eases with Their Signs, Signals and Symptoms,* for now the syndrome starts with hydration.

The First Contributing Factor of H.O.N.S.T.E.C. is:
H - Hydration or the lack thereof

"Water water everywhere yet not a drop to drink." I don't remember who said that and in what context, but I can imagine the speaker adrift on the ocean with no drinkable water on board.

Recently I went out to dinner with some friends and the waitress offered me a glass of water. I kindly declined, yet I was thirsty. My friends know me well enough, so they didn't ask why I refused to drink tap water. It's simple: tap water is toxic. It has chlorine, fluoride and anything else our "trusted" government wants to dump. Knowing that chlorine can cause cancer and even instantly kill you if inhaled as a gas, was my cause for rejection. But since fluoride is more insidious, it is a "horse of a different color."

The Internet and libraries throughout the country contain information concerning the truth about fluoride. Not the rhetoric the American Dental Association (ADA), metal companies and our government are putting out, but scientific, factual truth.

According to the research found in *Clinical Toxicology of Commercial Products*, 5th edition, 1984, lead has a toxicity rating of 3 which equals a *moderate* toxicity. Fluoride, more specifically sodium fluoride the form of fluoride put into our water and toothpaste, has a toxicity rating of 4, which equals a *very* or *high* toxicity.

Fluoridated toothpaste is so toxic the Food and Drug Administration (FDA) mandates that all toothpaste manufacturers using fluoride put a warning on their label. It states, **"If you accidentally swallow more than used for brushing, seek professional help or contact a *poison* control center immediately."** They go on to say that consuming half of the tube of that sweet-tasting, creamy, delicious, addictive toothpaste your child loves, can kill them. Are you surprised? You shouldn't be. After all, its a poison.

Sodium and fluorosalicic acid fluoride are used in rat poison and insecticides. The only difference between rat poison and your toothpaste is the parts per million (ppm). At a lower dose you won't die, at least not right away. Alarmingly, as little as 2 mg of fluoride per day can produce crippling skeletal fluorosis in a person's lifetime. Along with toothpaste and tap water, we also consume fluoride in soft drinks and other products using tap water.

The *United States Public Health Services* has stated that 50% of one's daily fluoride intake is eliminated, with the other 50% being absorbed in calcified tissues such as the bone and teeth. They also state that fluoride makes the bones more brittle and the dental enamel more porous. Tragically, mottled teeth, also called dental fluorosis, affects 1 out of every 5 children in the United States.

In the early part of the last century, fluoride was recognized as a dominant industrial pollutant. It was and still is a waste product from iron, steel, aluminum, copper, lead and zinc manufacturing operations and is a by-product of fertilizer.

Rather than pay to dispose of this toxic waste, the above manufacturing companies simply turned the public image of fluoride around from being an industrial pollutant, to being something that helps prevent cavities. In order to do this they had to fund "research" validating their claim. Since money talks, the claim was easily made with the help of the ADA. Americans bought this lie hook, line and sinker.

The promoters of toxic fluoride always state that fluoride is found in the earth and so it can't be harmful. Of course they don't differentiate between their sodium fluoride and the natural, harmless calcium fluoride found in the earth. They say fluoride is fluoride. As my dear late friend, Ruben Johnson, would say, "My word, something smells a little fishy." When it comes to fluoride, it's not a little fishy - it is down right rotten.

We and our children are being duped into believing this toxic drug has some kind of dental benefit. Even if this were partially true, you must ask yourself, at what cost? Is it worth not having a cavity in exchange for neurotoxic damage and subsequent sickness, dis-ease and premature death?

In 1990, the *National Cancer Institute* found and stated that commercial fluoride was carcinogenic. In 1992, they found a 6.9% increase in bone cancer was absolutely linked to fluoridated water. Other studies have revealed an increase in hip fractures, brain damage, osteoporosis, arthritis and other abnormalities.

Although there are no reliable studies conducted under legitimate, ethical research guidelines that indicate any benefits of fluoride application through water and toothpaste, there are however, more than 500 studies that indicate adverse health effects.

Even though, Jeff Green of the *Citizens for Safe Drinking Water*, has traveled throughout the United States from city to city educating local governments about the dangers of fluoride in public drinking water, our politicians simply supercede the voice of the people and mandate toxic fluoride be dumped in our public water supply. Ask yourself, "Why would they do this?" Of course it doesn't have anything to do with the fluoride manufacturing companies donating money to the elected's campaign fund. Right.

If you really want to know the history of fluoride, I suggest you research I.G. Farben on the Internet.

CoralWhite® Tooth Treatment

Because of my concern, I formulated the only all natural tooth treatment, not only fluoride free, but containing a mineral complex that has been proven to help re-enamelize teeth. It is called ***CoralWhite***® and is made by Coral, LLC. For more information see Index E *Resources* at the back of this book.

In 1971, I read a book by Dr. Allen E. Banik entitled, *The Choice is Clear*. Of all the types of water available to us today, from so-called mountain spring, well, artesian, purified, filtered, to reverse osmosis, only *distilled water* is recommended by Dr. Banik. Even one of my mentors, Dr. Paavo Airola, who once stated distilled water was toxic, later came around and claimed it to be the only purified water left on the planet.

The closest thing to the purity of distilled water was rain-water. If fact, rainwater *is* distilled water. The sun heats the earth and waterways, including the oceans, and pulls moisture up into forming clouds. Because today's rainwater passes through our current polluted skies, it is contaminated with the particles floating in the air. There are locations of pristine water still on earth, but as you can imagine, nowhere near civilization. The only solution is to make or buy your water.

Of course selling water is like selling anything else. Each manufacturer looks for a "hook" to make their product better than the other. If they can't build theirs up, they try to put their competition down. Because distilled water is pure H2O, it does not contain any minerals and therefore with continuous consumption, it may leach minerals from the body. For this reason, competitors have said it is unhealthy. In recent years, with the advance of computers and microscopes, competitors have claimed that the process of distilling water also damages the molecular structure of water thus making it unhealthy. The eminent Dr. Masaru Emoto a researcher from Japan, has scientifically proven the structure of water thereby providing validity to this claim.

Fortunately, I was taught over 30 years ago how to make my own pristine water. I call it charged distilled water. It is very simple and inexpensive to make.

To put minerals back in distilled water, take one-half teaspoon of sea salt and mix it into one gallon of distilled water. Although you could use any sea salt, I only use **Zeta Crystals®** by QCI Products® because of the mineral content. The other reason is because it electrically charges the water, enhancing the *zeta* potential. In so doing, it reconfigures the molecular structure of the water back to its crystallized pristine state. I am sure those making the expensive designer waters will disagree. However, as I said in the beginning, this book is for those with "eyes to see" and "ears to hear." The mind is like a parachute. It must be opened to work.

The Miracle of Water

The following pictures from Dr. Emoto's book, *The Message of Water,* offer fascinating insights to the energy of water. (See Index E-Re*sources* for more information on his book.)

Dr. Emoto sampled different sources of water from around the world. After freezing one molecule from each source he then took a collection of pictures using darkfield microscopy.

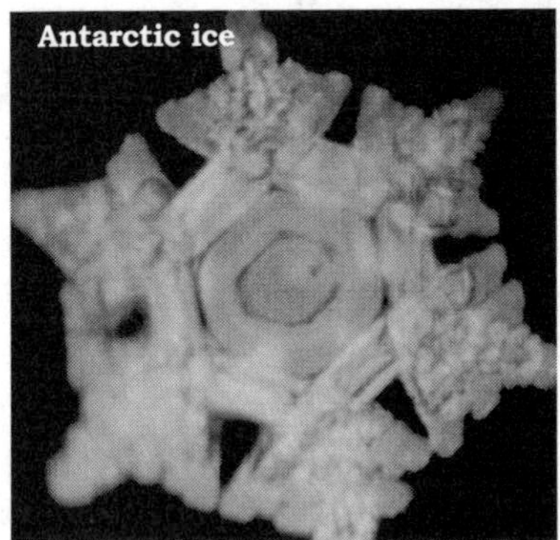
Antarctic ice

In this first picture on the left, we see what pristine water looks like from Antarctic ice. Notice the crystalline structure of the water. This water was taken at a depth representing 370,000 years ago. (These pictures show the HADO in water. HADO signifies energy related to consciousness or "Chi.")

The next picture below and to the right, was taken from a non-polluted spring in Japan. The structure is unmistakably clear. It has a vibratory energy that holds form and field. For those of us who believe in God or nature, it holds mystery and awe. What created such beauty? How can simple water be so geometric? These answers are still part of the Great Mystery.

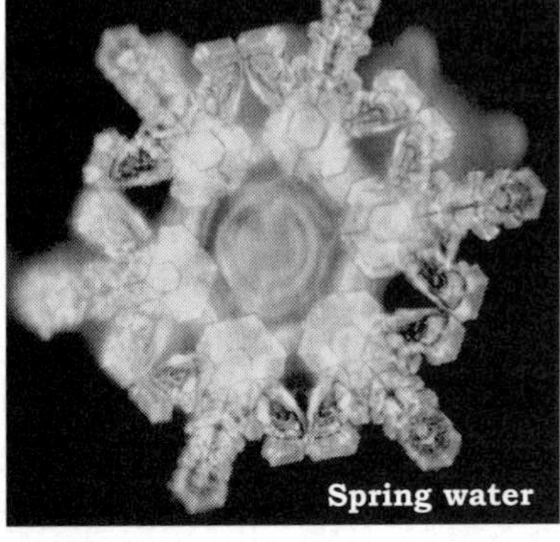
Spring water

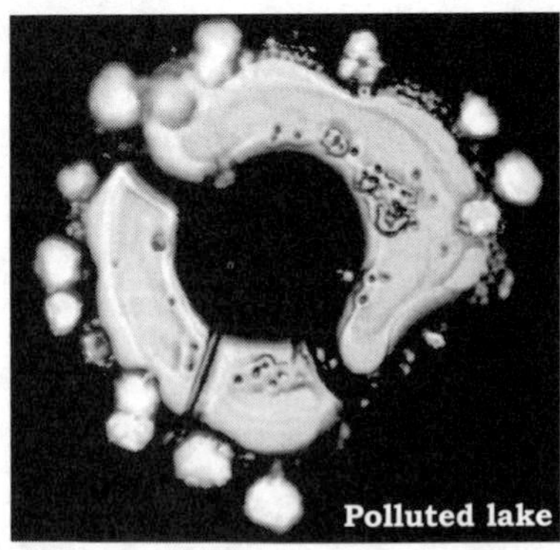
Polluted lake

The final picture to the left was taken from a polluted lake in Japan. This lake has dioxins, PCBs, petrochemicals and other toxins in it. Notice how mutated it appears. Is this what our tapwater looks like?

According to Dr. Emoto, all tapwater contains chemicals which alter the crystalline structure, thus lowering the life force or HADO.

Is there any doubt to his findings? I don't think so.

Dis-ease is defined as lack of ease or harmony, it is NOT the same as "disease," a medical term for illness treated by medicine. *NEVER* attempt to stop or reduce your medication without the supervision of your medical doctor.

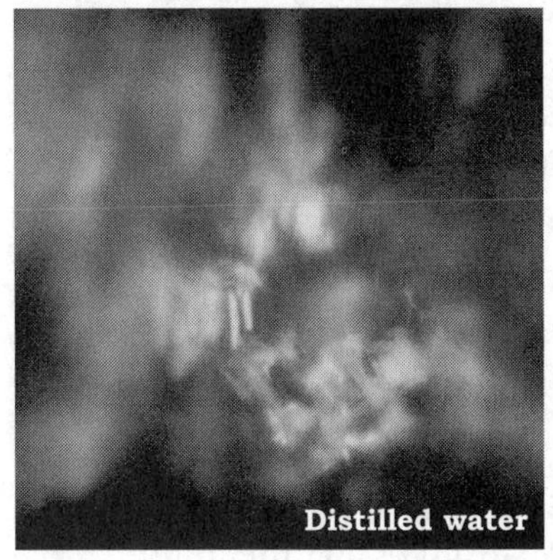

The most fascinating part of Dr. Emoto's research is what you are about to see. Although distilling water changes the crystalline structure, it seems to totally lose its shape and form. Although the picture on the left is blurred, there is no mistaking the difference between pristine water and distilled. I believe its the energy and minerals that give water its shape. This is one reason why I put *Zeta Crystals®* in my charged distilled water.

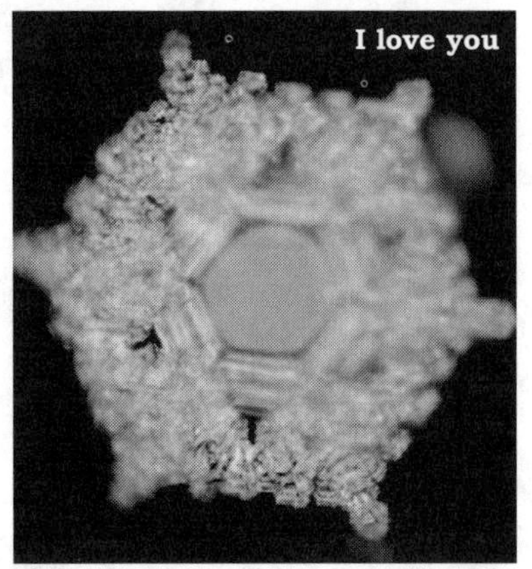

Dr. Emoto took a bottle of distilled water and placed a label stating, "I love and appreciate you" on it. Within days, the mutated-looking distilled water above, changed to the beautiful crystalline water to the right. Do you understand the significance? Just writing words on the bottle changed the water!

Using the same distilled water, Dr. Emoto wrote the words "I hate you." Within days the distilled water changed to an even more mutated shape seen on the left. What does all this mean?

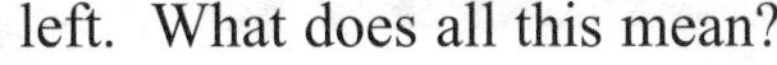

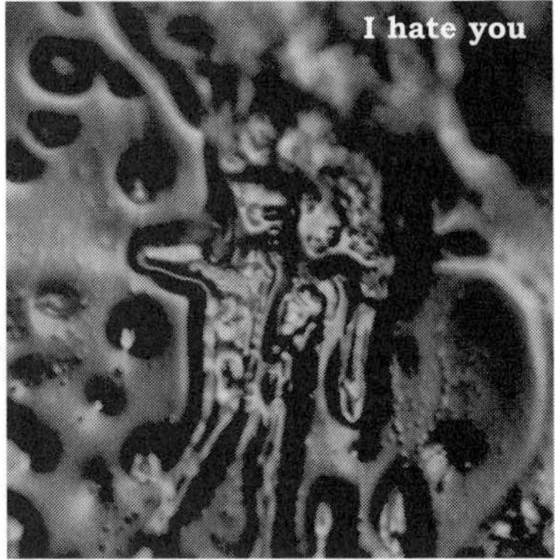

Dr. Emoto tested music, light and sound, all with the same results. Remember, we become what we think about all day long. If both written and spoken words can change the molecular structure of water outside the body, what do you think they can do inside the body?

Dis-ease is defined as lack of ease or harmony, it is NOT the same as "disease," a medical term for illness treated by medicine. *NEVER* attempt to stop or reduce your medication without the supervision of your medical doctor.

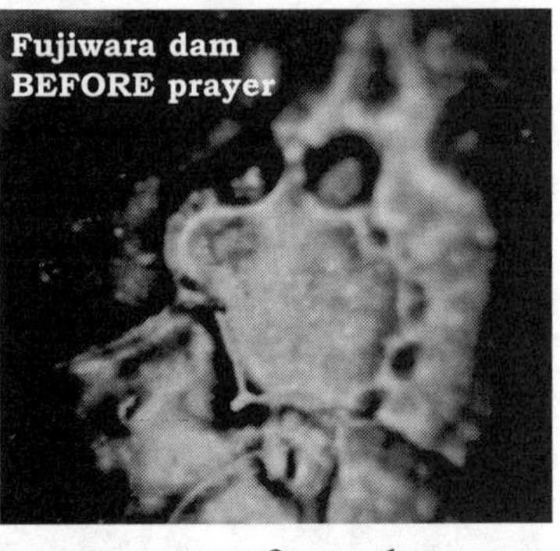
Fujiwara dam BEFORE prayer

I have saved the best for last. Finally, for the first time in my experience, we have unequivocal proof of the power of *effective* prayer. The picture on the right was taken from a water sample at the Fujiwara dam in Japan, a known toxic water supply. This is *not* distilled water, this is a polluted water way.

The picture below is the exact same water from the same location placed in a bottle. The only difference is this picture was taken after a group of people prayed for a healing. Not unlike when we either pray or have someone pray for us. However, I believe the key difference between how the typical American prays and how the Japanese prayed has to do with *effectiveness*.

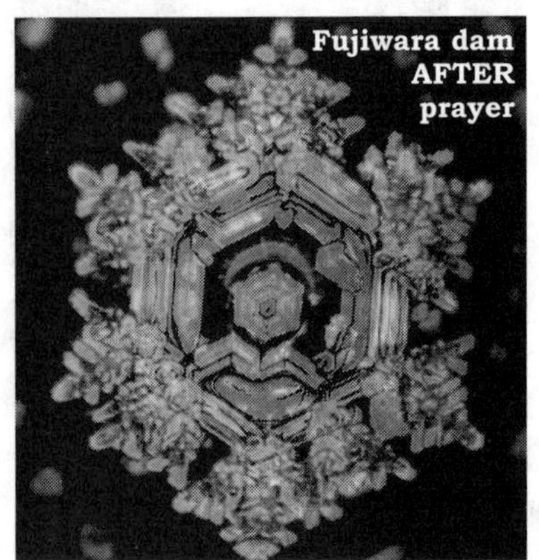
Fujiwara dam AFTER prayer

If we *demand* from God a list of requests, we are *not* following the proper "code of procedure." It is my understanding, we are to be quiet, still and listen for the Great Mystery knows what we want and need *before* we even ask.

If you can believe the pictures here are real, then you can also believe there are no incurable dis-eases. Fact: the human body is 75% water. The brain is 85% water and "we become what we think about."

Apparently, we have the ability to reconfigure vibratory chaos or scrambled molecular forms. However, *MOST OF US DO NOT KNOW HOW*. For those of us *not* spiritually mature enough to transmute dis-ease in an *instant*, in the interim, we need to practice the principles of good nutrition, hygiene, exercise, forgiveness, rest and relaxation found in this book. One day, there may be no need for the mundane replaced by the sublime.

Dis-ease is defined as lack of ease or harmony, it is NOT the same as "disease," a medical term for illness treated by medicine. *NEVER* attempt to stop or reduce your medication without the supervision of your medical doctor.

The key behind proper hydration is not only drinking pristine water, but drinking *enough* of it. Herein is another opportunity for those spewing misinformation to confuse you. They will say that "all the water you need is in your food. Drinking additional water has no value." In light of the human body being 75% water/fluid and the brain being 85% water/fluid, why would anyone say that? I guess everyone has a right to their own level of ignorance and they are simply demonstrating theirs.

The body loses water on a daily basis from respiration (breathing), perspiration (sweating), urination (kidneys), and defecation (colon). Dehydration is one of the major contributors to aging, illness and death. Water is so important, that we can only live days without it.

After consulting with more than 10,000 people, I found the majority demonstrated dehydration. Their internal organs were literally drying and shriveling up. This can easily be proven by darkfield microscopy, a low light/heat microscope. For that reason alone, I believe dehydration is one reason why we age and die prematurely. After all, wrinkles not only demonstrate oxidative decomposition, they clearly show how skin changes when it loses its moisture from a lack of water and oils.

According to natural healing, we must drink at least half of our body weight converted to ounces, daily. As an example, if you weigh 128 pounds and divide it by two, it equals 64. This means you need 64 ounces or eight, 8 oz glasses of water daily just to replace what you are losing from the above pathways.

Dr. Banik believed that nearly all "disease" developed from dehydration. As important as water may be, I believe the lack of it is only one factor in the cause of dis-ease.

Water is used to regulate temperature and to act as a solvent. It carries waste products from the body and dissolves food substances so they can be assimilated into every cell.

From Dr. Banik to Drs. Paul Bragg, Airola, and everyone in between, pristine water is always recommended for optimum health and longevity.

Water *IS* oxygen

According to Dr. Patrick Flanagan, a health researcher, most people believe water is the same everywhere. H20 is H20. Yet, there are significant differences beyond the obvious ones of taste, appearance and hardness. The kind of water you drink determines how efficiently your cells will absorb nutrients and expel toxins and free radicals. Not all water hydrates the cells.

If the water you drink is ordinary tap water with *high* surface tension and little or no electrical charge, nutrients will not be efficiently transferred. Most tap water lacks trace minerals and essential electrolytes. The surface tension of the water is greater (thicker) than our bodily fluids, which means there is very little cellular exchange of nutrients going into the cells and waste products coming out. Since cellular fluid has a *lower* surface tension than ordinary tap water, the body has to work harder to make this tap water more bio-available.

Some warning signs of cells beginning to dry up and suffer from dehydration are stiffness, loss of flexibility, dry wrinkled skin, tendons that tear more easily, brittle bones and loss of lung flexibility. The quality of our water has a great effect on the quality of our life.

Proper hydration and oxygenation of the body is essential for optimum health and is dependent upon the quality of the water we drink. When we drink "dead" water, the process of cellular exchange - nutrients in and toxins out, is inhibited. As we get older, our cells begin to suffocate in their own waste products and nutrients are blocked from entering the cells. One answer to health and longevity lies in the efficient circulation and removal of these toxins from the body, thereby paving the way for nutrients to enter the cells uninhibited.

Remember, the *lower* the surface tension the wetter the water and the more effective will be nutrient absorption. By "charging" your water (see page 29), it not only lowers the surface tension, it maintains a negative net electrical charge.

The negative charge is one of the key factors in the healthful effects of water and the ability to retain an electrical charge is known as zeta-potential.

If the zeta-potential (negative electric charge) is low, toxins cannot be suspended; separated for elimination and the whole system becomes clogged. Chemists say that zeta-potential is what keeps the billions of cells in the body in circulation. Unhealthy foods or high toxic levels in the blood, poor oxygen intake and other factors cause the blood cells to clump together, called rouleau. This impairs the transfer of energy and the flow of nutrients through the system.

One more comment about zeta-potential. Every cell in the human body is like a little battery. It has an electrical (zeta) potential ranging from 70 to 90 millivolts. When we don't feel well, this electrical potential diminishes. From 70 to 90, it drops 60/80, 50/70 and so on. When we are really ill, it can drop to 35. Cancer patients can drop to 15 or lower. Losing our electrical potential is synonymous with dying. It is extremely important to keep one's zeta-potential to a maximum level. When you drink charged distilled water with a substance called *stabilized oxygen*, increased electric charges are found on blood cells.

The Second Contributing Factor of H.O.N.S.T.E.C. is:
O - Oxygen/Tissue deprivation

Oxygen, carbon, hydrogen, nitrogen and sulfur are the five basic elements of all life. Nitrogen plus oxygen and carbon plus hydrogen creates *proteins.* Carbon plus oxygen plus hydrogen creates *carbohydrates.* Oxygen plus hydrogen creates *water.* Oxygen is the most abundant element of earth, however it is slowly depleting. Although it comprises 55 to 62% of the earth's crust and currently 18 to 20% of dry air, this colorless, tasteless and odorless element, so essential to life, comprises 65% of the elements of our body, including blood, organs, tissues and skin.

Oxygen helps to create energy, digest food, metabolize fat and carbohydrates, transport gases across cell membranes, manufacture hormones, proteins and other chemicals, regulate pH, incite the body to breathe, clean and detoxify toxins from the body, eradicate virus, amoebae, parasites, fungus and bacteria and maintain a healthy and strong immune system. Through breathing, oxygen turns sugar into energy, a process called oxidation. After oxidation, the most important effect of breathing is oxygenation. Oxygenation involves saturation with oxygen, as in the aeration of blood in the lungs.

The average person needs some 200 milliliters (1 cup) of oxygen per minute while resting and nearly 8 liters (2 gallons) during periods of strenuous activity. It is estimated that we breathe about 2,500 gallons of air each day. Therefore, oxygen is paramount to our health and survival.

According to Dr. Otto Warburg from Germany, a three-time Nobel Laureate, cancer and other dis-eases thrive on little to no oxygen. He found that all cancer starts and grows in an acid pH and low oxygen medium. In fact, there is a definite correlation between the rapid loss of planetary oxygen and the increase of cancer and other dis-eases.

This discovery is extremely important for it answers the question why we have more drug resistant infectious organisms and cancer today than ever before. As we continue to lose oxygen in the air we breathe, the opportunistic anaerobic bacteria, virus and cancer proliferate. Unquestionably, one reason why we have an increase in cancer and other dis-eases worldwide is because we are destroying our oxygen generating capabilities through clear cutting our forests and jungles and burning fossil fuels in our gasoline and oil combustible engines. When I started my natural healing career over 34 years ago, one out of ten people acquired cancer, that's 1 out of 10! As of 2004, one out of every two and a half were getting cancer. That's 1 out of 2.5! What is so frightening is that anaerobic and pathogenic organisms, including cancer, proliferate in direct proportion to our loss of oxygen. In other words, as we continue to lose oxygen, cancer, bacteria, virus and other dis-ease-related organisms grow. Listen to what a few *informed* researchers have had to say about the importance of oxygen:

1. "All chronic pain, suffering and diseases are caused from a lack of oxygen at the cell level." **- Arthur C. Guyton, M.D.**

2. "Virtually all heart attacks come down to a failure to deliver oxygen to the hardworking heart muscle."

- Phillip Stavish, M.D.

3. "Lack of oxygen clearly plays a major role in causing cells to become cancerous." **- Harry Goldblatt, Ph.D.**

4. "Hypoxia or lack of oxygen in the tissues, is the fundamental cause for all degenerative disease."

- Steven A. Levine, Ph.D.

5. "Oxygen plays a pivotal role in the proper functioning of the immune system." **- Paris M. Kidd, Ph.D.**

6. "It is the lack of oxygen in proper amounts in the system that prevents oxidation and oxygenation, which energizes the cell to biological regeneration. These processes are the foundation of life and death." **- Stephen R. Krauss**

7. "If the body is being starved of oxygen, then to avoid illness, the oxygen must be supplemented by nutritional supplements such as stabilized oxygen." **- John Muntz, D.O.**

What about just doing some vigorous exercise? Although exercise is vital for health and longevity and will be discussed in *Chapter 6 - The Chappell Protocol for Health & Longevity*, exercise alone will *not* help.

In 1996 two researchers drilled into an Antarctic ice cap at the level that represented 150 years ago. In analyzing the ice, they discovered the oxygen content of the atmosphere at that time was between 38 to 40%. The researchers then tested the current oxygen content in several cities of the world. Over all, the earth's level of oxygen was then 18 to 20%. This was a 50% drop in oxygen in the last 150 years. In addition, they found cities like Mexico, Tokyo and Chicago ranged from 13 to 16%. This is most alarming especially when considering the fact that at 6%, all oxygen breathing organisms will suffocate and die. Frighteningly, we are fast approaching our own extinction.

Besides losing oxygen from toxic hydrocarbons from industrialized societies,' we are clearing thousands of oxygen-producing acres of rain forest every day. From Brazil to Mexico, wherever there is suitable land, trees are cut down. What for? For *you*. For *you*, if you eat commercial meat, specifically beef.

With the onslaught of fast-"food" restaurants on every corner serving a *"Super-Size-Me"* hamburger, fries and soda, the meat industry had to find a place to raise cheap beef. As with most other "*Made-in-America*" products, "American" beef has simply been outsourced to third world countries.

The indigenous people are driven off their land by human rights violators and then their forests are decimated. Where there once was a world of vegetation and thousands of animal species, there now is only grazing land for cattle and other animals we consume. The end result of this gluttonous practice is the continuous loss of our precious oxygen and natural habitat.

Oxygen Deficiency Signals

The problem with most people having been indoctrinated into the Western mindset of "disease," is that they cannot differentiate between clinical and pre-clinical *signals* or corollaries of dis-ease. Typically, only when one has a full-blown illness will they seek medical advice or help. Pre-clinical *signals* of that dis-ease go unabated for months or even years.

Initial *signals* of oxygen deprivation may include overall weakness, acid stomach, bronchial complications, irritability, memory loss, depression, dizziness, irrational behavior, fatigue, poor digestion, muscle aches and pains and circulation problems. Instead of knowing the significance of these *signals* of oxygen deprivation, we write them off as normal or age-related. When we become somewhat concerned, we might try one of hundreds of over-the-counter symptom-treating drugs. For an acid stomach it might be Rolaids® or Tums®. For irritability or depression one might try something over-the-counter or even Prozac®. For poor digestion and gas it might be Bean O® and for aches and pains, of course it is Aspirin, Motrin® or something similar. Since the cause of the problem is not being addressed, only temporary relief (if any), will be realized. Once an over-the-counter symptom-treating drug is no longer effective, one might seek medical help for stronger drugs.

Because the most successfully advertised and promoted medical union in America is the American Medical Association (AMA), which has the full support of the pharmaceutical industry and the United States government's Food and Drug Administration (FDA), most uninformed people will seek an orthodox symptom-treating medical doctor (medic).

MDs have at their disposal a litany of highly powerful, symptom-treating drugs. Unfortunately, these drugs merely mask the symptoms. It is not unusual for a medic to be concerned with only *treating* symptoms. If doctors were concerned about the cause, they would *not* use symptom-treating drugs. As we know, if you do not address the core *issue* of dis-ease, eventually it will raise its ugly head and let you know it never went away.

Getting to One *Cause* of Dis-ease

As stated, oxygen energizes cells so they can regenerate. Additionally, our body uses oxygen to metabolize food and to eliminate toxins and waste through oxidation. Our brain needs oxygen each second to process information. In fact, all of our organs need a great deal of oxygen to function efficiently. It is quite obvious, oxygen is not only a critical nutritional component to our survival, but is crucial to achieving optimum health.

Tissue hypoxia or not enough oxygen is a major *cause* of *all* dis-ease. Thanks to a product I developed, a *stabilized oxygen* I call **Stable 'O,'** oxygen deprivation is one cause we can rapidly do something about. **Stable 'O'** comes in a easy-to-use liquid dropper bottle Placing 10 to 20 drops in an eight-ounce glass of charged distilled water (Zeta Crystals®) provides all the oxygen you need to bring your body back to balance. It is part of my all inclusive Lifepack System®.
(See *Chapter 4* for more information concerning the my lifepack system for optimum health and longevity).

Dis-ease is defined as lack of ease or harmony, it is NOT the same as "disease," a medical term for illness treated by medicine.
NEVER attempt to stop or reduce your medication without the supervision of your medical doctor.

The Third Contributing Factor of H.O.N.S.T.E.C. is:
N - Nutritional deficiencies and/or excesses

In the sixties, we said, *"You are what you eat."* In the seventies, we said, *"You are what you eat AND more importantly, what you assimilate."* Finally, in the eighties, we said, *"You are what you eat, assimilate and most importantly, DON'T eliminate."*

If this is true, we better eat all organic, pesticide-free, live food and we better have a digestive system that is able to breakdown and absorb it. We also *must* have an elimination system able to remove and expel our waste.

One key to balancing these systems is *not* eating more than our body has the ability to process. From digestion, absorption to elimination, what we don't eliminate, we become. Putrefied, toxic food not eliminated is reabsorbed. Unhealthy food makes the consumer, unhealthy. As you'll read, under the auspices of nutrition, digestion and elimination are just as important.

Nutrition

My father was in the vegetable-growing business. He was a *commercial* grower, selling produce to Safeway Markets and others, including the U.S. Army. As a young boy, I would work in the fields picking crops during the summer to make a little extra money. One day I asked him why the soil didn't have any worms or bugs in it. He said, "Bugs kill plants so I use insecticides to kill them first." He also said, "You can work the fields forever, if you just put some fertilizer back in." He didn't believe there was a need to *rest* the soil every seventh year as our forefathers suggested. He used a product called NPK, which stands for nitrogen, phosphorus and potassium to keep his crops growing.

My father said, "If food looks, tastes and feels good, people will buy it regardless. It doesn't matter if it is nutritious or not. It just has to pass the *'buy me'* test." He believed in "Better living through chemistry®."

Commercial farmers today still practice this strategy of sterilizing soil and using NPK. After all, the name of the game is profit. They may have fancier equipment, genetically engineered seeds and more powerful insecticides, but it is basically the same.

So what's wrong with this approach? Nothing, if you don't care about your health and you want "Frankenfood."

Anyone born *prior* to the 1940s most likely grew up on organic food. It wasn't until the 1950s, we really started the "Better living through chemistry" push. It doesn't take much to figure out why Americans and other fast-food nations are constantly struggling with sickness and dis-ease. Our food supply may look, taste and feel "delicious," but it has very little real nutritional value.

When we overwork the soil, we deplete its mineral content. Devitalized soil produces demineralized food. It may look good, but there is no comparison to the taste of *real* organically grown food. Especially when the grower practices sustainable farming.

The end result of commercial growing is a nation starving to death. We are not starving in the sense of being emaciated. To the contrary, 66% of all American's are overweight to obese, but we are literally undernourished, overfed and poisoned by our food. As a matter of fact, I usually say most of us get sick or die from food poisoning. Think about that for a minute; "You are what you eat." If your food has been sprayed with toxins, you are that, as well.

Food is supposed to represent *vital* nutrients; vitamins, minerals, enzymes, amino and essential fatty acids. We eat to acquire these nutrients. If these nutrients are not in our food, we will eat more in our attempt to satiate our needs.

I have a theory that some may want to call it a conspiracy. If I were a profiteer within the food industry and I wanted people to eat more of my product, why couldn't I genetically engineer less nutrients, specifically those that satisfy the appetite center of the brain? I could also add chemicals like MSG to really hook you. The more people eat my yummy tasting "food" stuff, the more they'll want. I might even come up with a slogan like, "I bet you can't eat just one®." Between my advertising propaganda and the actual addictive ingredients, I think I could make millions. Oh well, it's just a theory. I'm sure no one could ever do it. Right!

The tobacco industry has been adding addictive chemicals since Phillip Morris rolled his first "coffin nail." So maybe my theory isn't to far fetched?

It was easy to include the classification of nutrition or the lack of it into The H.O.N.S.T.E.C. Syndrome. We know the body must have building blocks to optimally perform its functions. These building blocks should come from our food, air, light and water, when they don't, we get sick.

Fast "food" causes the body to burn and store more calories. Calories are stored as fat. The end result of eating fast "food" and other convenience "food" is obesity, illness and premature death.

Just as I am writing this section, the *Los Angeles Times* announced the death of McDonald's Restaurant CEO Charlie Bell. Mr. Bell died of colon cancer. He was just 44 years old. It was only seven and half months from the time he was diagnosed until his death. What a tragedy. The current chairman of McDonald's board, Andrew J. McKenna, was quoted as saying, "Even during his hospitalization and *chemotherapy*, Charlie led this company with pride and determination." With that, we know Mr. Bell wasn't incorporating natural healing or at least *not* exclusively. Maybe he was using one of the new *complementary* medical approaches mixing healing herbs with toxic drugs?

Mr. Bell was chosen to replace James Cantalupo, who died of a sudden heart attack in April 2004. He had been working and eating at McDonald's for years, he was just 60 years old.

I am sure Bell's death shocked the world. How could a young man, only 44 years old die of colon cancer? Again, the answer is, respectfully, why not? He started working for and most likely ate McDonald's "food" since 1975. At nineteen years of age, he was one of the youngest store managers the restaurant giant ever hired. At that age, he was still in his formative growing years. Even *experimental* orthodox medicine has stated there is a *higher* risk of developing colon cancer with the consumption of eating red meat. Apparently, the AMA doesn't want to believe this or they would be screaming it at the top of their lungs.

Two Worlds

Unfortunately, we live in two worlds. On one side we have 'People of the Earth.' They live with nature or as close to it as possible. They know about natural healing and the power of food, water, air, light, sound, forgiveness and *effective* prayer. They are *not* aggressive people, rather choosing to be peaceful. Whether primitive or aboriginal, they are living off the land or oceans, making their shelters out of available materials. If and when they leave an area, you would never know they were there. They only use what they need and never waste any of God's bounty for they have the utmost respect and reverence for all of nature's creatures and the earth for which they feel responsible for.

They eat to live, NOT live to eat. With few exceptions, they eat little meat and always free-range, truly wild or organic. Their body fat ratio is ideal and they get plenty of fresh air and sunshine.

Then we have 'People of the World.' Most of us in "civilized" society fall into this category. In a nutshell, we are a complete antithesis of the natural order. We live in violation of natural laws. If we want something, we acquire it either with money or warring confiscation. We believe mankind has "dominion" over the earth and all of its creatures. Misquoting the Bible, we justify experimenting and torturing animals for drugs, cosmetics and medical research.

We know nothing about the healing effects of food, water, air, light, sound, forgiveness or *effective* prayer. For the sake of profit, we have created synthetic, processed "food" stuffs, made from petro-chemical derivatives and waste products. Animals that once roamed freely on ranges, prairies, woods and forests, are now restricted and confined to contaminated mud-hole feed lots. Their nutritional staple of wild grass, plants and berries have been replaced with genetically engineered, pesticide sprayed grains and rendered animal. To prevent dis-ease and encourage "Frankenstein" growth, our food animals are injected or fed massive doses of antibiotics and synthetic growth hormones. Those that cannot endure this filthy inhumane treatment, get sick and die on the spot. Their bodies are *rendered* in large grinders and either fed back to the herd or sent to be used in our pets food. (For more details see Index-E *Resources* under Farm Sanctuary)

As 'People of the World' proliferate and contaminate more and more of this planet, our land, air, forests, lakes, rivers and oceans are left with visible evidence of our parasitic aftermath. Are you really surprised that we, the 'People of the World,' are dying from dis-eases unheard of by our ancestors?

I know what you're thinking. If it weren't for modern medicine we'd still have polio or the plague. I suggest you do a little research on that.

As the number of polio cases was reportedly going down from our government-sponsored vaccination programs, aseptic spinal meningitis was going up. According to the figures from the *Los Angeles County Health Index Morbidity and Mortality Rates,* in 1955, prior to the introduction of mass vaccination, 273 cases of polio were reported and 50 cases of aseptic meningitis. By 1966, there were only 5 cases of polio reported, but oddly enough, there were 256 cases of aseptic meningitis. Since both conditions are known to be interchangeable, apparently someone wanted to prove that vaccines had value, hence they manipulated the statistical data.

Yes, but what about polio today? According to the *Center for Disease Control* (CDC), from 1973 to 1983, over 87% of *all* polio cases reported were *caused* by the vaccine. From 1983 to 1989, 100% of all cases of polio were caused by the vaccine. Of course you'll never hear that on the evening news.

Do I recommend being vaccinated? Not on your life. Remember, **"Only sick people get sick."** If you don't want polio or the plague, stop doing all the things known to contribute to illness and start doing all those things known to keep you well.

Since we have certain religions forbidding the use of drugs, vaccines and other experimental medical treatment, you do not have to vaccinate your child if you sign a waiver for religious or even personal reasons. In addition, no government agency can bridge the separation of church and state.

(For more information concerning vaccines, see Index E *Resources* in the back of the book).

Digestion

Although the body produces digestive enzymes to help breakdown our food, these enzymes are designed to work with the enzymes contained *within* the food.

Aboriginal natives eat mostly *raw* food, even raw meat and fish. Their food is often fresh picked and eaten immediately. We on the other hand, eat mostly processed, package and/or prepared *cooked* food, bought at our local market that could have been made or picked days or even weeks before. Cooking destroys food enzymes. This puts extreme stress on our digestive system. Our bodies were not designed to produce the levels of enzymes *cooked* food demands.

Because of our continued diminished ability to breakdown our food, we simply develop poor digestion, absorption and subsequent malnutrition. A *sign* of this H.O.N.S.T.E.C. component is what your medic calls acid reflux "disease." Of course, they have a drug you can take to mask the *signal*, but as you know, it does nothing to address the *cause*.

Eventually, after years of bloating, gas, "heartburn" and so-called acid reflux, we either develop ulcers, cancer or some other "mysterious" dis-ease. However, there is nothing mysterious about it. It is simply *cause* and *effect*.

Elimination

If it isn't bad enough that we, the People of the World, eat mostly cooked junk "food," through lack of hydration, exercise, stress and self medication, our elimination is deplorable. Only those in "civilized" society have bowel habits like ours.

Humans and animals in the wild will typically have a bowel movement cycled around their intake of food. In other words, if we eat three *healthy* meals per day, we will usually have three *healthy* bowel movements per day. However, unhealthy junk "food" changes our natural pattern.

Dis-ease is defined as lack of ease or harmony, it is NOT the same as "disease," a medical term for illness treated by medicine.
NEVER attempt to stop or reduce your medication without the supervision of your medical doctor.

A clear *sign* of a sluggish intestinal transition time is the size and texture of one's feces. 'People of the Earth' have large bowel movements between 12 and 14" or longer. They are usually the same circumference of their colon or about 1-1/2 to 2" for an adult. There was no time to think, let alone read a magazine (if they had one) when an aboriginal is squatting to have a bowel movement. It is fast and to the point. Depending on their diet, their feces are usually soft, fibrous and would float if deposited on water.

Again, 'People of the World,' are just the opposite. We usually have one bowel movement per day, regardless of how many meals we eat. Our feces are 6 to 8" long and looks like dried compressed rocks as we force it out our anus, often tearing our tender mucous membranes. Because of our diet, our feces is hard and heavy as it sinks to the bottom of the toilet bowl. Since we sit in an unnatural position as opposed to squatting, the time it takes to eliminate our waste causes our hemorrhoidal veins to bulge and sometimes rupture. The *sign* of poor elimination is often called hemorrhoids or piles. Medication is only of temporary benefit. Therefore, surgery is the orthodox medical treatment of choice.

Long before my mother developed colon cancer, she had multiple hemorrhoidal surgeries, a clear indication of delayed intestinal transition and constipation. Which brings us back to the late Mr. Bell and his colon cancer.

In my 34-year career, I have noticed the *experimental* orthodox medical system is consistently about 50 years behind times. In reality, when it comes to herbal medicines, the AMA and their union members are hundreds, if not thousands of years behind established *traditional* (natural) medical knowledge.

Within the same month of Mr. Bell's passing, The *American Cancer Society* announced the results of a 20-year study stating, *"Those who eat the most red meat; beef, and/or pork and/or processed meat products get colon cancer 30% to 40% more often than those who eat these foods only once in a while."*

The study went on to say that eating one hamburger daily, the size of your palm, raises cancer risk.

Dis-ease is defined as lack of ease or harmony, it is NOT the same as "disease," a medical term for illness treated by medicine. *NEVER* attempt to stop or reduce your medication without the supervision of your medical doctor.

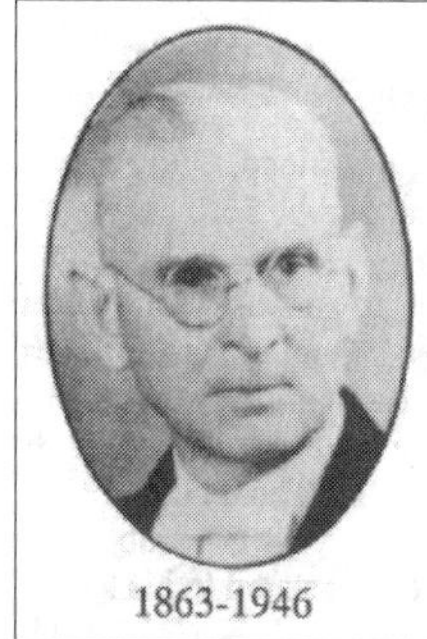

1863-1946

Unfortunately, the American Cancer Society, the AMA and their union members ("doctors") have not heard of Jethro Kloss.

Jethro Kloss is one of my heroes. He lived from 1863 to 1946. In 1939, after 50 years of serving humanity as a natural healer and minister, he wrote one of the most definitive books on natural healing ever written entitled, "*Back to Eden.*" I would not know half of what I know today without my *900-page* copy of his classic.

Reverend Kloss had a sanitarium, a health food company, a health magazine, a mercantile supply company and was known as a medical evangelist and herbalist. He personally *cured* many cases of cancer, including colon, breast, stomach, skin, ovarian and uterus.

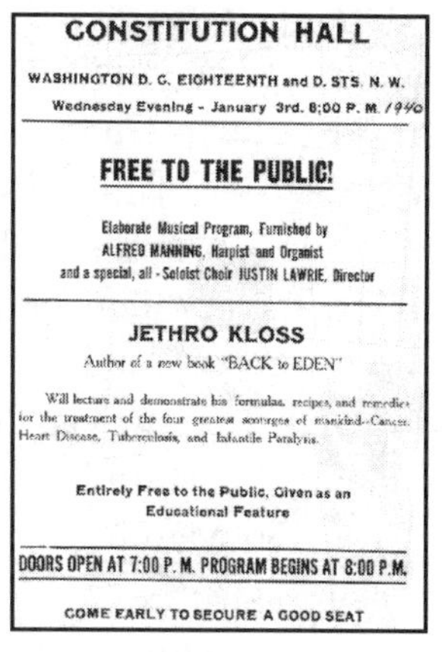

Over 115 years ago, Rev. Kloss taught and wrote about how to *cure* colon cancer. Over 65 years ago, 21 years before Mr. Bell was born, *Back to Eden* was released. For over 34 years, I have been teaching people about natural healing principles based on Rev. Kloss' experience and of those before and after him.

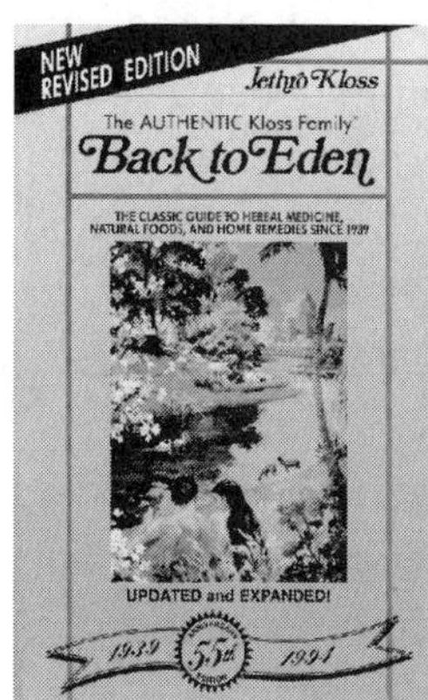

Many of the remedies in my book were first taught by Rev. Kloss in his book. Because, in this day and age, we have even more contributing factors to sickness and dis-ease, additional protocols have been added. However, the truth about natural healing never changes.

Over 100 years *before* the above *latest* medical "discovery," Rev. Kloss said, *"Cancer would be rare if no meats and devitalized foods were eaten."*

In addition to whole, pure food, herbs and other recommendations, Rev. Kloss used hydrotherapy as shown below in 1907.

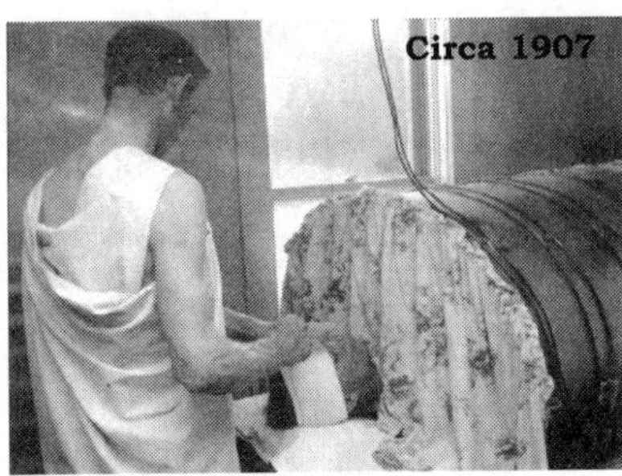

Jethro Kloss giving a hydrotherapy treatment at The Home Sanitarium. The Home Sanitarium was open from 1907 to 1912.

When asked what his secret cancer *cure* was, Rev. Kloss replied, *"To cure cancer you need correct food, herbs, water, fresh air, massage, sunshine, exercise and rest."* As simple as that sounds, what worked then still works now with a few additions.

Rev. Kloss also said, *"Cancer can <u>not</u> live in a system where all the mineral elements are present."* In my booklet, *The Miracle Elements: Fossilized Stony Coral Minerals* and in Chapter 4 herein, I explain the importance of minerals and their relationship with the pH of the blood and body. Without proper minerals, as Rev. Kloss has stated, the pH of the body will be acid. As we know, cancer thrives in an acid pH. Shifting the pH to alkaline decreases one's risk of getting cancer and helps to destroy it if you are afflicted. Oneway of doing this is to take fossilized stony coral minerals. (See Index E - *Resources* at back of this book).

On March 27, 1939, after treating thousands of patients for a litany of illnesses, Mr. Kloss offered to teach the *National Cancer Research Institute* and the *American Medical Association* his entire anti-cancer protocol free. As expected, both declined his generous offer, saying they were *not* in a position to accept.

This is nothing new. Dozens, if not hundreds of natural healers have been willing to give their remedies to the AMA and OMIC. However, if you can't get a patent on a product, remedy or treatment, the *powers to be* are simply *not* interested. For them, it's all about money.

From hydration, increased oxygen utilization to effective nutrition, including complete digestion and proper elimination, one can see why and how The H.O.N.S.T.E.C. Syndrome is the *real* underlining *cause* of *all* dis-ease.

The Fourth Contributing Factor of H.O.N.S.T.E.C. is: S - Spinal/Structural/Neurological aberrations

CHART OF THE NERVE SYSTEM

Every part of the body is controlled by nerves, and every one of these nerves connects directly or indirectly with the spine. This chart was compiled from over a dozen standard medical text and reference books.

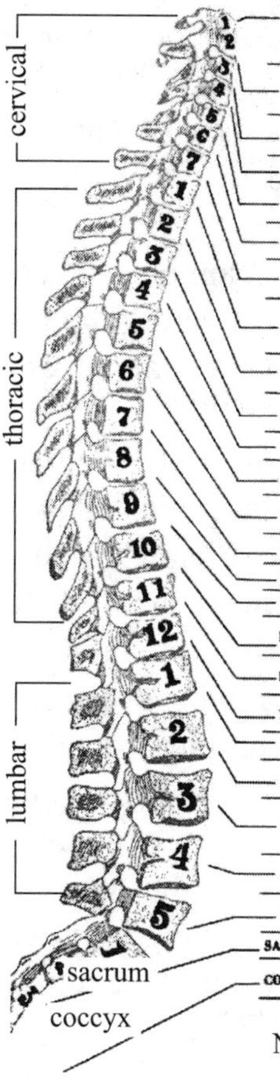

	AREAS KNOWN TO RECEIVE NERVE FIBERS FROM THESE NERVES.	SOME OF THE CONDITIONS THAT CAN FOLLOW A PRESSURE ON, OR INTERFERENCE WITH THESE NERVES.
1 C	Blood supply to the head, the pituitary gland, the scalp, bones of the face, the brain itself, inner and middle ear, the sympathetic nervous system.	Headaches, nervousness, insomnia, head colds, high blood pressure, migraine headaches, mental conditions, nervous breakdowns, amnesia, sleeping sickness, chronic tiredness, dizziness or vertigo, St. Vitus dance.
2 C	Eyes, optic nerve, auditory nerve, sinuses, mastoid bones, tongue, forehead.	Sinus trouble, allergies, crossed eyes, deafness, erysipelas, eye troubles, earache, fainting spells, certain cases of blindness.
3 C	Cheeks, outer ear, face bones, teeth, trifacial nerve.	Neuralgia, neuritis, acne or pimples, eczema.
4 C	Nose, lips, mouth, eustachian tube.	Hay fever, catarrh, hard of hearing, adenoids.
5 C	Vocal cords, neck glands, pharynx.	Laryngitis, hoarseness, throat conditions like a sore throat or quinsy.
6 C	Neck muscles, shoulders, tonsils.	Stiff neck, pain in upper arm, tonsillitis, whooping cough, croup.
7C	Thyroid gland, bursae in the shoulders, the elbows.	Bursitis, colds, thyroid conditions.
1 D	Arms from the elbows down, including the hands, wrists and fingers, also the esophagus and trachea.	Asthma, cough, difficult breathing, shortness of breath, pain in lower arms and hands.
2 D	Heart including its valves and covering, also coronary arteries.	Functional heart conditions and certain chest pains.
3 D	Lungs, bronchial tubes, pleura, chest, breast, nipples.	Bronchitis, pleurisy, pneumonia, congestion, influenza.
4 D	Gall bladder and common duct.	Gall bladder conditions, jaundice, shingles.
5 D	Liver, solar plexus, blood.	Liver conditions, fevers, low blood pressure, anemia, poor circulation, arthritis.
6 D	Stomach.	Stomach troubles including nervous stomach, indigestion, heart burn, dyspepsia.
7 D	Pancreas, islands of Langerhans, duodenum.	Diabetes, ulcers, gastritis.
8 D	Spleen, diaphragm.	Hiccoughs, lowered resistance.
9 D	Adrenals or supra-renals.	Allergies, hives.
10 D	Kidneys.	Kidney troubles, hardening of the arteries, chronic tiredness, nephritis, pyelitis.
11 D	Kidneys, ureters.	Skin conditions like acne, pimples, eczema, or boils.
12 D	Small intestines, Fallopian tubes, lymph circulation.	Rheumatism, gas pains, certain types of sterility.
1 L	Large intestines or colon, inguinal rings.	Constipation, colitis, dysentery, diarrhea, ruptures or hernias.
2 L	Appendix, abdomen, upper leg, cecum.	Appendicitis, cramps, difficult breathing, acidosis, varicose veins.
3 L	Sex organs, ovaries or testicles, uterus, bladder, knee.	Bladder troubles, menstrual troubles like painful or irregular periods, miscarriages, bed wetting, impotency, change of life symptoms, many knee pains.
4 L	Prostate gland, muscles of the lower back, sciatic nerve.	Sciatica, lumbago, difficult, painful, or too frequent urination, backaches.
5 L	Lower legs, ankles, feet, toes, arches.	Poor circulation in the legs, swollen ankles, weak ankles and arches, cold feet, weakness in the legs, leg cramps.
SACRUM	Hip bones, buttocks.	Sacro-iliac conditions, spinal curvatures.
COCCYX	Rectum, anus.	Hemorrhoids or piles, pruritus or itching, pain at end of spine on sitting.

cervical thoracic lumbar sacrum coccyx

Note: Thoracic is also known as the Dorsal area.

The above chart is used by many chiropractic, naturopathic and natural healers today. It demonstrates how every spinal nerve and trunk supplies different organs, muscles and glands. Since it is difficult to read, I have outlined it from page 52 to 55.

As you can see, there are 7 vertebrae in the cervical spine (neck), 12 vertebrae in the thoracic (back) area, 5 vertebrae in the

Dis-ease is defined as lack of ease or harmony, it is NOT the same as "disease," a medical term for illness treated by medicine. *NEVER* attempt to stop or reduce your medication without the supervision of your medical doctor.

lumbar or lower back, 5 unified segments in the sacrum and 4 segments in the coccyx (tailbone). There are approximately 600,000 (six hundred thousand) nerve fibers exiting from each segment. That's over 19 million nerves connecting throughout the body. Every part of the body is controlled by nerves and every one of those nerves connect directly or indirectly with the spine.

More and more people are going to body workers, chiropractors, traditional naturopaths, acupuncturists, Rolfers, DMT (Deep Muscle Therapy) practitioners and others that understand the holistic principles of health and longevity. If just for pain alone, the above healers are very effective.

How many of you have ever had sciatic pain or sciatica? It is not only painful, it can be crippling. As the name implies, it involves the sciatic nerve coming from the lumbo-sacral plexes and traveling down the leg.

In the 1980s, I became one of the first doctors to incorporate liquid crystal thermography in my clinic. It was a simple devise made of liquid crystal "pillows" applied to a patient's area of complaint. The theory was that whenever there is a nerve-flow problem, there will also be a corresponding blood-flow change directly within the same pathway of the challenged nerve. The "pillow" registered blood flow changes in color indicating normal, hot or cold and a camera would take a picture of these colorful images similar to the picture above.

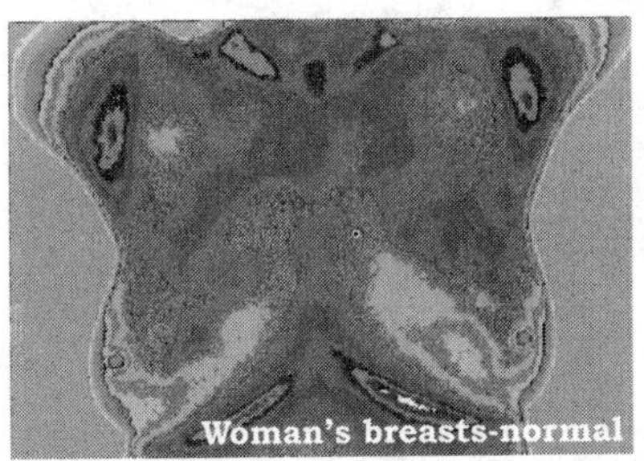
Woman's breasts-normal

Today, liquid crystal thermography is obsolete. It has been replaced with computerized thermography, a much better and efficient system that can even detect lumps and tumors of the breast 5 to 10 years before a mammogram, and without the use of radiation. Since the patient is never touched, it doesn't compress or hurt the breast as a mammogram does.

In my research and *prior* to buying several of these units, I discovered that the science and art of thermography was *not* new. Hippocrates (464 to 370 B.C.), the "Father of Medicine," who *never* used a drug (he was an herbalist), was actually recorded as one of the first individuals to use the *concept* of thermography. Even Hippocrates knew the intimate relationship of the spine, nerves and viscera. Although medics take what they call "his" oath, few practice it and fewer understand it. (See Chapter 5)

One day, as the story goes, a man came to Hippocrates for help. Apparently, he had fallen down and was now experiencing severe pain generally coming from his low back spreading out across his buttocks and down the back of his leg to his ankle. Although I don't know what it was called in those days, today we would call it sciatica.

During his examination, Hippocrates asked his patient to strip to expose the area of concern. He then applied wet mud to the entire back, buttocks and affected leg. The results were remarkable. Because blood flow is affected when nerve flow is compromised, heat is usually generated within the same pathway of pain. Hippocrates observed the mud drying in the exact pathway the patient had complained of. He then traced the origin of pain from the ankle to the precise vertebrae in the low back *causing* this problem. With herbal fomentations, compresses and massage to the muscles of the spinal vertebrae, the patient fully recovered.

I witnessed this same *cause* and *effect* thousands of times in my clinic. This may be a mystery to *experimental* orthodox medicine, but "bone setters" have been around since 2,700 B.C. in China and over 110 years in America thru chiropractic.

Although I never had a medical doctor refer a patient to me for fear of losing them to the natural healing approach, I had several medical doctors come through the back door of my clinic for sciatica problems. This was in the days when medics were vehemently opposed to natural healing. Now that natural healers are more popular than the drug doctors, they want to embrace us with what they call *complementary medicine*. This is interesting.

Dis-ease is defined as lack of ease or harmony, it is NOT the
same as "disease," a medical term for illness treated by medicine.
NEVER attempt to stop or reduce your medication without the supervision of your medical doctor.

How can there be such a thing as *complementary* medicine? Natural healing is *traditional* medicine, it can never complement drugs, surgery, radiation and chemotherapy. To the contrary, if incorporated properly, natural healing *prevents* sickness and dis-ease, thereby negating the need for most *experimental* orthodox medical treatments.

The following outline clearly lists each vertebral segment with its corresponding influence on the body. Every vertebrae emits nerve fibers going to their mentioned areas and more. Any structural-spinal-neural compromise may contribute to the referenced condition(s). From chiropractic, acupuncture to massage and Rolfing, each practitioner understands the nervous system and corresponding meridians.

Cervical Outline Based on Nerve Chart

C1 - Blood supply to the head, the pituitary gland, the scalp, bones of the face, the brain itself, inner and middle ear, the sympathetic nervous system.

May contribute to: Headaches, nervousness, insomnia, head "colds," high blood pressure, migraines, mental conditions, nervous breakdowns, amnesia, sleeping sickness, chronic tiredness, dizziness or vertigo.

C2 - Eyes, optic nerve, auditory nerve, sinuses, mastoid bones, tongue, forehead.

May contribute to: Sinus trouble, allergies, crossed eyes, deafness, eye problems, earache, fainting spells, certain cases of blindness.

C3 - Cheeks, outer ear, face bones, teeth, trifacial nerve.

May contribute to: Neuralgia, neuritis, acne or pimples, eczema.

C4 - Nose, lips, mouth, eustachian tubes.

May contribute to: Hay fever, catarrh, hard of hearing and adenoids.

C5 - Vocal cords, neck glands, pharynx.

May contribute to: Laryngitis, hoarseness, throat conditions, swollen neck glands.

C6 - Neck muscles, shoulders, tonsils.

May contribute to: Stiff neck, pain in upper arm, acute tonsillitis, whopping cough, croup.

C7 - Thyroid gland, bursae in the shoulders, the elbows.

May contribute to: Bursitis, "colds," thyroid conditions.

Note: If you have any of the above conditions, they may be merely *signs* and *signals* of a neuro-spinal compromise. Going to your *experimental* orthodox medical doctor for anyone of the above ailments will *never* get to the cause.

Thoracic Outline Based on Nerve Chart

T1 - From the arms to the elbows down, including the hands, wrists and fingers, also the esophagus and trachea.

May contribute to: Asthma, cough, difficult breathing, shortness of breath, pain in lower arms and hands.

T2 - Heart including its valves and pericardium, also coronary arteries.

May contribute to: Functional heart conditions and certain chest pains.

T3 - Lungs, bronchial tubes, pleura, chest, breast and nipples.

May contribute to: Bronchitis, pleurisy, pneumonia, congestion, influenza.

T4 - Gall bladder and common bile duct.

May contribute to: Gall bladder conditions, jaundice, shingles.

T5 - Liver, solar plexus, blood circulation.

May contribute to: Liver conditions, fevers, low blood pressure, anemia, poor circulation, arthritis.

T6 - Stomach

May contribute to: Stomach troubles including nervous stomach, indigestion, "heart burn," dyspepsia.

T7 - Pancreas, islets of Langerhans, duodenum.

May contribute to: Diabetes, ulcers, gastritis.

T8 - Spleen, diaphragm.

May contribute to: Hiccoughs, lowered resistance .

Dis-ease is defined as lack of ease or harmony, it is NOT the same as "disease," a medical term for illness treated by medicine.
NEVER attempt to stop or reduce your medication without the supervision of your medical doctor.

T9 - Adrenals or supra-renals.

May contribute to: Allergies, hives.

T10 - Kidneys

May contribute to: Kidney troubles, hardening of the arteries, chronic tiredness, nephritis, pyelitis.

T11 - Kidneys, ureters.

May contribute to: Skin conditions like acne, pimples, eczema or boils.

T12 - Small intestine, fallopian tubes, lymph circulation.

May contribute to: Rheumatism, gas pains, certain types of sterility.

How many of you have gone to your medical doctor because you had pain from your arm to your hands, shortness of breath and difficulty breathing only to find out after thousands of dollars worth of tests, exams and visits, you were told "Everything looks okay." As you have read, if the nerve supply coming from your First Thoracic vertebrae is compromised, you can easily have any one or all of those *signs* and *signals* just described.

Did your new *complementary* doctor refer you to a chiropractor or acupuncturist? I didn't think so. Why would they? Referring a patient affects their income and livelihood.

Remember, Spinal/Structural/Neurological Aberrations are only *one* component of The H.O.N.S.T.E.C. Syndrome, however, they are *very* important.

Lumbar Outline Based on Nerve Chart

L1 - Large intestine or colon, inguinal rings.

May contribute to: Constipation, colitis, dysentery, diarrhea, ruptures or hernias.

L2 - Appendix, abdomen, upper leg, cecum.

May contribute to: Appendicitis, cramps, difficult breathing, acidosis, varicose veins.

L3 - Sex organs, ovaries or testicles, uterus, bladder, knee.

May contribute to: Bladder troubles, menstrual troubles like painful or irregular periods, miscarriages, bed wetting, impotency, change of life symptoms, many knee pains.

Dis-ease is defined as lack of ease or harmony, it is NOT the
same as "disease," a medical term for illness treated by medicine.
NEVER attempt to stop or reduce your medication without the supervision of your medical doctor.

L4 - Prostate gland, muscles of the lower back, sciatic nerve.

May contribute to: Sciatica, lumbago, difficult, painful or too frequent urination, backaches.

L5 - Lower legs, ankles, feet, toes, arches.

May contribute to: Poor circulation in the legs, swollen ankles, weak ankles and arches, cold feet, weakness in the legs and leg cramps.

Sacrum - Hip bones, buttocks.

May contribute to: Sacro-iliac conditions, scoliosis and other spinal curvatures.

Coccyx - Rectum, anus.

May contribute to: Hemorrhoids or piles, pruritus or itching, pain at end of spine on sitting.

The above information and chart, is *not* my opinion or that of the chiropractic or naturopathic profession. It is a respected anatomical and neurological document. Unfortunately, medics refuse to accept the truth. They still claim spinal manipulation (also called spinal "adjustments") is appropriate only in some lower-back cases of mild sprain or strain. Perhaps they should go back to medical school and learn anatomy and neurology again or maybe for the first time.

Even the eyes have nerve fibers that can be traced to the carotid plexes, postganglionic fibers, superior cervical and thoracic ganglion to the first and second thoracic vertebral level.

Basically, this means the nerves coming out of our spine at the first and second thoracic level lead to our eyes. We also have nerves coming from the second cervical vertebra to our eyes. If we are experiencing vision problems or any other neurological aberration, we *must* rule out neuro-spinal *causes* first. Having a chiropractic or acupuncture evaluation is paramount to getting to the **Spinal/Structural/Neurological** *cause* of dis-ease, the fourth contributing factor in The H.O.N.S.T.E.C. Syndrome.

The Fifth Contributing Factor of H.O.N.S.T.E.C. is:

T - Toxic waste accumulation

"For the first time in the history of the world, every human being is now subjected to contact with dangerous chemicals, from the moment of conception until death." **- Rachel Carson**

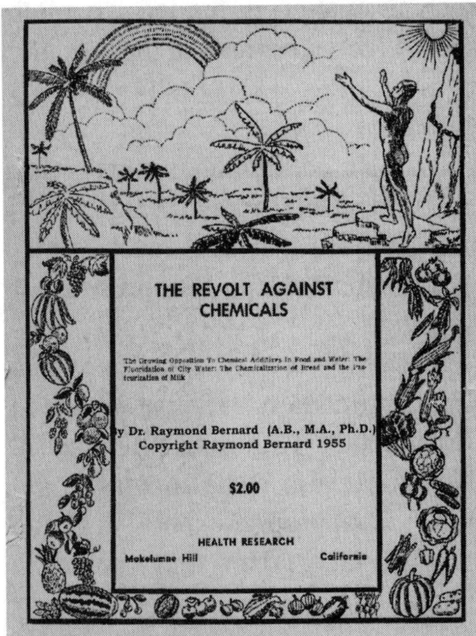

In 1968, I bought a copy of *The Revolt Against Chemicals* by Dr. Raymond Bernard written in 1955. Obviously his warnings concerning the dangers of toxic chemicals have been suppressed and ignored. We have more toxins today than ever in the history of the world.

Remember, we are what we eat, assimilate and don't eliminate. Anything that is toxic and is *not* removed from the body, will make us toxic. Unless of course you believe what your *experimental* orthodox medical doctor tells you, then this is just a bunch of non-sense, pure quackery.

Let's read some of this nonsense, we natural healers have been talking about forever:

Air

In 1998, T.J. Woodroff wrote an article for the *Environment Health Perspective* entitled, *Public Health Implications of 1990 Air Toxin Concentrations Across the United States.* In this report for 1990, the EPA conducted a comprehensive survey, measuring outdoor concentrations of 148 toxic contaminants. They found concentrations of hydrocarbons greater than the EPA's desired cancer-*causing* levels in more than *90%* of the 60,000 regions studied. Two hundred areas had concentrations of pollutants that exceeded their recommended levels by *10,000%* or more. This report was released in 1990!

During the year 2000, more than six billion pounds of toxic waste were released directly to the air, land and water in the United States alone. I am not talking about a few million pounds, I said over *6 BILLION POUNDS!* As of this date, we have hundreds, if not thousands of toxic contaminant's affecting our air quality throughout the world, not just the United States.

Indoor air pollution can be several to more than 100 times higher than the outdoors. From cooking and heating fumes, commercial household cleaners, tobacco smoke, pest-control products, out gassing from building materials (plywood, kitchen cabinets, carpets to radon), we are ingesting contaminants day in and day out. This is not just a theory it is a fact.

For one of the most complete lists of household toxins and what safe products you can replace them with, read Dr. Hulda Clark's, *The Cure to All Dis-eases* or go on the Internet searching under "Safe Household Cleaners."

Water

Water and hydration were covered under the first factor of The H.O.N.S.T.E.C. Syndrome, however, as we know, most water of the world today is contaminated. We *must* filter our water going into our homes or at least at the sinks and bath/shower. Washing dishes and clothes in clean water is important, but the water we drink and bath in is also vital.

How can we sit in a tub of chlorinated water and not absorb this toxin directly into our skin? Women especially are vulnerable since the vaginal mucous membrane is easily exposed. In addition to chlorine being toxic, it is extremely de-hydrating and will lead to premature wrinkling, aging and illness. Placing a simple chlorine filter on the tub or showerhead, should eliminate this problem. Do not drink tap water. It is toxic. By drinking charged distilled water you circumvent this problem.

Land

The same toxins found in the air settle to the earth. Petro-chemical derivatives in pesticides, insecticides, fungicides, herbicides and fertilizers, are all known to *cause* health concerns. From a simple skin rash to cancer, these chemicals are toxic and dangerous.

In 1998, the *American Journal of Industrial Medicine* reported that oil refinery workers suffered *increased* rates of mortality (death) from cancers of the lip (384% over normal), stomach (142%), liver (238%), pancreas (151%), connective tissues (243%), prostate (135%), eye (407%), brain (181%), and leukemia (175%). From golf course workers, gasoline attendants to "sick building" syndrome, we are reaping what we have been sowing. The good news is, we can still do something about the onslaught of toxins found in our environment. Besides finding other fuels to burn in our industrial plants and automobiles, we can detoxify our bodies on a regular basis. (See Chapter 6 for more information).

Food

Although I discuss food in Chapter 4, relative to toxins and food, you just read over *6 Billion pounds* of toxic chemicals and contaminates were released in our air and/or land in the year 2000. From airplanes dropping poison pellets to kill rodents in orchards, to direct spraying of pesticides and insecticides on all commercial crops, consumers in "civilized" society are unknowingly being poisoned every day.

When I worked for my father picking crops during the summer, beside picking, I also mixed and applied a green wax preservative used on green peppers and cucumbers. Have you ever wondered what the waxy substance was on your apples and other vegetables? It's a toxic chemical to give the appearance of freshness. All shinny textured fruits and vegetables can be sprayed with a colorized wax containing insecticides to keep "bugs" and other pests from eating it. It also extends shelf life by keeping mold and fungus at bay.

Many of our crops are kept in storage warehouses where they are placed in harmful gas chambers waiting to be shipped to market. Some chambers are pressurized to ensure complete chemical penetration. Of course there are no regulations mandating public notice to this affect.

It is estimated a minimum of five different toxic chemicals are applied from field to table to every commercially grown crop in the United States. The food industry, agricultural chemical groups and our own bought and paid for government will tell you that washing will remove these toxic chemicals. They even sell a "special" food chemical remover. Unfortunately, they don't tell you how readily their chemicals are absorbed through the roots of plants and trees or directly through the crop's skin.

Washing will only remove heavy chemical residue. It will NOT remove the pesticides, insecticides and other toxins within the food. The only way of ensuring you do *not* consume these toxins is to eat all organic. When you cannot, you must remove these toxins before they cause serious damage. I *will* show you how.

Electromagnetic Radiation

We live in an invisable ocean of electromagnetic radiation. From computer monitors, cell phones, hair dryers, electric razors, waterbed heaters, electric blankets, televisions, video games, stereos, alarm clocks to everything in between, including the wiring in our homes, cars and especially in airplanes, we are swimming in that which is unseen. In addition, we have *towers* for cell phones, television, radio stations, satellite transmitters and unknown government radar, HAARP and other technologies.

Although no one wants to admit it, electromagnetic radiation *causes* DNA damage and this damage *causes* dis-ease. It's fairly simple. We are not physically *tuned* for the frequencies bombarding us. I suppose if the manufacturers of these appliances and devises accepted responsibility, they would have to accept liability. However, this is not going to happen in the near future.

Humans resonate, oscillate or function within the Earth's eight (8) Hz cycles per second. This is known as the earth frequency. Even though we are innately programmed to thrive on this frequency, alternating current at 60 cycles per second; 60 Hz and cell and portable phones at nine-hundred (900) cycles per second. cause damage. This type of electromagnetic radiation has been proven to mutate our genetic make-up.

There are steps we can take to limit our exposure. We can sit at least 5 to 10 feet away from our televisions. We can install a filter on our computer screens. If you must use an electric blanket, turn it on high thirty minutes before you go to bed. Once in bed, turn it off. Make sure you are wearing socks to keep your feet warm. If your feet are warm, your body will stay warmer. If you still need the blanket, roll it down to cover only your feet. At least you won't be radiating your entire body.

I own a Motorola® cell phone and wireless headset with *Bluetooth* technology. It allows me to place my cell phone thirty feet away from me. Using the voice activation system, hand dialing is not necessary. In the car, unless I want to see every incoming number, I keep the phone in the glove box.

In Dr. Emoto's book, he shows the same pattern of molecular destruction or healing reconfiguration from different types of music. From Bach to Beethoven, heavy metal to jazz, the frequency of sound determines our molecular integrity.

Heavy-Metal Pollution

I am not talking about music. I am referring to actual toxic metals that have been shown to increase free-radical activity, a known cause of accelerated aging and severe illness.

Arsenic, beryllium, cadmium, cobalt, nickel, aluminum, lead and mercury are all heavy metals found in nature. By impeding the body's ability to recover from DNA damage, they become carcinogenic. Compromising the immune system, heavy metals make it extremely difficult to overcome health challenges. From fatigue, mood disorders, poor concentration to hair loss, heavy metal contamination must be ruled out first.

Of all the toxic metals, aluminum and mercury are the most prevalent.

Aluminum is found in cookware, food additives, medicine, especially antacids, cosmetics, and in the air we breathe. Research has shown that aluminum binds to DNA, is deposited in the neurofibrillary tangles in the brain and inhibits the enzyme hexokinase. Although Alzheimer's and Parkinson's "diseases" are recognized conditions relative to aluminum toxicity, the following *signs* and *signals* are of equal importance:

Ulcers in the mouth, spasms of the esophagus, stomach disorders, duodenal ulcers, appendicitis, colitis, kidney infections, constipation, blood clots, eye weakness to blindness, dementia, migraine headaches, upper respiratory infections, allergies to general fatigue. With just four (4) parts per million (ppm) aluminum can cause blood to coagulate.

Mercury is particularly toxic. Methylmercury, the form of mercury found in seafood, is a known neurotoxin. Wild Pacific salmon, haddock, blue crab, croaker and shrimp have the least amount with halibut, shark, swordfish, sea Bass and Gulf Coast oysters the greatest amount.

We are also exposed to mercury from "silver" amalgam dental fillings, which are 50 percent mercury. In time, the body absorbs this dental metal. This is one reason why most natural healers will recommend having all your amalgam fillings replaced with other composite materials such as ceramic or gold.

Lead and Cadmium are also dangerous toxic metals found in our environment, within the body. From automobile exhaust to cigarette smoke, these toxins must be removed.

Toxic metals can be removed with oral and/or IV chelation, a process of introducing binding agents into the body such as activated charcoal and slippery elm (orally) and/or EDTA intravenously. I have a compound that draws toxic metals.

Hair toxic metal mineral analysis, urine provocation testing and blood tests may all determine heavy metal toxins. Again, how will drugs ever address the *cause* of your problem if it is coming from toxic metal poisoning? Drugs *never* cure anything, they just treat and mask symptoms.

The Sixth Contributing Factor of H.O.N.S.T.E.C. is:
E - Emotional/Energetic (blocks or release)

In his 1956 book, *The Stress of Life*, Dr. Hans Seyle defines the term *homeostasis*, as that which seeks balance and harmony. The following chart demonstrates stressful imbalance and the different biological reactionary phases we go through after being challenged by stressors, such as surgery, infections, wounds, burns, crush injuries, immunological and allergic insults, severe exertions, *strong emotions*, malnutrition and severe exposures; heat, cold and sun.

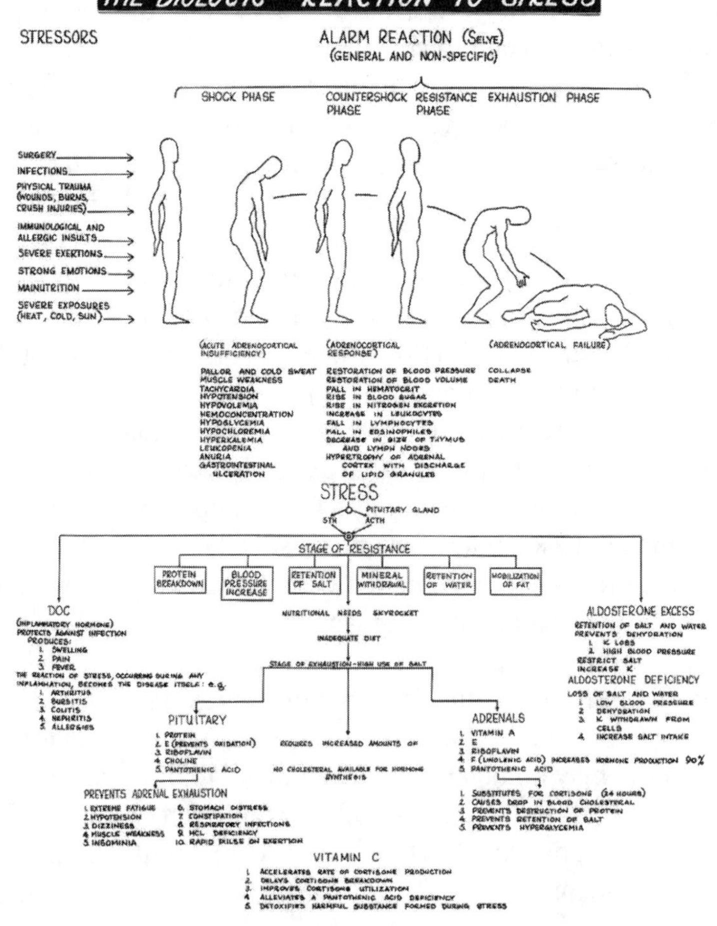

Dis-ease is defined as lack of ease or harmony, it is NOT the same as "disease," a medical term for illness treated by medicine. *NEVER* attempt to stop or reduce your medication without the supervision of your medical doctor.

Notice there is a Shock Phase illustrated by the body figure, second from the left, hunching forward. In this phase there is an acute adrenocortical insufficiency. Basically the adrenal glands are compromised. In the Counter Shock and Resistance Phase, the adrenals respond with corticosteroids (hormones) bringing the body back to a strained, but pre-stress state. In this phase there is protein breakdown, blood pressure increase, retention of salt, mineral withdrawal, retention of water and mobilization of fat. Nutritional needs skyrocket.

If the cause of one's stress is not determined, the final stage: the Exhaustion Phase, may lead to adrenocortical failure, collapse and death.

Dr. Seyle correlates the effects of stress with dozens of physical disorders, stating, "There is a healing force of nature which *cures* from within. It is our perception of stress that impedes it." Perception is the key here. It is not stress but how we perceive and then handle it that becomes the causative factor in sickness and dis-ease.

Stress is often related to our emotions. Emotion is Energy-in-motion. As vibrational thoughts and feelings come to and through us, we are energized. Good or bad, it is still energy. When the same vibratory frequencies do not pass through, but are blocked or locked within, we create vibratory chaos settling in our weakest areas. Vibratory chaos leads to dis-harmony or dis-ease. The key to emotion is releasing and keeping these vibrations in motion.

When a loved one dies, it is normal to grieve. Mourning the *perceived* loss of someone is healthy, providing it is not extended into a length of time that causes psychological or physical problems for the mourner. It's all about balance.

My mother never released her emotions. From fear to hate, she kept them inside. She felt guilt and shame for saying or doing something that was a mis-perception of reality. She believed in things that were not based on fact, the first being death.

Whenever I had an opportunity to be with the loved ones of someone who transcended this dispensation (died), I would either demonstrate or explain the process of boiling water. In this case, the water represents the human body.

If you take a pot of water and put it on the stove with the heat turned on high, the water will boil. As the water begins to boil, steam rises. This represents transition. Eventually the steam disappears as the hydrogen and oxygen gases separate. Does this mean the water is dead or did it simply transform from a liquid to a vapor to hydrogen and oxygen gases we can no longer see?

Humans are spiritual beings having a human experience. When we "die" we merely transform back to the essence of who we have been all along. "Ashes to ashes, dust to dust," we simple leave the confines of the physical body, releasing our radiating spiritual body as a wisp of pure love and energy.

Kirlian Photography

Many years ago, I saw a documentary showing several people being filmed while sleeping. What made this film unique was that they filmed the sleepers using Kirlian photography. Kirlian photography captures auraic heat signatures in color. The auraic field radiates out from the body in different colors and distances depending on state of mind or physical condition at the time.

In the film, participants went to sleep around 10:00 P.M. The most interesting part took place between 2:00 and 4:00 A.M. During this time, a wisp of white-ish blue light emanated and separated from the head and traveled directly up into the ceiling. Within an hour or two, coming from the ceiling, the same wisp of light, returned to the head in the exact place where it exited.

As intriguing as this may sound, it gets even more so. After this phenomena was observed, the researchers decided to see what happens when someone "dies." They placed a dying person in a thermostatically controlled room on a large, bed-size stainless-steel scale covered in a warm blanket. Much to their amazement, at the exact moment of "death," they not only witnessed the auraic field leaving the feet first, traveling towards the head, but at the moment the total wisp of light (auraic field) left the head, the scale dropped eight to ten ounces. This test was repeated several times with the same results.

What does this prove? First, part of our energy, auraic or spiritual field appears to leave and return every night. Where it goes is anyone's guess. But it does go somewhere. Second, at the moment of our perceived "death," this same field starts diminishing from the feet towards the head leaving the body dark as it moves up. When the field leaves from there, it does not return and the life form is now what we call "dead." However, energy never dies and this test proves neither does our spirit.

When my daughter Sydney was just three or four years old, she came into my bathroom while I was taking a shower. This was unusual behavior for her. However, she was angry.

As I came out of the shower, I was shocked to see her. While she threw a towel at me, she said, "I want to talk to you Daddy. I want to talk to you now." I asked her if she was okay and what the problem was. With her little hands on her hips, she said, "Daddy, before I was born, I was in Mommy's tummy. And before I was in Mommy's tummy, I was with God. And you know, when I was with God, I was talkin' to you but you couldn't hear me. How come?"

I was so surprised at my little girl asking such a profound question, I immediately called for her mother. Composing myself, I got dressed and tried to explain the differences between humans and angels. After all, she was my little angel so the story made sense.

The bottom line is and relative to The H.O.N.S.T.E.C. Syndrome, emotions play a major contributing factor in sickness and dis-ease. Stress is not as important as how we *handle* it. Our perception of reality, of good and evil, right from wrong, guides our emotions. Perhaps we need to learn to *not* take life so seriously. As my friend Dr. James Murray says, "We are *not* here for a long time, but we are here for a good time."

[The following is EC Wyndham's explanation of what emotion is. I think it says it all.]

Emotion

by

Eric C Wyndham

It's everywhere, can you feel it?
It's in the air, this thing called Energy.

It vibrates at every frequency with sounds heard and unheard.
It's the color of the rainbow and that of light unseen.
It's the warmth emanating from your hands and the language of Love.

As it passes to and through us, we amplify it. We give it physical form, motion and movement, purpose and meaning, joy and happiness.

Energy in motion is the E-motion we feel and convey for those of us willing to express it. It's the symphony of blissful peace when we chant, I love You. Can you feel your love projecting out and coming back to you ten-fold?

Yet when we don't, that is emote, we *block* it. We keep it from returning to the Source of life wherein it finds new life, a new charge within a charge returning to revitalize us.

These blocks of Energy of E-motion, cause dis-harmony, dis-trust and dis-ease. They cause ill circumstances to be, in our mind and body in you and me.

So surrender to it. Breathe deep. Feel, see and be the sights and sounds of Energy in motion. For without it, we merely exist watching life go by...

Dis-ease is defined as lack of ease or harmony, it is NOT the same as "disease," a medical term for illness treated by medicine. *NEVER* attempt to stop or reduce your medication without the supervision of your medical doctor.

The Seventh Contributing Factor of H.O.N.S.T.E.C. is: C - Creation Consciousness

Of all the *causes* of dis-ease, I saved the most significant for last. Not only does *Creation Consciousness* have to do with our spiritual essence, our divine beingness, but it is the most controversial. It hits at the core of our traditional religious beliefs and spiritual paradigm.

I am not *anti*-religion nor am I *pro*-religion. I approached understanding religions in the same investigative manner I used for health and dis-ease. Simply, I looked for commonalities or common denominators in the different religious orders.

Most religions have a deity, involve worship, fellowship, obedience, dogmas, doctrines and rituals. There seems to be a systematic order to achieve nirvana, bliss or "going to heaven."

It is the concept of *doing something* to achieve, nirvana, bliss, acceptance or heaven, that I will be addressing. In addition, I want to discuss dualistic misconception or our perception of separation from God or The Great Mystery.

As you have read, my mother felt God punished her for being a bad person. Although she never divulged all she did that was so bad, I do remember one incident.

I went to see my mother a couple of weeks before she died. She was in bed crying. I asked if there was anything I could do, thinking she was in pain and perhaps I could get her some more medication. She said it wasn't the pain; it was going to hell that scared her. When I asked her why she thought she was going to hell, she said it was because she lied to her priest. Like most Italians, my mother was a Roman Catholic.

Catholics were told they could not eat meat on Friday. Perhaps you are old enough to remember that? In fact, it was a "sin" to eat meat on Friday. Fish was okay, but no other form of animal protein was sanctioned by the Vatican, Pope or local priest.

My mother ate beef on a Friday and then went to confession the following day. Confession is the act of confessing your "sins" to a priest to expunge them.

When the priest asked her if she had "sinned," she mentioned everything but eating meat. According to my mother, her "sin" was compounded or elevated to a mortal "sin" status. Lying to a Catholic priest is very serious to believers. My mother thought there was no way out. She was about to die with a mortal "sin" on her soul which meant she was going straight to hell.

From the time of her "sin" to her final days, the Pope had a revelation. Eating meat on Friday was now acceptable. Whether it was God notifying the Pope of His new plan or the American Cattleman's Association putting a little pressure on - as they did when they sued Oprah Winfrey, I do not know. The bottom line, meat was in.

My mother was Italian, stubborn and angry. There was very little anyone could do to change her mind. I informed her of the new Catholic policy regarding eating meat, but she didn't care. I asked her if she knew what happened to all those individuals now in hell for eating meat on Friday since the rule had changed. She didn't know. I said I would find out.

The next day, I went to our local Catholic church and spoke with a priest. I asked him if the individuals currently in hell for eating meat on Friday and not confessing their "sins" were being let out now that the Pope changed the rules. He said he didn't know.

I explained my mother's condition and how she was *tormented* with fear of going to hell. I asked him to immediately go to her house and tell her she was *not* going to the fiery pit. He was reluctant at first, but I emphasized how important it was as one Italian to another and offered him a fifty-dollar bill to make it happen. He went the next day. I'm sure I will go to hell for bribing a priest (if there is such a place), but at least my mother won't be there suffering for all eternity.

What is a "sin" anyway? There is evidence to suggest that the English word "sin" came from the old English archery term *syn* or to miss the mark. In that light, we may all be syners, since we may all be missing the mark. However, we need to know what the mark is in order to be missing it.

In archery there is a round target with different circular colors, the center circle in black is called a bull's eye. If you miss that mark you *syn* up, down, left or right. Anything that misses the bull's eye is a *syn*. From that archery term, we have extrapolated a vivid, colorful doctrine of hell, fire and damnation. Perhaps a time-line of Biblical history is in order.

Note: Verification of authenticity was not provided, including what the "word" of God means:

Timeline of Bible *Translation* History

1,400 B.C. - The first written "word" of God. The Ten Commandments delivered to Moses.

500 B.C. - Completion of all original Aramaic (ancient Hebrew) manuscripts, that which make up the 39 books of the Old Testament.

200 B.C. - Completion of the Greek manuscripts that contain the 39 Old Testament books and 14 Apocryhpha books.

1st Century A.D. - Completion of all original Aramaic manuscripts that make up the 27 books of the New Testament.

[Note: Jesus spoke ancient Hebrew called Aramaic. His scribes wrote and spoke Aramaic as well. Even the King James Bible left Aramaic words in its translation].

382 A.D. - Jerome's Latin Vulgate manuscripts contained all 80 books: 39 Old Testament, 14 Apocryhpha and 27 New Testament.

500 A.D. - Scriptures were translated into over 500 languages including Latin.

600 A.D. - Latin was the only language allowed for scriptures.

995 A.D. - Anglo-Saxon (Early roots of the English language) translations of the New Testament were produced.

1384 A.D. - Wycliffe was the first person to produce a hand written manuscript copy of the complete Bible; all 80 books.

1455 A.D. Gutenberg invents the printing press. Books may now be mass-produced instead of individually hand written. The first book ever printed is the Gutenberg's Bible in Latin.

1526 A.D. - William Tyndale's New Testament; the first New Testament printed in the English language.

1535 A.D. - Myles Coverdale's Bible

1537 A.D. - Tyndale-Matthews Bible

1560 A.D. - The Geneva Bible: First Bible to add numbered verses to each chapter in all 80 books.

1609 A.D. - First complete English Catholic Bible translated from the Latin Vulgate (80 books).

1611 A.D. - The original King James version of the Bible had the 14 Apocryhpha books included. This version was a 1. translation of a 2. translation of a 3. translation of a 4. translation of a 5. translation of a 6. translation of a 7. translation of a 8. translation of a 9. translation of a 10. translation of a 11. translation of a 12. translation of a 13. translation of a 14. translation of a 15. translation. Each translation contained subtle changes.

Note: One Aramaic scholar, Dr. George Lamsa, counted over 12,000 *mis-translations* in the King James Bible when comparing it to the oldest available (464 A.D.) Aramaic manuscripts called the Peshitta. Dr. Lamsa spent over 35 years translating the Aramaic texts directly into English. His work is known as *The Peshitta, The Authorized Bible of the Church of the East.*

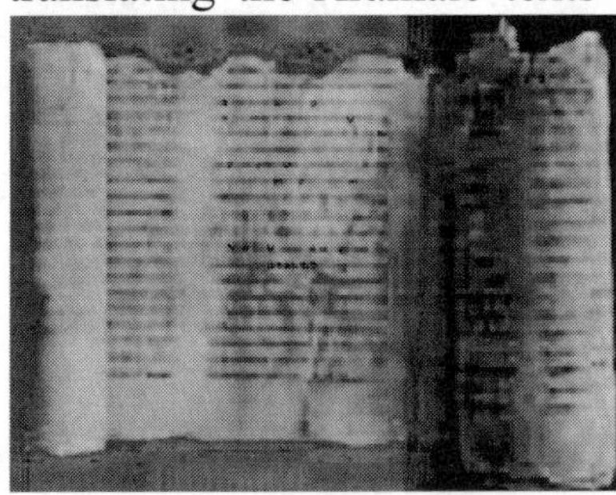

I spent over eight years studying with Dr. Lamsa's protege, Dr. Rocco Errico. During that time, I was privileged enough to learn the seven keys to finally understanding the Torah. From Aramaic, idioms, mysticism, culture, ancient psychology, symbolism; metaphors, parables and poetic philosophy to Eastern amplification, the Peshita is a fascinating book of inspiration and wisdom. It is well worth reading.

If you are interested in obtaining a copy of The Holy Bible by Dr. Lamsa call Harper Collins Publishers at 1-800-331-3761.

1885 A.D. - The English revised version of the King James Bible with the 14 Apocryhpha books was ordered removed.

1901 A.D. - The American Standard version of the King James Bible.

1971 A.D. - The New American Standard version taken from the American Standard version.

1973 A.D. - The New International version was printed.

1982 A.D. - The New King James version.

2002 A.D. - The New English Standard version.

Somewhere between the original Aramaic manuscripts and the King James version, *syn* became "sin." My mother never knew the truth concerning God's "word." How could she? It has changed hundreds, if not thousands of times since Moses came down from Mt. Sinai.

I hope you realize that religion is based on doctrines, dogmas and rituals that tend to *restrict* our spiritual growth through fear and control. True spirituality is about freedom of spiritual awareness, not constriction or regulation.

Another issue my mother had was her concept of God healing her. She always felt God did not heal her because she was not worthy and deserved to suffer and die. She felt separate from God, as taught in her Catholic church.

Many religions imply God is something "out there" resting in the heavens or heaven. This Grand Architect of the universe is referred to as Him, He or Our Father. Those that dare to portray God as Father, Mother God are seen as "New Agers," one that blasphemes Christianity and possibly other religions.

It is the concept of dualism or separation that contributes to our fear. It is our belief system that has kept us from realizing our own divinity or true spirituality. It is this loneliness under Creation Consciousness that contributes to our health or lack of it.

Many years ago, I watched a program on the National Geographic Channel about a specific black fly in the Amazon river. Apparently, the fly larvae lives in the mud for two years. Upon hatching it swims to the surface of the water and exits its wet world for one of sun, air and sound. Flying no more than three feet above the water and no more than three feet in any direction where it once exited, this insect hovers for up to eighteen hours before it "dies." On the way down back to their now watery grave, the males mate with the females, releasing their eggs to the mud below, and the cycle starts all over again.

While watching this program, I had an epiphany. One of those moments that bring you to your knees with a sense of awe and wonder. In a flash of awareness, I saw the purpose of life.

We are physically here to live and express this life, to procreate as a consequence of intimate relationships, to have fun and succeed in meaningful endeavors. However, we are spiritual beings having a human experience. Spiritually, we are here to re-discover our divinity by learning from the opportunities God or the Great Mystery has set before us.

Most importantly, we are here to *teach by example* and help others find their divinity, as well.

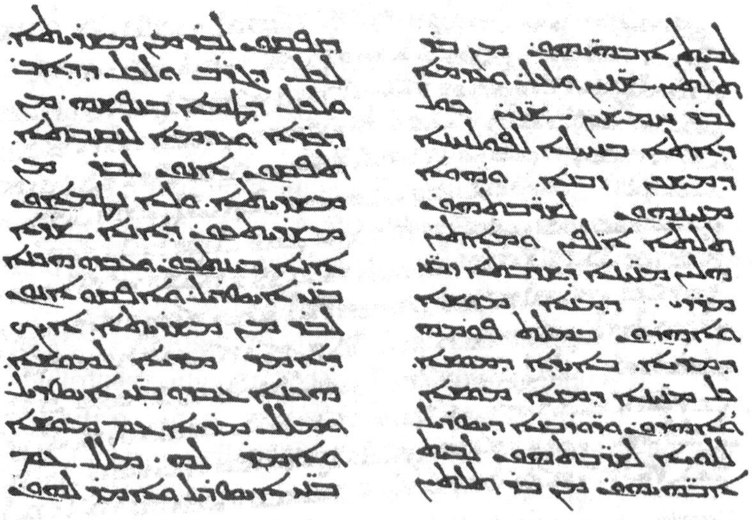

PLATE I

CODEX AMBROSIANUS — 5TH CENTURY

(Ambrosian Library, Milan, Italy.)

[Aramaic text. 5th Century A.D. Used by Dr. George Lamsa]

Dis-ease is defined as lack of ease or harmony, it is NOT the same as "disease," a medical term for illness treated by medicine.
NEVER attempt to stop or reduce your medication without the supervision of your medical doctor.

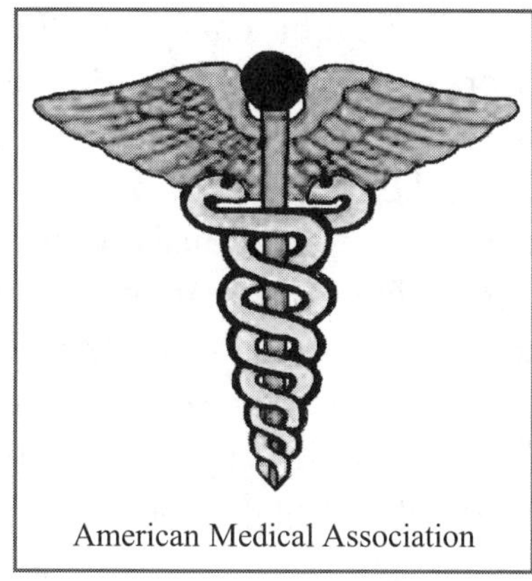

American Medical Association

CHAPTER 3 - TOP TWELVE DIS-EASES WITH THEIR SIGNS, SIGNALS AND SYMPTOMS

"Disease. If you call it something long enough, true or not, the masses will believe it. Just give it enough time." **- Sagarius**

1. **Cancer**	5. **Diabetes**	9. **Parkinson's**
2. **Heart Dis-ease**	6. **Hepatitis**	10. **Alzheimer's**
3. **Strokes**	7. **Obesity**	11. **Lupus**
4. **Emphysema**	8. **MS**	12. **Chronic Fatigue**

What is the difference between a *sign*, *signal* and symptom? Not much. However, there is enough of a difference to *kill* you.

Since the beginning of time, humans have had health challenges. Even Adam and Eve were not without pain and suffering, especially after the apple episode. But at least we can blame that on the evil, conniving snake. Odd. Isn't the snake the symbol of *experimental* orthodox medicine?

One key to differentiating a *sign* and *signal* from a *symptom* is whether or not it is attached to a so-called "disease." Take for example sexual dysfunction, depression or mental illness. The H.O.N.S.T.E.C. Syndrome can easily *cause* hormonal imbalances which can then *cause* the above conditions. Once the *signs* and *signals* are listed as *symptoms* these conditions are then classified as "diseases," treatable by *experimental* orthodox medicine.

Dis-ease is defined as lack of ease or harmony, it is NOT the same as "disease," a medical term for illness treated by medicine. *NEVER* attempt to stop or reduce your medication without the supervision of your medical doctor.

If your endocrine (hormonal) glands are not being fed proper nutrition, are dehydrated, hypoxic (low oxygen) or neurologically compromised, they will not be working properly. Once hormones are out of balance, they may *cause* a list of conditions erroneously classified as "diseases" such as clinical depression, Adult Attention Deficit Disorder, Bi-polar Disorder and numerous other physical problems.

Hormonal *balance* is critical to the health and integrity of the entire body. Before we go into the *Top Twelve Dis-eases,* let's learn a basic understanding about several major endocrine glands:

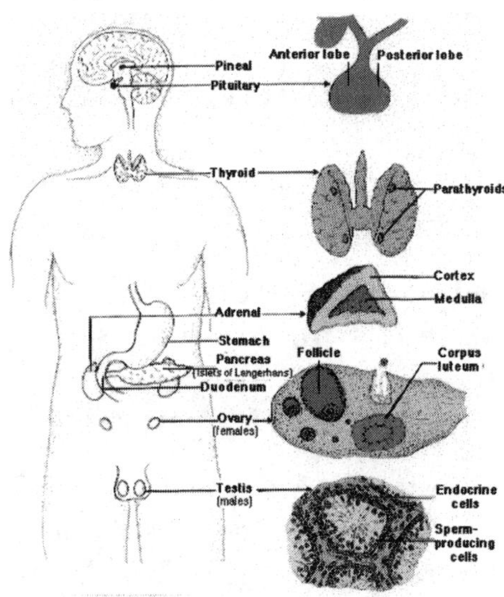

Hormones

Hormones are vital chemicals produced in the body by the endocrine (ductless) glands or other various substances that have a specific regulatory or functional effect on the activity of other organs or cells. Target glands or organs are those specifically influenced by a hormone. The word hormone originally meant to *arouse* or *excite.* Hormones are carried by the blood where they cause a response. Hormones serve *three* major functions:

1. Reach all the cells of the body and permit different tissue groups to act as a whole in response to internal or external stimuli.

2. Play a vital role in the maintenance of the internal environment.

3. Control the rate and type of growth of the organism.

The key to hormonal balance is always relative to the health and integrity of the gland or glands responsible for its production, not using a synthetic hormonal drug to mask the imbalance.

Problems occur when the endocrine organ or gland becomes unhealthy and the hormones they produce are either excessive or diminished. This can create a virtual cascading (domino) affect whereby one problem leads to another. A loss of hormonal balance plays a major role in one's health or lack of it.

From the *pituitary*, pineal, hypothalamus, *adrenals, thyroid*, parathyroid, thymus, *ovaries*, *testes*, *pancreas*, kidney, skin, heart, liver, fat cells and small intestine, there are forty-five vital hormones influencing the entire body. Only six endocrine glands will be discussed in this section.

The first, most influential endocrine gland is the pituitary. However, the key to understanding endocrinology is realizing the importance of hormonal *balance*. Poor nutrition can cause hormonal problems. Hormonal problems can then cause organs, glands and other body processes to function abnormally thus effecting the way we metabolize nutrients. This cycle continues on and on.

The **pituitary** gland has two lobes (anterior/posterior) and is known as the master gland. Located at the base of the brain in a small bony "saddle" of the skull, it is part of and just behind the sphenoid sinus (nasal) called the sella turcica. It is called the master gland because it has a wide influence on many other tissues and glands. From the ovaries, testes, skin, bone, adrenals and thyroid, the pituitary provides a different hormone for each.

The anterior portion produces Thyroid Stimulating Hormone (TSH) (thyroid), Follicle Stimulating Hormone (FSH) (ovaries/testes), Luteinizing Hormone (LH) (ovaries/testes), Prolactin (PRL) (ovaries), Somatotrophin or Growth Hormone (GH) (bones) and Adrenocorticotrophic Hormone (ACTH), all of which help to regulate the adrenal glands. From the time a child is born, the pituitary is sending its Growth Hormone (GH) into the bloodstream, so that the child increases in stature and weight. If there is a disorder in the pituitary, the child will either stop growing or attain abnormal height. The anterior portion also secretes Lactogenic Hormone without which milk would not form in the mammary glands.

The posterior portion of the pituitary does not actually produce any hormones, but functions in storing two hormones; Antidiuretic (ADH/vasopressin) and Oxytocin (Pitocin). Pitocin stimulates the uterus to contract at the time of childbirth and acts on the smooth muscle of the pregnant uterus to maintain labor. ADH promotes water retention and stimulates smooth muscle of blood vessels and the digestive tract.

As a master gland, pituitary abnormalities caused by any one or more of the H.O.N.S.T.E.C components, can influence secondary glands, organs or areas. Some of the direct signs of pituitary challenges are:

- Excessive urination
- Left side head pain, left cervical
- Headaches - chronic, at level of eyes
- **Abnormal weight size**
- Seizures - especially at night
- **Type II diabetes**
- Loss of libido
- Weak ligaments, bone or tendons
- Mental illness

Again, the ovaries, thyroid, testes, thymus, spleen, adrenals and even the digestive function are strongly influenced by the pituitary.

As you know, my mother developed Type II diabetes. Could her pituitary gland have contributed to her diabetic condition? How many of you have the above signs and signals of a pituitary challenge and yet you are taking a drug for a so-called "disease" when you don't even have it?

We become what we eat, absorb and don't eliminate. Our organs and glands are only as healthy as what we feed them. If they are not fed properly, they suffer imbalances, deficiencies and over-production, and so will the rest of the body. Everything is related to everything else. The concept is just the *opposite* of what my mother was told to believe by her medical practitioners, but it is undeniably true. How can anyone be healthy without their hormones being balanced? And how can your hormones be balanced without giving them the building blocks (nutrients) they need for health?

The **adrenals** are located above the kidneys. They are known as the fright, fight or flight glands. The cortex portion produces androgens (testosterone), glucocorticoids (*cortisol*; *hydrocortisone*), mineral-corticoids (*aldosterone*), and estrogen/progesterone (estradiol). The medulla portion produces adrenaline (*epinephrine*) and noradrenaline (*norepinephrine*).

One of the most important glands, the adrenals were a key in my mother's early illnesses. As you will see, no matter what kind of a health program you are on, if you are "*stressed to the max,*" you will adversely affect your adrenals, hence they are called the *stress glands.*

As fight or flight glands they provide a burst of strength and energy. In primitive humans, when being threatened with danger as when being attacked by a vicious animal, the hypothalamus (brain), signals the pituitary gland (brain) to produce ACTH, which in turn stimulates the adrenal cortex to produce cortisol. Cortisol is carried in the bloodstream and causes a dramatic but temporary increase in metabolism (energy) and stimulation of the body to move more quickly. In addition, adrenaline (epinephrine) and norepinephrine are released. Adrenaline gives the body tremendous strength.

These hormones have a dramatic effect on the body. They nearly halt the digestive process and increase blood pressure, cholesterol levels, blood sugar and the rates of breathing and heartbeat.

During primitive times, the flood of these necessary hormones would be oxidized (burned) in the process of fighting or fleeing leaving the individual either energized or exhausted. But this is no longer the case for Westernized society.

While few of us are rarely attacked by wild animals, we are being subtly "attacked" by bills, problems and pressure. Just driving on the freeways will cause the same adrenaline and cortisol release - as with an actual animal attack. The problem is we have no process for oxidizing these stress-related hormones. We may want to fight or get away, but we are stuck in traffic, so we internalize our frustrations. We are holding on and storing stress hormones. The *signs* and *signals* we receive will depend on where they are stored. Hormones are normally meant to be used, not stored once secreted. What once was a healthy substance has now become a toxic one.

Primitive man found ways of respite. They were not always being attacked by vicious animals and therefore had moments of rest and relaxation. Modern man, especially those in Westernized society, has created a way of life that continuously stimulates their adrenals with virtually no oxidizing mechanism in place. There is no rest from our onslaught of stimulus. The end result is a toxic overload and accumulation of displaced adrenal hormones. This is why exercise is so important. It is one proven way of burning off these stored hormonal substances.

The continual and persistent activation of this pathway is a major contributor to what the medics call heart "disease," Type II diabetes, stroke, cancer, rheumatoid arthritis, depression and accelerated aging. Adrenal overload puts the body in a constant state of emergency. The adverse effects of which become chronic.

When we are under a continuous stressful experience, toxic or malnourished, our adrenal glands become exhausted and out of balance. The *signs* and *signals* include the following: (I have noted my mother's complaints in ***bold***).

Low blood pressure
Loss of hunger
Diarrhea
Dizziness
Bronchitis
Sinusitis
Weak heart
Impotency
Depression
Mental instability
Impaired digestion
Asthma

Dis-ease is defined as lack of ease or harmony, it is NOT the same as "disease," a medical term for illness treated by medicine. *NEVER* attempt to stop or reduce your medication without the supervision of your medical doctor.

Fatigue
Weight loss/**gain**
Nausea
Nervousness
Hypoglycemia
Insomnia
Neuromuscular problems
Hypertension

If you suffer from allergies, hay fever, angina, arthritis, heart palpitations, shaking, pain just below the rib cage in the center front and in the back, kidney problems, salt cravings, motion sickness, alcohol or sugar addiction, you are demonstrating an adrenal problem. These conditions are merely indicating a H.O.N.S.T.E.C. process. The focus of which may be the adrenals.

As you read, my mother experienced devastating losses, insecurity, abandonment and confusion, which lead to anger, resentment, lack of forgiveness and hatred. Coupled with her smoking and alcohol addictions, poor diet and lack of exercise, her adrenals were exhausted at an early age. Without proper nutrition to support and heal them, she acquired most, if not all of the above classical *signs* of adrenal insufficiency.

As mentioned, the medulla portion of the adrenal gland produces adrenaline (epinephrine) allowing one to meet a fright, fight and flight challenge. This hormone will normally, temporarily elevate blood sugar. However, if your adrenals are compromised, you may have an overproduction of epinephrine and hence a continuous elevation of blood sugar. For those dividing the body into a system of individual parts as an orthodox medical doctor will do, they won't see the correlation. For those of us that understand synergistic relationships, it is obvious.

How many of you are being treated for any one or more of the above *signs* and *signals* of adrenal exhaustion under a so-called "disease?"

Do you take medication like Viagra for erectile dysfunction or impotency? Your adrenals may be simply trying to tell you they are out of balance not your libido. Are you being drugged for a weak heart or for acquired hypertension? Did your doctor check your adrenals? More importantly, did she look for the *cause* of why your adrenals are out of balance? How about Type II diabetes?

The constant production of adrenaline causes a continuous elevation of blood sugar. Have any of your doctors suggested stress-releasing techniques?

The Physician Desk Reference (PDR) lists thousands of drugs for every known *symptom* just waiting for you to walk into your drug doctor and get on board the sleepy train. But not one of those drugs will ever get to the *cause* of your problem. Until, if and when you address the *real* problem, you will only be treating the effects, *not* the cause.

In addition to lifestyle changes, good food, fresh air, proper exercise and seeing life as a *choice*, there are whole-food vitamins, minerals and herbs paramount for nourishing the adrenal glands. In fact, water-soluble nutrients are easily destroyed when under stress, or while smoking or drinking alcohol, so we really need to replace them daily. The minerals sodium and potassium are equally as vital, but do *not* take isolated nutrients or individual vitamins and minerals. If you do, only take them at a low dose and for a short period of time.

Isolated nutrients, whether organic or not, work like drugs and throw all the other nutrients out of balance. The best form of nutrition has always been organic whole-food and whole-food supplements. For those requiring it, I also recommend taking an adrenal extract for a specific length of time, not indefinitely.

It is important to note: Whole-food nutritional supplementation may be consumed on a regular basis just like good food. When you have a specific condition, nutraceuticals, herbal extracts and/or homeopathics may be used, but only for a specific amount of time. Isolates may be used, but only if you are already taking a whole-food supplement first. (For more information go to Chapter 4).

Life by Choice

By the way, did you notice I said "life as a *choice*?" Life by *choice* is an interesting concept. Most of us have a "*have to*" approach to life. We *have* to go to work, *have* to go to the store, *have* to pay rent or other bills, *have* to "work out," *have* to pay taxes, *have* to go see the doctor, *have* to let the dog out, *have* to do EVERYTHING. The truth is, we don't *have to* do anything. Everything we say we *have to* do is really a *choice* to do.

Do you have to go to work? No, not really. One reason why people go to work is to *earn* money so they can pay their bills. (The only people that really *make* money work in a government mint, all others must *earn* it). If you don't have any bills or any other reason for using money, you don't have to go to work. You also don't have to pay your bills, instead you could throw them away and be thrown out of your house, lose your car and all other "things" you think you own. The truth is we choose to live the way we do and therefore need money, but it is our *choice*. We could choose to live in the desert or jungle, forests or off the land. After all, aboriginals throughout the world don't use or need any money, unless of course they want something we offer. Then they need to exchange something of value, like their land, water, oil and mineral rights. We could either pay them for it or wait until they die from Westernized "diseases" like what happened to the Hawaiians after Captain Cook introduced them to syphilis or the American Indians when the British brought them tuberculosis.

Once you realize life is about *choices* and there is nothing we *have to* do, the emotional stress and adrenal exhaustion that comes with the *have to's* diminishes.

Another example of *choice* was when I decided to write this book. I set a goal to finish the manuscript within months, not years. Although it took me twenty years of research with another fourteen years of experience before that, I gave myself two months to write over 400 pages. I even accepted an advance from my publisher, so I was really under pressure. What was I thinking?

Did I have to finish this book or did I choose to finish this book? In reality, *I chose to have to*. Get it? **We are in control of our out-of-controlness.** If I feel pressure to perform, it's because I am allowing it. I could have given the money back and sat on the beach watching the birds fly. I also could have demanded more time. But the message is clear: We choose to do what we want and, therefore, should accept the consequences of our *choices*.

The net result of seeing life as a *choice* simply means our life is in *our* control and hence our adrenals are less affected. We then can truly live more of a stress-free life.

The **thyroid** is located in the front and base of the neck below the "Adams Apple" or hyoid cartilage. It has two lobes lying on either side of the trachea or tube that goes to the lungs. It produces the hormones *thyroxine* (T4) made of four atoms of iodine and the amino acid tyrosine and *calcitonin*, a polypeptide made from 32 amino acids. Passing through the liver, T4 is converted into *triiodothyronine* or (T3). Thyroid hormones increase basal metabolic rate and increase the rate and strength of the heartbeat. One factor that influences the thyroid is TSH or Thyroid Stimulating Hormone released from the anterior lobe of the pituitary gland. TSH stimulates T4 production in the thyroid.

When the thyroid is <u>under</u> producing due to The H..O.N.S.T.E.C. Syndrome, you may experience *hypo*thyroidism with the following signs and signals:

- ***Hypo*thyroidism**
- Weight gain, particularly upper body
- Mental dullness, cannot work under pressure, stress or strain,
- Coarse hair, thick skin, brittle nails
- Lowered temperature, cold hands and feet
- Numbness, tingling sensations
- Lethargic personality, at times dull
- Basal Metabolic Rate (BMR) temperature below 97.8

Conversely, when the thyroid is <u>over</u> producing due to The H..O.N.S.T.E.C. Syndrome, you may experience *hyper*thyroidism with the following *signs* and *signals*:

- ***Hyper*thyroidism**:
- Fast heart rate
- Tremors, particularly of the protruding tongue
- Sweating, moist skin and palms of hands
- Weight loss, increased appetite

- Vertigo (dizziness)
- Intense personality, strong drive,; at times frightened in appearance
- BMR temperature above 98.2

A thyroid challenge may cause problems with kidneys, sinus, high triglycerides, bulging eyes or puffiness, general edema and lethargy. In addition, since the liver is associated with thyroid conditions you may also experience gallbladder dysfunction, colitis, inability to digest fats, poor resistance to infection, pain under right rib cage, pain anywhere on the right side of the body, pain between the shoulders, arthritis, obesity, dry or oily skin, sexual hormone problems, jaundice, excessive gas, flatulence, bloating, spastic colon, diverticulitis, hemorrhoids, hypoglycemic symptoms, eczema and menstrual problems and other complaints.

In a nut shell, without sufficient iodine, the amino acid tyrosine, 32 other amino acids and a well-functioning liver, your thyroid may not be working properly. Of course if your pituitary gland is not producing enough TSH, you might also be demonstrating *signs* and *signals* of a thyroid challenge, but it is really a pituitary problem *caused* by The H.O.N.S.T.E.C. Syndrome.

The answer is NOT taking a drug to make up for a deficiency or to lower an excess. The best approach is to always "peel the onion" until you get to the *core* of the problem. In *Chapter 7, The Cure to Diabetes,* I discuss the holistic approach to health and healing, including the thyroid. Suffice it to say, the thyroid is the third endocrine gland of vital importance to keep one healthy.

The **ovaries** are located at either side of the uterus in the lower abdominal cavity and are the primary organs producing *estrogen* and *progesterone*. At birth they contain all of the immature eggs, also known as follicles, that will mature and be released during a woman's fertile life. As the egg follicle grows, it releases *estrogen* (estradiol) into the blood. *Estrogen* generates the changes that take place at puberty; the growth of breasts, the development of the reproductive system and the shape of a woman's body. It also enables the uterine mucous to become more profuse, thinner, wetter and clearer.

The ovaries also dramatically increase their output of *progesterone* at the time of ovulation. *Progesterone* production leads to a refinement and 'ripening' of tissue and blood in the uterus. The rise of *progesterone* causes a rise in body temperature of about one degree Fahrenheit and is a measure often used as one of the indications of ovulation. When *progesterone* peaks, there is about 140 times as much *progesterone* as *estrogen*. This is a very important point, which I will explain later. Just remember, *there is more progesterone than estrogen.*

Progesterone is the hormone necessary for increased libido, not *estrogen* as is commonly believed. It is also associated with the increased sense of well-being that many women feel during the third trimester of pregnancy. Decreased secretion of *progesterone* leads to menstrual irregularities in non pregnant women and spontaneous abortion in pregnant women.

Estrogen proliferates the growth of endometrium (inside the uterus) tissue and *progesterone* facilitates its further maturing. Contrary to popular belief, the ovaries do not shrivel up; nor do they cease functioning. They just change in their production level. Even the post-menopausal uterus is actually the main site for the production of the hormone *prostacyclin* which protects women from heart "disease" and unwanted blood clotting.

A normal thyroid has a lot to do with the function of the ovaries. With a hypothyroid condition, menstruation may not appear normal though the ovaries and uterus are normal. If medical doctors were to practice natural healing, they would always seek to find the *cause* of dis-ease and, therefore, would always consider the thyroid when evaluating the ovaries.

During the formative years of a young girl's life, it is paramount that she have proper nutrition to support and nurture these most precious and important endocrine glands. As you have read, my mother didn't have a chance of having a normal puberty.

When she developed *signs* of a hormonal imbalance - mood swings, depression, hot flashes and sleeplessness, her medical doctor prescribed Premarin®, a synthetic estrogen made from the urine of pregnant mares (horses). Premarin® has a totally different composition of estrogens than those found naturally in the human body. The three estrogens found naturally in women are estriol (90 percent), estradiol (7 percent) and estrone (3 percent). Premarin® contains almost *no* estriol, but lots of estrone (75 percent) and estradiol (5 to 15 percent). In addition, horses have a number of estrogens unique to their species, most notably equilin (6 to 15%).

The real travesty is that the above *signs* and *signals* of an ovarian imbalance were in fact demonstrating a progesterone deficiency and not an estrogen one.

First and foremost, we live in a world of xeno-estrogen mimickers. Organo-phosphates, fertilizers, flame retardants, plastics and pesticides, are all converted into synthetic estrone. This fake hormone increases a women's risk of breast cancer and other cancers. Breast cancers are estrogen sensitive, however, it is not the estrogens that women naturally produce. If that were true every women producing estrogen would be at risk of developing breast and other cancers. It is The H.O.N.S.T.E.C. Syndrome, in combination with xeno-estrogens and synthetic hormone replacement therapies like Premarin® that have increased ovarian, breast and other cancers in women in the United States.

How many of you are taking birth control pills, Hormone Replacement Therapies (HRT) or other synthetic drugs and chemicals? Like my mother, you may have no idea how dangerous these *experimental* drugs are. You are not alone. My mother was one of millions just as naive. For a complete explanation of female hormones and the role they play in optimum health, I suggest you read *Hormone Heresy* by Sherril Sellman.

The **pancreas** is a large, lobulated gland resembling the salivary glands in structure. It has both exocrine (external) and endocrine (internal) functions, secreting externally through a duct and internally into the blood or lymph. Digestive juices are examples of an exocrine function. The digestive secretions are collected by the major pancreatic duct and emptied into the small intestine. The enzymatic constituents of the pancreatic fluid are trypsin, chymotrypsin, carboxypeptidase, amylase and lipase.

The endocrine part of the pancreas consists of million of tiny cells called the pancreatic islets or the Islets of Langerhans. They produced two vital hormones: insulin and glucagon.

Pancreatic secretion is under control of the hormones, secretin and pancreozymin, which are released from the duodenal mucosa (intestines) and carried to the pancreas by the blood. They function in pH regulation and digestion. These two hormones are secreted by the mucosa as a result of stimulation by the acid gastric contents in the duodenum when chyme (liquefied food) from the stomach enters the duodenum (intestines).

This is worth repeating. Acid pH food (chyme) detected in the intestines stimulates the mucous membrane to produce secretin and pancreozymin which control pancreatic secretions. Simply, the more we consume animal protein, starch (bread, pasta, grains), sugars, soda, pastries, candy, ice cream, junk "food" and even medications or anything else that creates acid in the body, the more the intestine will signal the pancreas to produce its hormones and enzymes.

It is obvious with the current diabetes epidemic in the United States, the pancreas is in trouble. It just can't keep up with the demand. For a more detailed explanation of the pancreas, see its role in diabetes below.

Mis-diagnosed

Instead of my mother's doctors recognizing the above *signs* of a hormonal imbalance, her General Practitioner (GP) sent her to a cardiologist for her weak heart, a psychiatrist for her depression, a pulmonolgist for her smoke-induced chronic cough, an internist for her hypo and hyperglycemia, a neurologist for her nervousness and dizziness and a proctologist for her hemorrhoids.

Each "doctor" prescribed medication without ever considering what could be *causing* her symptoms. She went from bad to worse. After her cancer diagnosis, two other doctors, an oncologist and an opthalmologist (she was going blind) were added to her team of individual "specialists."

Having excellent insurance, every doctor in town wanted in the loop. Strangely enough, treatment often stops when the insurance runs out or the patient gets well. Since wellness is not taught or practiced in orthodox medicine, that is unlikely.

In my mother's case, treatment, tests, drugs, surgery, radiation, and chemotherapy were all *experimentally* used to "see how she does." What happened was the so-called "scientifically" based orthodox medical approach to medicine was an *experiment* and actually *hastened* her death.

If baby boomers can remember and recite the song, "The knee bone is connected to the hip bone," why can't medical doctors remember? Is it so difficult to conceptualize that every part of the body is connected physically and etherically? The human body is not only inter-related and inter-dependent, so is the planet and universe. We are all connected within the matrix of thought and consciousness.

Below are the Top Twelve Dis-eases most people are concerned with. If your dis-ease is not listed don't worry. It doesn't make any difference what you call your condition, when you detoxify the entire body, balance the immune system, nourish every cell and forgive the unforgivable, you have set the foundation to *curing* the incurables.

Please do not forget, only a *holistic* approach to health and healing will prove to be of any long-term benefit. Quick fixes will not pass the test of time.

In order to avoid medical incompetence from happening to you, let's find out together what may be done to prevent sickness and dis-ease and how to detect the red flags early on.

For a complete explanation on how to heal yourself, go to Chapters 4 & 6.

Top Twelve Dis-eases #1

Cancer -

About 150 people per hour, 24 hours per day, seven days per week, were diagnosed with cancer in the United States in 2004. Currently, Americans have a 50/50 chance of acquiring cancer.

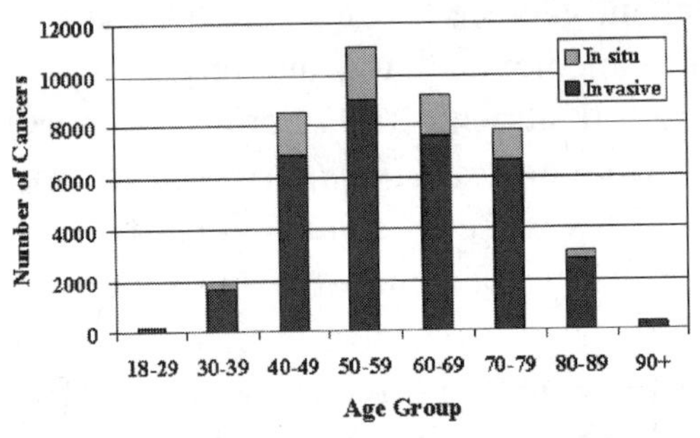

More than 560,000 of us *die* every year because of it. In 2003, Seventy-seven percent of all cancers were diagnosed in those over 55 years of age. The most common malignancies and the number of cases diagnosed annually, (2004), in the United States were as follows:

Lung (1,200,000)	Stomach (876,000)
Breast (1,050,000)	Liver (564,000)
Colon/Rectal (945,000)	Cervix (471,000)

If you listen to the AMA and the National Cancer Institute, we are winning the battle. Unfortunately, the statistics don't agree and the statistics are getting worse.

The Internet is filled with thousands of articles concerning cancer and the "new" findings of what *causes* it.

There is no mystery about cancer. Natural healers have known the *cause* and *cure* of cancer since its inception. Even though mainstream medicine now recognizes diet and environment playing a part, they still have their head in the sand.

Tobacco

Don't look to your government for any help either. As you can see, lung cancer rates are higher than all other forms of cancer. Yet, the United States government continues to subsidize the tobacco industry in spite of statistics showing over 400,000 people per year die from cigarette smoke and lung dis-ease.

Why would this country allow almost 35,000 people per *month* to commit "smokers" suicide and even help them by subsidizing the system used? The answer is simple. It's all about money. The facts are clear: Cigarette smoking contributes to the *cause* of cancer. Period. The United States government allows this toxic substance to be sold. Period.

According to the U.S. Department of Agriculture, there were 410,000,000,000 (four hundred and ten billion dollars) cigarettes sold in the United States in 2003. At an average retail cost of 20 cents each ($4.00 per pack), the tobacco industry received $82,000,000,000 (eighty-two billion dollars) in revenue. They paid the U.S. government $6,000,000,000 (six billion dollars) in tobacco taxes and state taxes of $8,300,000,000 (eight billion three hundred thousand dollars). Tobacco companies also contribute an average of $10,000,000 (ten million dollars) every campaign cycle in Washington to their favorite representatives. Although the FDA can take a herb like chaparal off the market with no evidence of mortality, a known killer like tobacco, remains. Why does the United States government allow tobacco? It's simple. It's all about money! A lot of money.

Petroleum

Our government also allows over 100,000 different chemicals to exist in our environment, most of which have *never* been tested for toxicity. Why? It's all about money. Petrochemical companies earn billions and billions every year. They too, make sure their candidates are well placed in Washington, including oil rich presidents from Texas.

Drugs

The Physicians Desk Reference (PDR) is a 3,000-page book listing every known drug currently being prescribed and each drug's side effects. From liver, kidney and heart failure to coma and death, the PDR is the drug *bible* of choice. Why would our Food and Drug Administration (FDA) allow toxic drugs to be on the market? Again, it's all about money.

Pharmaceutical companies make billions of dollars every year. Their stockholders make millions. Their political candidates are well financed and are easily re-elected. By now, you should realize, money makes the world go round. The FDA is in the loop by charging millions of dollars in fees to "approve" these drugs.

Cancer and the treatment of it, is all about money, too. The *cures* are here and have been for hundreds of years, however, only those in the "club" using their patented, expensive treatments of choice, are allowed to "legally" treat cancer patients. Like the *Mafia*, if you're not in the clan, you're out.

I saw the following information on a website. You may recognize some of the people. They all died of cancer. Their fortune, fame and position, made no difference. When compared to the 120-year life expectancy of the Hunzas in Pakistan or the Okinawans in Japan, these people died prematurely. In the end, nothing is more important than our health. Nothing:

Name	**Age of Death**	**Name**	**Age of Death**
Jimmy Dorsey	53	Gary Cooper	60
Dick Powell	58	Aldous Huxley	69
Rachel Carson	56	Nat King Cole	45
Edward R. Murrow	57	Buster Keaton	70
Walt Disney	65	Robert Taylor	57
Vince Lombardi	57	Edward G. Robinson	79
Betty Grable	56	Bud Abbott	78
Duke Ellington	75	Charles Lindbergh	72
Ed Sullivan	73	Susan Hayward	56
Ozzie Nelsen	68	Joan Crawford	69
Bob Marley	36	Ingrid Bergman	67
Andy Kaufman	35	Yul Brynner	65
Donna Reed	64	Desi Arnaz	69
Buddy Rich	69	Jackie Gleason	71
Gilda Radner	42	Jill Ireland	54
Michael Landon	54	Roger Miller	56
Audrey Hepburn	63	Frank Zappa	52
Dinah Shore	77	Jackie Kennedy	64
Mickey Mantle	63	Carl Wilson	51
Linda McCartney	56	Walter Payton	45
Jack Lemmon	76	Chet Atkins	77

The average age at death of the listed *forty-two* people is 61.4 years. How old are you? What are you doing to *prevent* cancer, heart dis-ease, stroke, diabetes, Parkinson's or Alzheimer's? If you don't take the time to be healthy, you will have to take the time to be sick. How much time do you think you have?

Read about someone that took the time to be healthy and her results. You be the judge on whether it was effective.

A Personal Case

It was in October of 1996, when I attended a fundraiser for a little 9-year-old girl named Sarah. She was apparently dying from a glioblastoma multiforma, a medically incurable brain cancer. She went through the best of what the renown doctors of UCLA and Children's Hospital in California could offer, including the most powerful drugs known to mankind; three sessions of chemotherapy, 10 weeks of high-dose radiation and even brain surgery, but nothing could stop the spider web growth of her Glio. At the fundraiser I assumed were all her family and friends, well wishers and those only there to satisfy their morbid curiosity.

I attended to donate money to the family and to see for myself whether she could be helped. One look in a person's eyes and with a touch of a hand, I can tell whether someone is ready or wanting to die. After seeing over 10,000 people in my career, I have developed the 'feel' for it, you might say. In fact, some people say I have been gifted with an insight similar to that of the prophetic Edgar Cayce. I'd rather think it's all about love.

As I approached Sarah, I saw a beautiful little girl struggling to live with a drug-swollen body, limping from the paralyzing effects of brain surgery and unable to focus both eyes as one now deviated into the distance. Her hands were cold and clammy and equally as swollen, obviously from lymphatic congestion, but one look and I knew I could help her.

I do not solicit. It is always better to be contacted by those seeking advice. I held Sarah's hand, placed my other hand on her shoulder and looked directly into her eyes. Without words, I told her I loved her and then left.

Sent Home to Die

It was almost a year before I was approached by a member of Sarah's family for help. In September of 1997, I entered Sarah's house and noticed she was much more ill looking then before. She had a muco-purulent discharge coming from her sinuses, eyes and ears. Her head hung forward and her eyes had the beginning stage of the glassy dying stare. Next to her was her dinner of pizza and a cola beverage. Her parents secretly told me the doctors at Children's Hospital said there was "nothing more that could been done" and sent her home to die. They gave her three months.

This prognosis was not new to me. Most of the people I consulted had been given a three-to-six-month death sentence. This is only after the medic's experiment with every toxic drug available, burn their patients with cancer producing radiation and cut vital body parts out.

This *experimental* orthodox medical treatment leaves many victims of "modern" medicine crippled and deformed. Instead of admitting to their limitations by saying there is nothing more they can do or that they know of, these self-proclaimed "gods" simply send their castaways home to die. By the time someone like me sees these bewildered people, many are financially destitute and extremely ill.

I can't blame only the orthodox medical profession or their trade union the AMA (American Medical Association). Medics are basically sales agents for the pharmaceutical houses which are owned, or at least controlled, by petro-chemical companies. These multinational globals control our news and entertainment media, insurance companies and governmental agencies such as the Food and Drug Administration (FDA). From birth, with their biological *experimenting* vaccines to their "legally" addicting toxic drugs, the organized industrial medical complex influences much in the way we live, breathe, eat and die. Their control is ominous, using the legal arm of government to eliminate all competition. Those caught treating cancer outside orthodox medical approval, are simply destroyed financially and sent to prison. It is for that reason, I never *treated* patients. I merely taught and still teach students as I am allowed to under the United States Constitution. (At least up to this time with Bush Jr. as president (2005)).

No Time to Lose

I knew from experience, we had no time to lose in trying to save Sarah's life or at least healthfully prolong it. As in all conditions of dis-ease, I needed to evaluate and correctly align Sarah's attitude and perception relative to her health challenge.

If you think you are going to die, you most likely will. After all, Earl Nightingale said many years ago, *"We become what we think about all day long."* I asked little Sarah if she knew what was happening to her. She said she had brain cancer. I asked her what cancer was. She said it was something growing in her body making her sick and would kill her if it doesn't stop. I asked her if she wanted to die. This is *not* a trite question. Some people, for a litany of reasons, want to die and will never recover. Sarah said she wanted to live. With that, I told her that it would take a lot of work, but I would be there with her all the way. She told me she didn't want to be hurt anymore - no shots, no surgery, no more tests. I told her I was *not* that kind of a doctor. She said she knew because her "Mommy said you are a healer and healer's don't hurt people."

Elimination Channels

The first thing I explained to Sarah and her family was how important it was to open up the elimination channels of the body.

The body always uses the colon, kidneys, lungs and skin to remove toxins. (See Chapter 6 for complete explanation). Once these organs are working to their full potential, it is then safe to detoxify. However, one should never proceed in a full body detoxification without depolarizing the blood and lymph.

Depolarization

Every cell in the body has a polarity. When that polarity changes, as in all illnesses, the cells start to attract each other. This causes the blood and/or lymph to thicken or congest. Since the lymph is the sewer system of the body, it is paramount for it to be completely clean and functioning. This can be accomplished through either biochemical intervention or electrical application. Only after the body is properly detoxified, can one then effectively normalize and rebuild the immune system.

Nearly Lost

It was 11 PM on the third night since I started helping Sarah. I had left her house around 9 PM after teaching her parents the importance of full body massage. The caller was Sarah's Mom. She was absolutely hysterical. Apparently, Sarah had just suffered a stroke. The left side of her body was now paralyzed. I could hear her in the background screaming and crying, calling for her Mother. I immediately returned.

Upon arriving, I rushed into Sarah's room where her parents were kneeling by her bed holding her limp little hands. Sarah was crying with a white foam coming out of her mouth. Her mother said Sarah was sound asleep, when all of the sudden she started screaming that she couldn't move. When I looked at her, she just kept repeating, "I don't want to die, I don't want to die. Mommy help me."

Again, from experience, I knew we only had about 48 hours to initiate oxygen therapy. Not just oxygen (O2), but only OZONE (O3) could save her now. Unfortunately, my ozone machine was being repaired. I immediately called a friend of mine in Oregon who manufactured ozone machines. I told him what had happened and he said he would fly his private plane down in the morning with a brand new ozone machine.

I assured Sarah and her parents that she would be okay. I told them that in the morning she would be able to use her left side a little better and after starting ozone therapy, she would completely recover. I didn't just think so or hope so, I knew it!

Sarah was given an enema to purge her liver and gallbladder and fell right to sleep.

First thing in the morning, my friend arrived as promised with a new ozone machine. I immediately taught Sarah's parents how to apply rectal insufflation. Within 24 hours, Sarah had total use of her left side again.

Education is Key

The key to true wellness is love, attention, education and taking effective action, *not* treatment. However, misinformation is everywhere. Book stores are filled with overnight so-called natural healing gurus, selling their 'how to' manuscripts prescribing everything from Tiger penis to pet rocks. Medics who spent their entire career promoting drugs, surgery and radiation, now retired, have become "wanna be" natural healing celebrities with their books, tapes, videos, seminars and T-shirts. Even alleged natural healers are using inferior products in an allopathic, symptom treating application. I have seen many of these people come and go along with their "miracle" cures. However, my students are taught how they acquired their illness and how not to re-acquire it. In the case of infants, parental education is mandatory for true recovery.

Healing Program

Because no two people are the same, no one protocol will work for everyone. Only after a thorough consultation will a student be directed to a program that will best serve them. There are some procedures and products I teach in general - from coffee or lemon water enemas, lymphatic massage, EMF protection, immune modulation, oxygen therapies, super whole-food nutrition to visualization, most people need the basics.

Sarah was no exception. She immediately was given organic vegetable juice, specific herbs, bioenergetic supplementation, coffee enemas, hydrotherapy and a host of other advanced healing protocols, including medical grade ozone therapy.

For her sinus exudate, I used a system I re-discovered that was used over 4,000 years ago in Egypt. It is called nasal irrigation. Not unlike a colonic, I bought her a water-pik tooth cleaning instrument and retro-fitted a special nasal tip. Using herbs and specific natural oils, she cleansed her sinuses daily. Within a week, her ears, eyes and sinuses were clear.

Eliminating chemical-laden dairy products alone stopped the mucous discharge building up in her body. With her colon, liver, kidneys, lungs and skin now working properly, she was ready to liquefy her blood and lymph. Red clover tea is a tremendous blood purifier. Drinking that with a little stillingia root cleans the lymphatic circulation as well. Had that not worked, I have a multitude of effective products at my disposal. One is 714X out of Canada. You may recall how a doctor in Kentucky helped a young boy named Billy Best with lymphoma by using 714X. Although I do not sell this product, students may order it directly from the company. (Cerbe Institute - Quebec: 1-819-564-0492)

Another way of depolarizing the lymph is by using a magnetic pulser. This instrument uses Beck's technology and is extremely effective. At a cost of only a few hundred dollars, it is truly worth every penny.

Results

After about six months of *intensive* therapy, Sarah was cancer free. She had an MRI every six months or so showing only the shadowing of the remnant of where her cancer used to be and where the surgeons removed part of her brain.

As with all "modern" medical treatment, the effects of toxic drugs, chemotherapy, radiation and surgery permanently disabled this precious child. If only people would trust natural healing first, perhaps we wouldn't have so many innocent victims?

Sarah's biggest challenge was keeping away from junk food at school and at her friends homes. For over six years, Sarah and her parents kept her cancer from returning. However, she eventually fell back to eating processed, devitalized junk "food." As so often happens, if one's cancer returns, it returns with a vengeance. Although we again tried everything we could, little Sarah passed away in 2004.

Sarah lived longer than any glioblastoma multiforma patient UCLA had ever seen. They had no idea how she lived so long when they gave her only three months to live. Her mother hinted that they were trying natural healing, but no one at the *UCLA Children's Cancer Center* cared enough to call and find out what we were doing. Does this sound familiar? Regardless of what the medics say, they can't *really* care. If they did, they would embrace *all* disciplines of the healing arts for the betterment of the patient. The proof is in the pudding.

Although others may have given up on her, Sarah never lost faith. Even when her medics gave her a "time-set certain" to die, she refused to believe it. I can't tell you how many "terminally" ill people I have consulted that died within days of their doctor's final decree. Each and every one of them circled the date on their calendar and counted the days. Remember, "We become what we think about all day long."

Whether you have brain, breast, liver or bone cancer, the body knows how to heal itself if given what it needs to do the job. In Chapter 6 you will learn how.

Top Twelve Dis-eases #2
Heart Disease

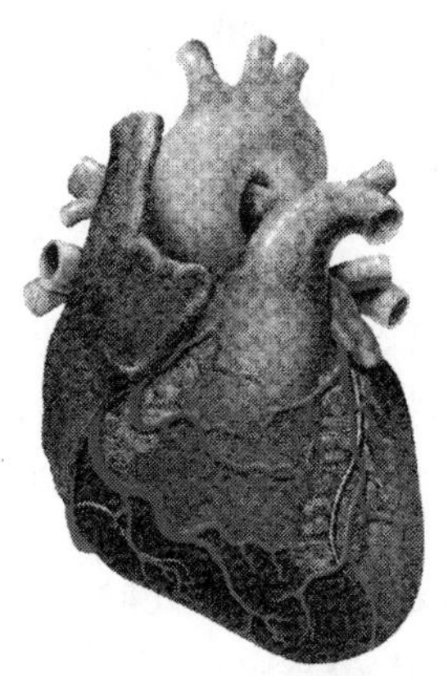

Recently, CNN covered a story where the AMA announced their latest findings concerning heart "disease" and arteriosclerosis. The report indicated that lowering cholesterol alone did not significantly lower one's risk of heart attack. The "news" indicated it is now believed that inflammation is the *second* factor in heart "disease."

The previous understanding of heart "disease" caused by LDL "bad" cholesterol clogging arteries, caused thousands upon thousands of unnecessary surgeries and ballon angioplasty. With a 6 to 7 percent chance of mortality, surgery is risky. However, there is an 80 percent chance of decline in mental function and mood in coronary bypass survivors. Of course we know these surgeries do not get to the *cause* of the problem. It is only a matter of time before the arteries clog again or one has a heart attack.

For over 30 years, I have lectured on the *cause* of heart dis-ease and that *cause* is inflammation created by The

Dis-ease is defined as lack of ease or harmony, it is NOT the same as "disease," a medical term for illness treated by medicine.
NEVER attempt to stop or reduce your medication without the supervision of your medical doctor.

H.O.N.S.T.E.C. Syndrome. The pathway is simple. Whenever anything causes the pH of the body, specifically the blood, to become acidic, it creates lesions within the vessel walls. Because the arteries contain a muscle layer that allows them to expand and contract with every heart beat, once a lesion has been infiltrated with LDL (low density lipoprotein) cholesterol, the vessels ability to expand and contract is greatly reduced. As the cause of arteriosclerosis continues, high blood pressure will force the infiltrated lesion to crack. Either additional plaque will "clog" the artery risking thrombotic occlusion or it will rupture causing a hemorrhage. Either way, the person has what we call a heart attack.

Risk Factors

High blood pressure is a *major* risk factor for heart attack. Smoking, diabetes, being over weight and of course The H.O.N.S.T.E.C. Syndrome, all contribute. Smoking accelerates the oxidation of LDL, the first step in plaque formation. Taking antioxidants helps to reduce oxidation. Elevated glucose from pre, Type I and Type II diabetes causes glycation: the binding of a glucose molecule to protein and DNA. Again, balance is the key. Too many advanced glycation end products (A.G.E.s) interfere with the proper functioning of proteins. This can cause a cross-linking with other proteins - causing a stiffness in tissues that were once flexible and elastic.

Orthodox Medicine Does Not Work

In most cases, bypass surgery replaces an artery with a vein. Veins are not able to adequately handle the high pressures of blood flow; therefore they tend to develop plaque more quickly than the original artery. Surgery does nothing to slow down plaque formation or get to the *cause* of the problem. This type of surgery gives one a false sense of security only buying a little time and making the surgeon a lot of money.

Angioplasty involves a balloon inserted into the suspect artery. As the balloon compresses obstructions, it actually damages tissue, causing either more plaque to form or a rupture. This accelerates the inflammatory process and risks a heart attack as a consequence of the procedure.

Arterial stents do nothing to remove plaque. In fact, this procedure causes a *strong* inflammatory reaction, which is counterproductive. The key is how plaque is created.

How Soft Plaque Is Formed

A. LDL cholesterol is normally used to repair vessel membranes. When there are a few areas to be repaired, it is not a problem. However, because of the increasing contributing factors from The H.O.N.S.T.E.C. Syndrome, there are more multiple areas requiring repairs than the body can handle. From toxic hydrogenated oils and fats to other acidic producing lesions, LDL plaque builds-up in the intimal layer of the vessel.

As mentioned, oxidation and glycation are contributing factors of LDL accumulating.

B. No longer appearing normal to the body, the modified LDL plaque is seen as a foreign invader. The endothelial (lining) cells in blood vessels will *signal* the immune system by secreting chemicals that warn of infection or invasion, which then seeks out, attacks and damages the invaders; plaque.

C. Monocytes are white blood cells that ingest dead or damaged cells, T-lymphocytes are white blood cells that attack foreign substances and germs, respond to the immune system going to the intimal layer of the vessel where the soft plaque has formed.

D. The monocytes are converted into macrophages, fully matured immune fighters, where they ingest the oxidized and glycosylated LDL molecules. As the macrophages become filled with fatty LDL, they take on the appearance of foam, hence they are then known as a "foam cell."

Together with T-cells they form "fatty streaks" in the blood vessel walls.

E. The above process, along with the acidic condition of the body, causes inflammation. The smooth muscle normally below the intima, now travels to the top of the fatty streak, where they form a fibrous cap. This adds to the size of the plaque.

F. As the process continues, the foam cells undergo

additional changes increasing the inflammatory condition. The new foam cells damage the fibrous cap causing it to rupture.

G. In its attempt to stop the hemorrhage from the ruptured cap, the macrophage foam cells secrete a substance called "tissue factor," which helps to form a blood clot or thrombus.

H. A coronary thrombus large enough to block a vessel results in a heart attack.

The process of soft plaque formation outlined above is associated with about 85 percent of all heart attacks.

As many times as I have said it, it bears repeating, **"Only Sick People Get Sick."** The key to avoiding a heart attack is to prevent one from ever developing. We must stop doing all things known to cause inflammation and an acid pH, including, but not limited to; smoking cigarettes, over indulging in food and alcohol and especially eating sugar. Keep your body fat down with sensible eating and exercising regularly. High emotions - anger, jealousy, hatred and lack of forgiveness all contribute to an acid pH and high blood pressure.

There are specific nutrients such as antioxidants; the Acai berry and natural vaso-dilators such as cayenne that will benefit the heart and body. For more details, see Chapter 4 & 6.

Top Twelve Dis-eases #3

Strokes

Every year over 700,000 Americans suffer strokes, the third leading cause of death after cancer and heart "disease." Even the vivacious American actress Sharon Stone and the youthful TV personality Dick Clark, have had strokes.

Also called cerebral vascular accidents or CVA, most strokes occur when a blood clot travels to the brain and lodges in a smaller vessel. This area then dies from lack of oxygen. The good news is, the death of brain cells does not occur instantly. In fact, there is a window of opportunity and a special treatment only natural healers employ, that if performed within 72 hours of a stroke, this procedure reduces the possibility of permanent disability or paralysis by 75%.

Many years ago, I received a frantic call from an Italian gentleman in Alabama. He had read an article I wrote about oxygen therapies, specifically ozone and how important it is to start this type of therapy within 72 hours of a stroke. Although his wife had a stroke, it only occurred within 48 hours of his call. After hearing the desperation in his voice, I immediately flew to Alabama.

When I arrived at his home, what struck me the most, was the size of his family. Gathered around the living room were over 30 friends, relatives and immediate family members. There was enough home-cooked Italian food to feed a small army. I was reminded of one of my mother's dinner parties. I was greeted as if I were a long-lost relative. Between the hugs and kisses, I thought I would never get to the patient. When I made a comment to that effect, one older woman said, "She's sleeping, she can wait. First, you must eat."

Entering the master bedroom, I found a beautiful, slim Italian woman lying peacefully in a rented hospital bed. Since I had no time to lose, I asked the women in attendance to help me give the patient a coffee enema. Not being familiar with natural healing, there was an instant chatter throughout the room, all in Italian of which I did not speak. When I explained the importance of evacuating the colon before anything else could be done, I immediately had a dozen volunteers.

Laying plastic and clean sheets on the bedroom floor, we gave the patient a high enema cleansing her entire colon. Returning her to bed, I ozonated her IV saline solution at 2.5%. I then injected 30 cc of 2.5% ozone IV. Finally, I gave her a vaginal and rectal insufflation of 3.5% ozone for approximately two minutes or until she started expelling the healing gas.

Later that evening, I repeated the entire ozone treatment and then went to bed in one of the guest rooms. The entire entourage spent the night on couches, the floor and on cushions.

I rose at dawn to check the patient. Upon entering her room, I found her sitting up looking out the window. She asked who I was. I told her and we embraced as she cried.

Within minutes, there were 30 people standing in the room, exclaiming and crying and thanking God for a miracle and for sending His angel.

I'd like to think I am an angel, however, I'm not that nice of a person. What actually took place was the *cause* and *effect* of using oxygen therapy in a timely manner. After several hours of teaching this wonderful family about natural healing and how to prevent a future stroke, I left the ozone machine with instructions on its application and flew home.

Within two weeks, my new friend had totally recovered from her life-threatening stroke with no side effects.

Status on Oxygen Therapies

For those unable to find a practitioner qualified to use medical grade ozone therapy or that do not have a home unit to at least do insufflation and water purification, hyperbaric chambers can be just as beneficial.

I encourage all concerned about their health to contact an ozone qualified natural healer or a hyperbaric chamber facility - *before* you need them. In the alternative, medical-grade ozone machines are available for personal use. I only endorse the **Oxy-Charge® Water Purification System** engineered in Germany, since I participated in its research and development.

Oxygen therapies are not only critical for stroke victims, they are paramount for preventing a litany of health challenges. Although legal to use in all states for water purification, IV application and rectal/vaginal insufflation may only be used in a few states, Nevada being one. [*Of course you can do what you want in the privacy of your own home under self treatment.*] In addition, Georgia, Texas, New York, New Mexico, Oklahoma, Alaska, Washington, Colorado and North Carolina, have protective alternative therapy laws that may allow ozone therapy.

If you live in the Los Angeles, California area, contact the *Hyperbaric Oxygen Clinic of Santa Monica* at 900 Wilshire Blvd., Suite 102 Santa Monica, CA 90401. Phone: 1-310-260-0033 or visit at www.HBOT.com. If you mention reading about them in my book maybe they will give you a discount as a courtesy.

The same mechanisms that adversely affect the heart, also affect the brain. Blood dyscrasias cause thrombi and ruptures. If the vessel is in the heart, you will have a heart attack. If the vessel is in the brain, you will have a stroke. Both are preventable.

Top Twelve Dis-eases #4
Emphysema

I originally started writing this sub-chapter weeks ago. However, just within the last three days one of the most influential television personalities ever to entertain the mass media, passed away from emphysema.

Like most of us, I grew up watching Johnny Carson and his *Tonight Show.* I just loved his style, demeanor and interaction with his guests. He always made me laugh and laughter is one way of releasing stress and anxiety.

If you watched the *Johnny Carson Show*, you know he was a chain cigarette smoker. He was part of my parents generation where most people learned to smoke at an early age. It was a time when the tobacco industry and cigarette companies were hiding the truth about *what* their government-protected-product was *really* doing to unsuspecting consumers.

We now know that smoking cigarettes not only causes cancer, heart disease, strokes and emphysema, it causes oxidative decomposition, which contributes to free-radical damage, DNA mutations and premature aging. In spite of these facts, hundreds of thousands of people die every year in the United States from smoking. In addition, it costs billions of dollars to take care of their healthcare needs.

On one trip to New England, I decided to take a late-night flight. By the time we took off from LAX, it was around 11:00PM. As I was just about to fall asleep, an older gentleman, possibly in his eighties, a couple of rows away, started to cough. He was actually gasping for breath. I noticed he had an oxygen tank helping him breathe. He obviously had emphysema.

After 10 or 15 minutes of listening to him hack, choke and cough, I realized I wouldn't be getting any rest on this flight if I didn't try to help him. Since I always carry a bottle of lobelia and fenugreek tincture with me, I decided to approach with my remedy.

At first glance, I noticed he had marked cyanosis, a dark blueish color of the lips and sometimes fingers, toes and face.

I introduced myself as a natural healing doctor. I told him that I thought I heard him coughing and that I just happened to have a cough remedy with me. I explained the effects of taking lobelia, specifically in small doses and how it *dilates* the bronchial tubes, making it easier to breathe. In a stronger dose, it works as an *expectorant* and will help break up and get rid of mucous. At an even stronger dose, it is an *emetic*. It will actually cause one to vomit from their lungs.

I told him he was gasping because his lungs were full of mucous, most likely a thick, black mucous. I suggested he follow me to the restroom where he could take the entire two-ounce bottle in one large dose. This would immediately cause him to vomit from his lungs. I'll never forget the way he looked at me and said, "What do I have to lose? I'm dying anyway. Lead the way."

We went back to the restroom where he swallowed two ounces of lobelia and fenugreek. Within minutes he expelled half a cup of black mucous. Instantly, he could breathe better and his lips were no longer blue. I walked him back to his seat and with tears in his eyes, he thanked me for helping him. I gave him the empty bottle and told him to buy more when he got home. I suggested he take a couple of eyedroppers three or four times per day as a maintenance dose to help him breathe a little easier.

I am thankful to say, both of us were able to sleep all the way to Boston.

According to the *World Health Organization*, over 5 million people throughout the world die every year as a result of smoking.

Just as my mother did, most claim they have a *right* to smoke. I suppose that's true, however, I have a right *not* to smoke. I believe in order not to violate *my* rights, smokers should *inhale* only. It is when they *exhale,* they contaminate the same air I breathe, thereby affecting *my* rights. As reported by the U.S. Environmental Protective Agency (EPA), over 6,000 people die every year from lung cancer caused by *second-hand* smoke. The *exhalers* are killing us.

It isn't just tobacco that causes lung and other health problems. Anything that we inhale that is toxic may have the same result. In addition to carcinogenic chemicals found in cigarettes, inhaling hot air has devastating effects.

Back in the 70s my hometown had a terrible fire. For days the mountains and hills were burning all around us. Animals were running wild down mainstreet to get away from the smoke and flames. At one point it looked like the skies just after Mt. St. Helen's, Washington erupted in 1980.

Black smoke and ash were everywhere. Breathing was nearly impossible. Eventually the fire was under control and everything went back to normal. Well, not quite.

Over the next few weeks, I saw several firemen at my clinic with lung problems, mostly pneumonia. Whenever we inhale burning air (smoke or no smoke), the hot air either paralyzes or singes the fine hairs in our lungs called cilia.

Normally, the cilia move mucous from the lungs up into the throat. This is one way of detoxifying the lungs of air borne contaminates. If we compromise this system of detoxification by inhaling any lit substance, lung problems will ensue. For this reason and others, smoking cigarettes, marijuana or any other substance can cause lung problems.

From a chronic cough, bronchitis, bronchiectasis, pneumonia, emphysema to lung cancer, our lungs are not designed to inhale toxic substances. The above conditions merely reflect the consequences of abusing them.

The answer to *preventing* emphysema is to never do anything that can cause it. If you have started abusing your lungs, stop now before it progresses to permanent damage.

I had a patient with severe emphysema. By the time she

came to see me, her condition was non-recoverable. On the day before she died, she asked me to come visit her at the hospital. I met her husband, daughter and son out in the parking lot. What struck me the most about this family was that they were all smoking. I looked at the husband with shock and disdain. He glanced at me and said, "We can't all live forever."

If you think living is difficult at times, try dying a slow, painful, torturous death while choking and gasping for air. When his time comes, it won't be so funny. What's worse is the legacy he and his wife have left their children and possibly their children's children. I believe everyone has a right to their own level of ignorance, however, children are very impressionable, they learn by the examples their parents leave.

Top Twelve Dis-eases #5

Diabetes

Sugar intolerance involves the body's inability to properly metabolize sugars. The end result is either hypoglycemia - low blood sugar and/or hyperglycemia - high blood sugar or diabetes. The gland responsible for maintaining healthy glucose levels is primarily the pancreas.

Located transversely in the upper abdomen in between the liver and stomach above the transverse colon, the pancreas has a head, neck, body and tail. The head has two parts similar to a two-prong fork. The part closest to the stomach is called the dorsal (top). The bottom part is called the ventral. The ventral portion of the pancreas contains the pancreatic duct (tube) that joins with the bile duct to transmit pancreatic fluids to the small intestine at the duodenum section.

The dorsal (top) branch of the pancreas contains the accessory pancreatic duct (tube), which also enters the small intestine, but is not joined with the bile duct (tube) and does not seem to transmit fluids on a regular basis.

The pancreas is a gland of both external (exocrine) and internal (endocrine) secretion. Its external secretion is conveyed by the pancreatic duct to the small intestine (duodenum) where its fluid (enzymes) aids in the digestion of proteins, carbohydrates and fats. Pancreatic enzymes are trypsin, lipase, chymotrypsin, carboxypetidase and amylase. The internal secretion comes from pancreatic alpha and beta cells located in an area called the Islets of Langerhans. The secretion contains either insulin (beta) and/or glucagon (alpha) hormones. Insulin is taken up by the blood stream and is an important factor in the control of sugar and fat metabolism. It is the production of insulin or lack thereof that is at the core of sugar intolerance and obesity.

Insulin/Glycogen

Depending on the pH of the intestine which is based on what was consumed, the duodenal mucosa secrete two hormones: secretin and pancreozyme. Soon after a meal, these hormones signal the pancreas to release digestive enzymes and insulin. Insulin lowers blood glucose by increasing the rate at which glucose is taken up by cells throughout the body. Glucose not immediately used is stored as glycogen. Once the body stores all the glycogen it can in the liver and muscle, it converts the rest into fat. Any significant reduction in normal blood glucose levels will cause the release of the hormone glucagon by the alpha cells of the pancreas. Glucagon stimulates the release of glucose stored in body tissues/cells and the cycle starts all over again.

A similar synergistic relationship is found throughout the body in all areas, glands and processes. As with all nutrients, balance is the key to homeostasis. Our body is truly a symphony of harmonious balance. However, the pancreas was never intended to be used to help digest the ever-increasing onslaught of refined carbohydrates, sugars and processed, devitalized junk "food." Excluding genetic pre-dispositional disorders such as juvenile diabetes or diabetes Type I, after years of a poor diet and emotional overload, sugar problems and Type II diabetes are likely.

Anger, fright, stress and poor diet may stimulate the release of epinephrine and corticosteroids by the adrenal glands to provide quicker breakdown of stored glucose (glycogen) for extra energy during increased need. From an improper diet and a stressful lifestyle, hypoglycemia and diabetes are common diseases.

Hypoglycemia

As the term implies, hypo literally means below or low. Glycemia means glucose or sugar, hence hypoglycemia is low blood sugar.

As we consume sugars, be it in a refined state such as found in pastries, candy, soda and other processed junk "food" or those sugars found in starch, pasta, bread, fruits and vegetables, the pancreas must produce enough insulin to metabolize it. If the pancreas overproduces insulin, we will go into a state of hypoglycemia that is really called HYPER-insulin-ism. It is the constant stimulation of the pancreatic beta cells or insulin-producing cells that leads to diabetes Type II or hyperglycemia.

Type I Diabetes

Type I diabetes was previously called insulin-dependent diabetes mellitus (IDDM) or juvenile-onset diabetes. Type I diabetes develops when the body's immune system destroys part or all of the pancreatic beta cells. This form of diabetes usually strikes children and young adults, although the disease can occur at any age. Risk factors for Type I diabetes include autoimmune, genetic and environmental factors. As of 2002, approximately 10% (1.8 MILLION) of all 18 MILLION diabetics in America have Type I diabetes. For those acquiring Type I later in life, poor diet and lack of exercise are the pre-requisites that seem to contribute the most to developing diabetes. In some cases after severe infection, the beta cells of the pancreas can become non-functional. As always, getting to the cause is very important.

Since insulin therapy is usually prescribed at an early age, it typically causes the beta cells to shut down. Therefore, it is very difficult to reactivate beta cells once atrophy (wasting away) has begun. However, it is not impossible, as you will see in the following pages. There is hope.

Type II Diabetes

Type II diabetes was previously called non-insulin-dependent diabetes mellitus (NIDDM) or adult-onset diabetes.

As of 2002, approximately 90% (16 MILLION 200 THOUSAND) of all diabetics have Type II diabetes. With Type II diabetes, insulin is being produced but not being metabolized properly.

Problems usually begin as insulin resistance, a disorder in which the cells do not use insulin properly. As the need for insulin rises, the pancreas gradually loses its ability to produce sufficient amounts.

Type II diabetes is associated with older age, obesity, family history of diabetes, prior history of gestational (pregnancy) diabetes, impaired glucose tolerance, physical inactivity, race, ethnicity, poor diet and lack of exercise.

Pre-Diabetes

When one has impaired glucose tolerance and/or impaired fasting glucose, they are said to be pre-diabetic. There are approximately 41 MILLION Americans (2002) that fall into this category - and they don't even know it.

Pre-diabetes is the state that occurs when a blood glucose levels are higher than normal, but not high enough for a diagnosis of diabetes. The current acceptable blood glucose range is 80 to 100 mg/dl. Normal fasting blood glucose is below 100 mg/dl. A person with pre-diabetes has a fasting blood glucose level between 100 and 125 mg/dl. If the fasting blood glucose level rises to 126 mg/dl or above, a person has diabetes.

Studies have shown that people with pre-diabetes can prevent or delay the development of Type II diabetes by up to 58 percent through changes in their lifestyle that include modest weight loss and regular exercise.

High Risk

If you have pre-diabetes, you are at a 50 percent increased risk for heart disease or stroke. 25 percent of very obese children and 21 percent of very obese adolescents have pre-diabetes. Obviously, weight plays a major role.

Some of the earliest signs of pre-diabetes are unexplained fatigue, weight gain and blurred vision. Again, there are over 41 MILLION Americans (2002) with pre-diabetes and most are not aware of it. If you have any of the above symptoms, I suggest you either acquire a glucose monitoring devise from your local pharmacy or see your doctor to have your fasting blood glucose checked. You may also buy one direct from QCI Products. (See Index E- *Resources*). Remember, if it is over 100 mg/dl you are most likely pre-diabetic. If it is over 126 mg/dl you are most likely diabetic.

If you have Type I or Type II diabetes, you not only will feel fatigued, maybe over weight and have blurred vision, but you may also experience general blood vascular circulatory problems affecting your feet and legs, heart and brain, kidneys and even your nervous system. Symptoms include but are not limited to, cold extremities, continuous infections, gangrene, atherosclerosis, high blood pressure, extreme thirst, frequent urination, dry and itchy skin, ravenous hunger, weakness, confusion, irritability, flu-like symptoms, dizziness, shortness of breath, aching type of pain especially at night, abdominal pain, loss of libido and impotence.

Eventually, diabetes can lead to heart attacks, stroke, diabetic retinopathy and glaucoma, blindness, extremity amputation and kidney failure. Although genetics, diet and lack of exercise are major contributing factors, smoking and alcohol abuse are known antagonists.

Facts Relative to Diabetes:

1. 65% of all diabetics will die from heart disease or stroke.
2. Up to 24, 000 new cases of diabetic blindness are discovered yearly.
3. 21% of all diabetics acquire kidney disease.
4. Up to 82,000 people per year lose their feet or a leg to amputation caused by diabetes.
5. 80% of all children diagnosed with diabetes are over weight.
6. 88 million disability days were caused by diabetes in 2002.
7. $182 billion was spent in 2002 on diabetes.
8. Diabetes is the 5th leading cause of death in the US.

Orthodox Medical Treatment & Prevention

Diet and exercise will not only lower glucose, but will also lower cholesterol, as well. This alone, will help the majority of those with pre-diabetes and even those with Type I and Type II. In addition, avoiding smoking and only drinking alcohol in moderation, will further contribute to improving one's health status and diabetes. If being overweight is a factor, by losing a modest amount of weight, like 5 to 10 percent of total body weight, the benefits maybe soon realized. Even a loss of 10 to 15 pounds can make a huge difference.

For those with Type I and Type II diabetes, diet and exercise alone will NOT be enough. There are two distinctive approaches to diabetes treatment: one is the orthodox method and the other natural healing. Orthodox medicine will usually start with oral medication. The drug of choice today is Metformin.

Metformin -

Unfortunately, Metformin has a litany of toxic adverse side effects as listed in the Physicians Desk Reference (PDR). They include but are not limited to: Lactic Acidosis, a serious condition that is FATAL in 50% of cases acquiring it; increased cardiovascular mortality (death), gastrointestinal reactions such as diarrhea, nausea, vomiting, abdominal bloating, flatulence and anorexia, and finally impaired renal (kidney) and hepatic (liver) function.

Insulin Injections/Pump -

If Metformin is not effective, the next drug of choice is insulin. The most common side effect of using insulin is drug-induced hypoglycemia. If this happens and it becomes severe, disorientation, unconsciousness, seizures and even death, can occur. Of course, once insulin has been used for a number of years, most beta cells still healthy enough to produce insulin will probably atrophy and cease to do so indefinitely.

The good news is there is now a much safer way to control and even *cure* diabetes for most pre-diabetics and even those with Type I and Type II. The formulae are discussed in *Chapter 7.*

My mother ate whatever she felt like eating. It was mostly refined carbohydrates, processed food, animal protein and anything sweet. I grew up on that diet.

I remember going to the dentist as a teenager, when he told my mother I had more cavities than teeth. From years of dental filings, I had thirty-one cavities with only twenty-eight teeth. Although I now eat differently, it is easy for me to go back to my childhood diet.

Safe and Effective

With a healthy diet emphasizing organic fruits, vegetables, nuts, seeds, sprouts, legumes, free range chicken, turkey and wild Alaskan salmon, drinking charged distilled water and taking only whole food nutraceuticals, the seven elements in Chapter 7 are paramount to slowing down, stopping, reversing and *curing* diabetes. If you are *only* interested in a diabetic cure, turn to Chapter 7 now.

Top Twelve Dis-eases #6

Hepatitis

The liver is the largest organ in the body and is located in the upper part of the abdominal cavity under the right front rib cage. Blood is transported to the liver from the digestive tract and spleen via the portal vein and from the aorta via the hepatic artery. The liver is a highly vascularized organ.

The liver destroys old and worn-out red blood cells and removes bacteria and foreign bodies from the blood. It also produces bile which is stored in the gallbladder. Bile aids in the production of an alkaline reaction in the intestine, in the breaking down and absorption of fats and in preventing putrefaction.

The influences of the liver on nutrition include production of bile, storage of glycogen, releasing it as glucose when needed; storage of oil soluble vitamins A, D, E and K, as well as B12 and certain other water soluble vitamins, and metabolism of fats, carbohydrates and proteins.

The liver is the organ most concerned with lipid or fat metabolism. When it has been compromised by any of the components of The H.O.N.S.T.E.C. Syndrome, it can easily be infected by a host of pathogenic organisms.

Since 'hepa' means liver and 'itis' means inflammation, hepatitis literally means inflammation of the liver. Orthodox medicine blames viruses and names them A, B, C, D, E & G. (I wonder what happened to F?). They also blame hepatitis on herpes simplex, cytomegalovirus and Epstein Barr virus. That's not to say someone with an inflamed liver will not have a concomitant viral infection, but as you know by now, viruses come as a consequence of The H.O.N.S.T.E.C. Syndrome and *do not cause* dis-ease. They are scavengers coming after the fact, attacking weak organs, glands, muscles and tissue.

The *signs* and *signals* of hepatitis are similar to many nutrient deficiencies and issues of toxicity. From dark urine, fatigue, loss of appetite, nausea, fever, vomiting, headache, abdominal discomfort, light stools, muscle pain, drowsiness, irritability, itching, diarrhea to joint pain, hepatitis can be troublesome.

As with all health challenges, there is a specific procedure to slow down, stop and then reverse them. It is as follows: 1. Open the elimination channels. 2. De and re-polarize the lymph and blood. 3. Detoxify the entire body and 4. Modulate the immune system.

Similar to other "diseases," hearing a diagnosis of hepatitis sends chills down one's spine. "Oh, my God. Are you sure Doc? Now what? Am I going to die?" I've heard people react the same way from hearing the words cancer, AIDS, lupus to Alzheimer's. I am always surprised at how *serious* people take hearing they may have a "disease." I suggest a little attitude adjustment is in order. Attitude determines your altitude. It is easier to get a clearer perspective on life from a higher advantage point. Reacting to words in a *fearful* and negative manner imprints one's consciousness releasing harmful neuro-peptides within our brain. Depending on how inclusive this reaction is, determines how well you recover from your health challenge.

Dis-ease is defined as lack of ease or harmony, it is NOT the
same as "disease," a medical term for illness treated by medicine.
NEVER attempt to stop or reduce your medication without the supervision of your medical doctor.

For a complete, step by step process on healing yourself from hepatitis, go to Chapter 6.

Top Twelve Dis-eases #7

Obesity

Being just 20 percent overweight triples your risk of high blood pressure and diabetes, doubles your risk of elevated cholesterol and increases your risk of heart "disease" by 60 percent. According to a report in the 2003 edition of the *Journal of the American Medical Association*, an obese 20-year-old man has a life expectancy 13 years *less* than others of normal weight. (I wonder if that is with medical treatment or without?)

As in most medical conditions obesity is veiled in mystery as if no one knows what causes this puzzling disorder. I believe one reason for this cloaking is because *common sense and logic has been effectively replaced with intentional misinformation.* Wait. Before you discount what I just said, consider a few facts:

1. Prior to 1912, before the creation of hydrogenated lard called *Crisco*, there was virtually no Type II, Adult Onset or Insulin Resistant diabetes. How could this be? It's simple; hydrogenated oils and fats seal cellular glucose receptor sites. keeping glucose out and insulin up. Hydrogenated fats and oils are not broken down in the body easily. These toxic lipids are deposited with the consistency of plastic. The net result is Type II diabetes.

Told by her medical doctor that butter was high in cholesterol and therefore bad, my mother immediately switched to margarine, a hydrogenated vegetable spread. The manufacturers of margarine spend millions of dollars putting out misinformation to convince the American people how "healthy" their synthetic, toxic, hydrogenated, trans-fatty acid, butter replacement product is. With the help of the *American Medical Association* and its union members, the all-knowing allopathic doctors, along with their subordinates, the registered dieticians, margarine became an instant hit.

2. In 1904, the average American consumed 5 pounds of refined sugar yearly, which equaled 1.35 teaspoons per day. As of

2004, the average American consumed 182 pounds of refined sugar yearly or 50 teaspoons per day. This is for only processed sugar not natural sugars found in our food. With an eight-ounce glass of fresh-squeezed orange juice containing equivalent to eight teaspoons of sugar, it doesn't take long to add up to pre-diabetes.

Prior to the chemical revolution of the 1940s and 1950s, we once consumed all organic fruits and vegetables, nuts, seeds, sprouts and legumes, free-range beef, pork, chicken, turkey and wild fish. We now eat mostly pesticide-sprayed, genetically engineered, irradiated, refined carbohydrates such as potato chips, french fries, bleached white bread and pasta, polished rice, sugar-coated cereals, processed ice cream, desserts, cookies, candy, chocolate, donuts, pastries, liquid-sugar sodas and commercial or farmed animal. Is there really any mystery to the cause of diabetes, let alone any disease? Consider the following *misinformation* our "doctors" are putting out:

Since the average medical doctor knows little to nothing about nutrition they depend on registered dieticians. Read what one dietician had to say about sugar in the December 2004 edition of Cooking Light: "*No body actually needs to avoid sugar, including people with chronic diseases or those trying to lose weight*," Dawn Jackson Blatner, R.D. Can you believe that? Sugar is okay, even if you're sick.

Then we have the *Institute of Medicine* stating in the same journal that they recommend each American consume 125 grams of sugar per day. That's 31.2 teaspoons daily, ten pounds of sugar per month or 120 pounds per year!

Of course, the *World Health Organization* is much more conservative. They recommend 50 grams of sugar per day or 12 teaspoons daily or a little less than 40 pounds per year! Why in the world would a known cause of diabetes, cancer and other diseases be recommended by anyone, especially these two "respected" organizations? I will answer that in Chapter 5. However, raw, organic sugar cane was consumed by the natives of Jamaica and Hawaii for centuries without ever causing tooth decay - let alone

*C*ancer and ***H***eart disease. (I wonder if that's what ***C & H*** sugar stands for?)

Unfortunately, during the processing of sugar cane, the nutrients and anti-cavity factors are destroyed. This once *food* has become another processed "drug" with devastating consequences. We not only have become accustom to the sweet taste of sugar, but it is one of the most addicting substances known. The food industry is well aware of this and hence puts it into everything they can. After all, it's good for business.

This is exactly the kind of justification my mother needed to continue her food and sugar addictions. She even sought out overweight doctors that smoked so they wouldn't condemn her for having the same addictions.

Those that typically offer *misinformation* have a vested interest in the outcome of their recommendations. If you follow the money trail, you will find the answer.

I realize I am selling this book and other information I have acquired through my years of research and experience. I also sell products I have developed. For those reasons I fall under the vested interest doctrine of caution. I'm not unlike, Jack LaLanne selling his juicer or George Foreman selling his grill or Tom Oreck selling his vacuum cleaner. For over 30 years, I have developed remedies for my patients. Using organic, whole-food extracts from the finest sources I can find, nothing comes close to the power of my products. For the first time, I am now offering these time-tested remedies to the general public.

Several years ago, I worked as a nutritional consultant for a health spa. It was more a weight-loss center. Each week I gave a seminar to a group of participants, teaching the basics of nutrition, health and longevity. I also offered computerized fat analysis. After two years of service, I was called into the owners office and notified of my termination. The reason was simple. Since I had been working, their repeat business was declining. It seemed fewer people were regaining their body fat and therefore did not need to come back.

What I taught was a different approach to eating and exercising. In my program eating was encouraged, not restricted. *What* to eat was more important than how much.

When we eat highly nutritious foods with plenty of vitamins, minerals and especially enzymes, the body easily reaches satiety. Junk and processed food keep the "I'm - hungry" signal firing until we eat so much, "bellies overlap belts."

Eating raw fruits and vegetables, nuts, seeds, sprouts and legumes provide "live" enzymes and tremendous bio-active nutrients. With any kind of increased mobility, commonly called exercise, exogenous obesity (fat), comes off with little extra effort. Adding thermogenic herbs like yarrow tea and ruling out a thyroid or adrenal imbalance, its easy to lose two pounds per week. The key is lifestyle change, not a diet. Above all, don't lament about being overweight. Stress, worry and anxiety only stimulate the need for pleasure satisfied by eating to overcome these emotions.

When I wanted to lose 10 pounds, I simply became aware of how much bread, pasta, dessert, sugar and alcohol I was consuming and then cut back by half or more. I'd like you to believe I am above reproach, but that is not the truth. I love to eat out and socialize with my friends as much as anyone.

Being Italian, I enjoy good, red wine. However, there is a difference between having a glass and a bottle, a scoop of ice cream and the full container, a piece of bread and the loaf, a couple of cookies and the entire package. Even eating all organic, we must practice moderation. Remember, balance is vital to health and longevity.

In addition, just chewing my food more thoroughly made a *significant* difference in my ability to lose weight. By slowing down, I learned to appreciate flavors and textures where before I swallowed my food to quickly. The faster you eat, the poorer your digestion will be. Poor digestion equals poor absorption. The fewer nutrients you absorb, the more food you will consume attempting to satisfy your nutritional needs.

In order to know where you want to be, you need to know where you are. There is a simple way of determining your frame size by measuring your wrist.

Assessing Frame Size from Wrist Circumference

	Small frame	Medium frame	Large frame
Adult Males	Under 6 1/4"	6 1/4 to 7"	Over 7"
Adult Females	Under 5 1/4"	5 1/4 to 6"	Over 6"

Unless you are *really* obese, 30% over your ideal weight, your wrists won't change size with weight, so their circumference is a good indicator of your natural build.

After determining your frame size, determine your optimal weight by the next chart (next page). Your *optimal* weight is at the bottom of the range. At 5'9" medium framed, my range is 148 to 160 lbs. My optimal weight should be 148, however, I feel best at around 158. Currently, I need to lose ten pounds.

Most of us sitting all day and weighing 130 to 160 lbs need 2,000 to 2,400 calories daily to maintain optimal weight. The more your optimal weight is the more calories you need to maintain it. If you are *moderately* active, you can add 20% more calories. If you are *very* active add 40%. (For more information on calories in food see *any* calorie-counting book.)

Diets never work. Let me repeat: **DIETS NEVER WORK!** The reason is simple. If you stop eating what you usually eat and then go on a diet until you lose the amount of weight you desire, then go back to eating what you did prior to, it's just a matter of time before you weigh exactly what you did. This is why people experience the up and down of gaining, losing, gaining and losing weight. If you don't change your lifestyle, nothing will ever improve. By changing your lifestyle and effectively addressing The H.O.N.S.T.E.C. components, once the weight is off, it stays off.

Remember, my mother developed obesity first. This lead to diabetes and both lead to cancer. If you are seriously overweight, perhaps you should implement an effective health and lifestyle program before it is too late. (See Chapters 4 & 6 for complete details).

This chart is a guide, not an absolute. Find out where your idea weight should be and strive to achieve it.

Height and Weight Table For Women

Height (feet/inches)	Small frame	Medium frame	Large frame
4'10"	102-111	109-121	118-131
4'11"	103-113	111-123	120-134
5'0"	104-115	113-126	122-137
5'1"	106-118	115-129	125-140
5'2"	108-121	118-132	128-143
5'3"	111-124	121-135	131-147
5'4"	114-127	124-138	134-151
5'5"	117-130	127-141	137-155
5'6"	120-133	130-144	140-159
5'7"	123-136	133-147	143-163
5'8"	126-139	136-150	146-167
5'9"	129-142	139-153	149-170
5'10"	132-145	142-156	152-173
5'11"	135-148	145-159	155-176
6'0"	138-151	148-162	158-178

Your wrist size:____ Your height: ____
Your weight range: ______to ______
Your current weight______ Amount to lose:______

Height and Weight Table For Men

Height (feet/inches)	Small frame	Medium frame	Large frame
5'2"	128-134	131-141	138-150
5'3"	130-136	133-143	140-153
5'4"	132-138	135-145	142-156
5'5"	134-140	137-148	144-160
5'6"	136-142	139-151	146-164
5'7"	138-149	142-154	149-168
5'8"	140-148	145-157	152-172
5'9"	142-151	148-160	155-176
5'10"	144-154	151-163	158-180
5'11"	146-157	154-166	161-184
6'0"	149-160	157-170	164-188
6'1'	152-164	160-174	168-192
6'2"	155-168	164-178	172-197
6'3"	158-172	167-182	176-202
6'4"	162-176	171-187	181-207

Top Twelve Dis-eases #8
Multiple Sclerosis also known as M.S.

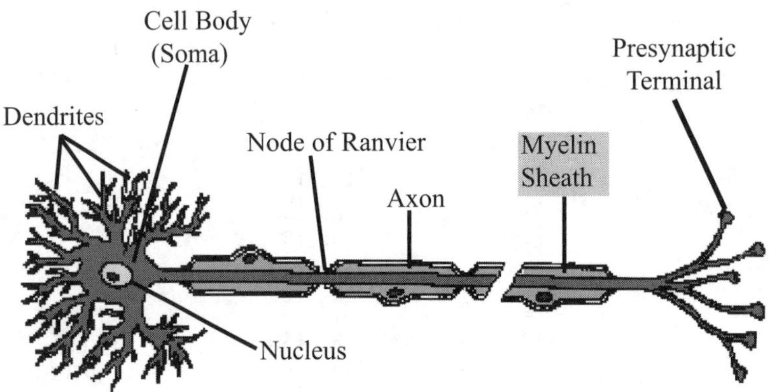

The basic unit of the nervous system is the neuron or nerve cell, which conducts an electrical impulse from one part of the body to another.

Neurons have two types of processes: axons and dendrites. An axon is a single, elongated cytoplasmic extension carrying nerve impulses *away* from the cell body. There is only one axon per neuron. Dendrites (tree-like) are processes that carry impulses *toward* the cell body.

Axons consist of four parts, one being the *myelin* sheath or covering (see above). This covering (myelin), encompasses the entire axon, except at its termination and at periodic constrictions called nodes of Ranvier. Most peripheral nerves are surrounded by a myelin sheath.

The term nerve fiber includes the axon and its myelin sheath. Larger fibers with myelin sheaths conduct impulses *faster* than smaller ones lacking the myelin sheath. There are also non-myelinated nerve fibers such as the nerve fibers in the gray matter (brain) of the central nervous system.

Multiple sclerosis is a penetrating demyelinating "disease."

The pathologic mark of this devastating disorder consists of areas of demyelination (plaques) that vary in size and location. The size and location will determine the corresponding *signs* and *signals* produced.

It is interesting to note, about two-thirds of all cases occur between ages 20 and 40 and women have a slight lead over males at 60% female, 40% male. Geographic distribution of the "disease" corresponds with higher latitudes. These high-risk areas include the northern United States, Canada, Great Britain, Scandinavia, northern Europe, New Zealand and Tasmania. People that move from a low-risk area to a high-risk area before age 15 have a high risk of developing MS. Those who make the same move after adolescence retain their low risk.

Studies have shown a strong negative association between a diet rich in animal and dairy products and the incidence of MS. Conversely, the more one consumes omega 3 oils from fish and flaxseeds, the lower the incidences of MS. *Deficiencies* of the omega 3 oils are thought to interfere with lipid elongation and permanently impair formation of normal myelin.

Early Warning Signs of Multiple Sclerosis

Type	Frequency	Symptoms
Motor	42%	Feeling of heaviness, weakness, leg dragging, stiffness, tendency to drop things, clumsiness.
Sensory	18%	Tingling, "pins and needles" sensation, numbness, dead feeling, band-like tightness, electrical sensations.
Visual	34%	Blurring, fogginess, haziness, eyeball pain, blindness, double vision.
Vestibular	7%	Light-headedness, feeling of spinning, sensation of drunkenness, nausea, vomiting.
G-urinary	4%	Incontinence, loss of bladder sensation, loss of sexual function.

In addition to taking whole-food nutraceuticals; vitamins, minerals, amino and essential fatty acids, proteolytic and digestive enzymes, antioxidants and stabilized oxygen, there are condition-specific nutrients that are helpful (see Chapter 6).

Acai is a berry that has been consumed by the aboriginals in the Brazilian Amazon rainforest for over 500 years. Prior to its discovery by western civilization, the highest rated antioxidant was the wolfberry from China with an ORAC (oxygen radical absorption capacity) rating of 875. Acai has an unbelievable ORAC rating of over 3,871!

The increased levels of lipid peroxides and other indicators of free radical damage in the central nervous system in patients with MS suggest the need for increased antioxidant support. Acai exerts positive effects on platelet function and has been shown to enhance nerve cell functions. Since it is the most powerful of all antioxidants I have ever used, I not only recommend it for MS, I recommend it for life! For more detailed information, go to their website at www.acaiforlife.com or call them at 1-714-731-0021. Mention my book and they will give you a 10% discount as a courtesy. (see Index E- *Resources* for Acai PLUS)

Top Twelve Dis-eases #9

Parkinson's - Named after an English physician, James Parkinson (1755-1824), this condition is characterized by a shaky hand palsy or tremor. There is a wide-eyed, un-blinking, staring expression with the facial muscles smoothed out and almost immobile. Saliva frequently drools from the corner of the mouth, which is usually slightly opened. The face skin is often greasy. The afflicted usually walks with slow, short, shuffling steps.

When the famous actor, Michael J. Fox first announced he had Parkinson's, the world was aghast. How could a young, vibrant man acquire this dreadful "disease?" As uncaring as this may sound, the answer is, why not? No one is immune to The H.O.N.S.T.E.C. Syndrome. Not you, nor I.

According to some of the latest "scientific" research, Parkinson's is now linked to one component of the "Syndrome," specifically toxic chemical contamination. Apparently, scientists discovered two genes that are responsible for handling protein that became mutated after the exposure to the toxic pesticide: *Rotenone*.

In addition, toxins also destroy dopamine cells. Dopamine is a neurotransmitter that carries messages from one nerve cell to another. In healthy people, it exists in balance with other neurotransmitters. In individuals with Parkinson's the area in the brain responsible for the manufacturing of serotonin, dopamine, and noradrenaline is damaged, hence the brain loses the ability to manufacture these chemicals. Loss of dopamine cells in the brain is a major *sign* of Parkinson's. Recent statistics indicate that 1 in every 200 persons over the age of sixty is affected.

Drugs for this condition have little to no effect. If the *cause* can be ascertained and the brain has not been permanently destroyed, the following condition specific nutrients and botanicals may prove to be a miracle:

1. Alpha -lipoic acid at 100 to 200 mgs, twice per day with meals.
2. Quercetin at 500 to 1,000 mgs, three times per day with meals.
3. Milk thistle in whole, organic herb form (*not* standardized) daily in a cup of red clover tea on an empty stomach.
4. Ginkgo biloba in whole organic herb form, again *not* standardized daily in a cup of red clover as above.
5. Wheat germ vitamin E at 400 IU three times per day.
6. Above-the-sea fossilized stony coral minerals minimum of 450 mgs, three times per day with or without meals.
7. CoQ10 at 120 to 240 mgs, twice per day with or without meals.

Top Twelve Dis-eases #10

Alzheimer's "Disease" (AD) - Named after a German neurologist, Alois Alzheimer (1864-1915) is a condition typically classified as presenile dementia: the deterioration of the mind's ability to relate, marked by loss of memory and cognition. Unfortunately, there has been a 1000% (ten-fold) increase in AD in this century. Even President Ronald Reagan fell victim to this horrific condition.

Without getting too technical, the brain develops plaque

and amyloid deposits. There's also a granulovascular degeneration. Amyloid is a starchy, glycoprotein. Granulo means granules of material. This basically means the brain is infiltrated with substances supposedly *causing* aberrant lesions. Since Alois Alzheimer discovered this phenomenon, it's called Alzheimer's.

As mentioned, *experimental* orthodox medicine has evolved from germs to genes. The most recent explanation for the increasing incidences of AD is blamed on genetic predisposition. However, it is interesting to consider the high rates of AD in relation to aluminum and/or silicon toxicity, environmental factors, neurotoxins, head trauma, free radicals and oxidative decompositional damage. In other words, The H.O.N.S.T.E.C. Syndrome.

As you have learned, according to the "Syndrome," chemical and/or environmental toxicities are contributing factors to dis-ease. When considering aluminum, it is best to avoid antacids, aluminum-containing antiperspirants (as a matter of fact, never use *any* antiperspirant only deodorant), cooking in aluminum pots and pans, wrapping food in aluminum foil, non-dairy creamers, baking powder and table salt. There also is a correlation between taking *calcium citrate* and an increase in aluminum absorption. Eating foods high in magnesium will prevent absorption of aluminum since magnesium competes with aluminum in the intestine and blood-brain barrier.

Taking antioxidants from Acai, CoQ-10, Quercetin, vitamin C to vitamin E, will help to neutralize free radical and oxidative decomposition damage. QCI Products makes an **Ultra C**, which is a whole food rain forest vitamin C-complex. They also make **Acai PLUS**, a whole food antioxidant complex containing CoQ-10 and Quercetin. One of the best forms of vitamin E is wheat germ and/or Kamut. There is plenty of current epidemiological evidence suggesting that antioxidant nutrients offer *significant* protection against AD.

Although thiamine or vitamin B-1, mimics acetylcholine, a very important neurotransmitter, B-complex, in general helps with brain function and health. One of the best sources of B-complex is Brewer's yeast.

Since zinc deficiency is one of the most common nutrient deficiencies in the elderly, it has been suggested that it may also be a major factor in the development of Alzheimer's "disease." In addition to taking **Coral Blend**, a fossilized stony coral mineral complex, you may want to eat organic sunflower seeds, since they are high in zinc and other nutrients.

Please remember, you do not want to take isolated vitamins and/or minerals. Although you may experience a temporary benefit from them, eventually isolated nutrients will cause an imbalance with other vital nutrients. The importance of supplementing one's organic diet with whole food nutrition can *not* be over emphasized.

Another element to consider is DHEA. DHEA is a steroid hormone secreted by the adrenals and to a lesser degree the testes and ovaries. It's levels decline dramatically with aging, actually peaking at about 25 years of age. Low levels of DHEA in the blood and brain are thought to contribute to many symptoms associated with aging. Declining levels of DHEA are also associated with diabetes, elevated cholesterol levels, obesity, heart "disease," arthritis and other age-related conditions, specifically dementias. DHEA is best taken under the supervision of your natural healing doctor. They need to monitor your levels making sure you do not overdose. However, taking 25 mgs per day, as an adult, is within a safe dose recommendation.

Finally, there is a moss that has been used in China for hundreds of years called Huperzia serrata or Huperzine A. It has been proven to be a potent inhibitor of acetyl-cholinesterase, an enzyme secreted in the body to metabolize (breakdown) acetyl-choline, a neurotransmitter.

People with Alzheimer's lose nerve cells as the "disease" progresses. By taking Huperzine A, acetyl-cholinesterase is partially blocked thereby elevating the levels of the neurotransmitter acetyl-choline, strengthening the nerve signals that remain.

As stated, "What we don't use we lose." This not only applies to muscles, but to the brain and mind, as well. A German team recently taught a group of young volunteers how to juggle. These individuals increased the size of the gray matter in specific areas of the brain over the course of their training, however the gains disappeared when they quit practicing. The key is to not give up and stay with a program that is effective.

Top Twelve Dis-eases #11

Lupus (Systemic Lupus Erythematosus)

When commenting on Lupus in 1999, one of the editors of the prestigious *Townsend Letter for Doctors & Patients*, Alan R. Gaby, M.D., said, *"The conventional view of autoimmune disease is that the immune system, for no good reason at all, goes awry and attacks the body's own tissues. But, considering the intimate connections that exist between the mind, the brain and the immune system, it might be pretentious to assume that the human system has no good reason for doing what it does. Perhaps it has a reason that we don't understand."*

I take it back. Not all medical doctors are fools. Dr. Gaby has admitted to something I very rarely hear anyone in the medical profession say, "Perhaps we don't understand?"

This touches the core of another issue I have with medics as they proclaim time and again, "There isn't anything more that can be done." Have you ever been told or know anyone that has been told that? Why can't they admit they don't *know* everything? Why can't they say, "There isn't anything more we know to do" or "There isn't anything more that can be done, that we know of."

I'll be the first to admit, I know very little. After all, anyone that only understands 10 percent of their own language is fairly ignorant, wouldn't you say? Supposedly, there are 600,000 words in the English language. A college graduate is assumed to know approximately 25,000 words. If you read as much as I do, perhaps you know 50,000 words. Even if you know 60,000 English words, you are still 90 percent ignorant of the total amount of words contained in our language. The point is, when a doctor tells a lupus patient or any other patient there isn't anything they can do or that their treatment is only for temporary relief, they have *imprinted* that patient with a deep-seated fear and hopelessness.

When I was actively seeing patients/students, my specialty was cancer and degenerative dis-eases. Every person, with *no* exception, came to me with a defeated, rejected, depressed attitude. They acquired this attitude from their medical doctor announcing a prognosis of pain, suffering and even death. Let's see how hopeless Systemic Lupus Erythematosus really is.

According to F. Batmanghelidj, M.D., in his book, *ABC of Asthma, Allergies & Lupus*, lupus is "medically" classified as a "dis-ease" of unknown etiology (no known cause). It is a chronic "disease" that involves several organ systems. It is classified as an autoimmune "dis-ease," a condition where the immune system attacks and produces a wide array of antibodies against some of the body's own tissues. Some antibodies attack the nucleus of the cell, some attack the membranes on or inside the cells; others attack the blood proteins and the structures inside the cells. The tissues most affected are the blood vessels in the kidneys, the lungs, the brain, the skin and the joints. When blood vessels are attacked, swelling, redness and even bleeding in the tissues can occur.

The diagnosis of lupus is based on clinical manifestations of any three of the following conditions, plus the appropriate blood tests confirming the dis-ease;

1. Extreme fatigue
2. Persistent headaches
3. Skin rash on the bridge of the nose and under the eyes that often looks like a "butterfly rash."

Dr. Batmanghelidj gives an excellent explanation of how lupus develops in the body. He also makes his suggestions for treating this condition, which includes drinking water with sea salt in it. This is exactly what I have suggested when I explained how to make charged distilled water using Zeta Crystals®.

Serious degenerative dis-eases call for serious remedies. In addition to my *intensive* protocol in Chapter 6, concentrated whole-food nutraceuticals, essential fatty acids, amino acids, green vegetables, fruits and copious amounts of the right water are critical for the lupus patient.

Lupus and other immune-compromised dis-eases, produce huge amounts of free radicals. As free radicals bombard the DNA, they cause the long strands of DNA to break. The more free radicals you produce, the greater the likelihood will be that you will eventually develop lupus or one of the other Top Twelve Dis-eases.

One of the most important systems neutralizing free radicals, thereby preventing DNA damage, involves cellular antioxidant enzymes and proteins. Glutathione is a special molecule found in every cell. L-cysteine, an amino acid found in high levels in garlic, increases the level of glutathione in the cells. You can either supplement your diet with glutathione products or eat organic garlic every day. I prefer non-dairy supplements. In addition, Alpha lipoic acid is not only a powerful antioxidant, it dramatically increases cellular glutathione. However, nothing is a more powerful antioxidant than Acai from Brazil.

Normally, our cell's DNA is exposed to 10,000 free radical impacts per cell every day. With a progressive dis-ease this can increase to 100,000 impacts per cell every day.

The H.O.N.S.T.E.C. components, including lack of hydration, toxic chemicals to emotional stress, all contribute to free radical damage. The good news is that we can do something about it.

Even though free radicals constantly attack our cells damaging the DNA, we have many antioxidant enzymes repairing up to 98 percent of the damage. Unfortunately, it is the 2 percent remaining that cause most of our genetic mutation problems.

As we age, these repairing antioxidant enzymes become less efficient. This is one reason why degenerative dis-eases such as lupus and cancer develop more in the elderly. The following ingredients improve the repair process:

1. Eat all organic food.
2. Take whole-food nutraceuticals: QCI's LifePack®

Part of QCI LifePack:

3. Acai - take two capsules three times per day with or with out meals.
4. L-carnitine found in Super Kamut
5. Zinc found in fossilized stony Coral Blend
6. B6 and B12 found in Super Kamut
7. Folate and niacin found in Super Kamut.

It is of special importance to avoid all red meat whether organic, free-range or not. Beef contains a large amount of iron, 60 to 70 percent of which is absorbable "free iron." Free iron is a very powerful generator of free radicals and lipid (fat) peroxidation.

Although broccoli and spinach contain as much iron as a comparable amount of beef, only a small amount of iron is absorbed from vegetables. By avoiding all those things known to make us ill and doing what is known to heal us, we can overcome lupus (See complete protocol in Chapter 6).

Top Twelve Dis-eases #12
Chronic Fatigue Syndrome (CFS)

I mentioned in Chapter 1 how my father used to beat me when I was a child and teenager. For many years, I had difficulty breathing from damage caused to my nose. In 1993, I decided to have nasal surgery to correct some of the damage. What was supposed to be a forty-five minute "piece of cake" surgery, turned out to be a five-and-a-half-hour nightmare. Upon awakening, I was told that I may experience a liver and/or kidney problem "for awhile," since I was under anesthesia "a little too long."

I came out of the hospital with an Epstein Barr virus infection, a compromised right kidney and a highly toxic liver. Within a few weeks, I had what was medically called Myalgic Encephalomyelitis (ME) or Chronic Fatigue Syndrome (CFS).

Besides being constantly tired, I literally had difficulty getting out of bed. I had "brain fog," loss of memory, depression, irritability, flu-like symptoms, insomnia, blurred vision and extreme allergies to everything tested. But at least I could breathe.

Like my mother, I surrendered to my doctors. I was a *zombie* acting like one. I had every conceivable test performed to rule out all known dis-eases. From an MRI, CAT scan, EMI, cardiovascular tread mill, blood tests to AIDS evaluation, there was not a sacred place left on my body. After weeks of being "medicalized," I final received a diagnosis: I had Chronic Fatigue Syndrome, plain and simple.

It seems that when you *can't* think, is when you *need* to the most. I was on a sabbatical from my clinical work at the time, so I wasn't required to think at that level of intensity. However, I became a guinea pig for *experimental* orthodox medicine.

There isn't a symptom known that they haven't created a drug to treat it. The first drug I left the hospital with was for pain. It in itself put me into a drug stupor. Next, was an all-powerful anti-biotic. Of course, this caused an intestinal yeast infection, so I was given Nystatin. Eventually, all I remember was sitting around the house, drooling on myself and going to an allergist every week for shots.

"But Dr. Chappell, I thought only sick people got sick? What about The H.O.N.S.T.E.C. Syndrome?"

What happened to me clearly demonstrates both The H.O.N.S.T.E.C. Syndrome and only sick people getting sick.

If you recall, T in H.O.N.S.T.E.C. stands for toxic chemicals. The toxic drugs they used in the hospital were designed for an hour operation, not a five-and-a-half. I was immediately given drugs to prevent bacterial infection and a couple for pain.

Pain medication not only effects your sensory nervous system, it effects your motor nerves as well, specifically the peristaltic action of the colon. The net result from taking pain pills is not only constipation, but toxemia. If you shut down one of the most important elimination channels you have, the body will reabsorb the toxins. This is called automatic intoxication or autointoxication.

This brings up another issue concerning pain medication and toxemia.

Although most of my cancer patients had chemotherapy, radiation and surgery and then were told, "There isn't anything more that can be done. You have six months to live," every once and a while I would see someone with less expected time.

I had an occasion to see a man that had only days left on his pre-ordained sentence. Using everything I knew to do, he seemed to be doing better. His appetite was returning, his weight was improving and his energy was increasing. However, on the seventh day, his cancer ate through his carotid artery and he hemorrhaged. He was rushed to the hospital for emergency surgery and the bleeding was stopped.

While in the hospital the doctors told his wife they could help him rest a little easier with a stronger dose of morphine. He was in pain, not only from the cancer, but from the surgery, so on the surface it made sense. But something didn't feel right to my patient and in his stupor, he asked me to get him out of there. The doctors refused to let him go. I told them he wanted out and I would help him. As we were attempting to leave, hospital security was called and I was detained and removed from the hospital.

I'll never forget his screams begging me to help. He was dragged back to his room, strapped to his bed and injected with morphine. Within 24 hours, he was dead.

Pain medication, especially morphine is often used to "keep the patient comfortable." I am not against comfort: I am against unauthorized euthanasia. When in the hospital, Caveat Emptor.

Everything that happened to me when I had my surgery, fell under The H.O.N.S.T.E.C. Syndrome. I not only had my immune system suppressed, I was infected with bacteria, viruses and other pathogens. It made me sick; therefore I became sick.

I couldn't think properly. I knew what needed to be done, but just like my patients, I was in a drug stupor. I simply allowed the medics free rein.

Once I came to my senses, I immediately detoxified my liver. This cleared up 99 percent of my allergies. The liver humanizes or de-humanizes every molecule entering the body.

If the liver has been compromised for any reason, it can attach a de-humanizing signature on everything. From celery to fish, sprouts to tap water, all allergies involve the liver. The first step to improving your allergic reaction to your environment and food, is to detoxify your liver.

I then followed my own protocol in Chapter 6. If you have so-called "Chronic Fatigue," stay away from toxic drugs and start a natural healing program to bring you back to life. It will work!

Conditions That *Can* Become Dis-eases

Hair

I remember when being bald was "not beautiful." Hollywood and the music industry now have celebrities with shaved heads making it popular, but there is a difference between a shaved head of hair and no hair.

I started losing my hair around twenty-one years old. Because of the way I lost my hair, they call it male pattern baldness. Although there are many factors involved, the most widely used explanation is a testosterone imbalance or genetic predisposition. That's why bald men say they are better lovers; they have raging male hormones.

I not sure if bald men are better lovers or not, I personally don't care, however, male pattern baldness is a contributing factor to one losing their hair.

Stress or the way we handle it, is also a contributing factor. Anything that can cause a vaso-constriction - reduced blood supply, which stress will do, will cause malnutrition. Since blood transports nutrients it's easy to see why malnutrition is a consequence of vaso-constriction.

Exercise is one way we move body fluids. It stimulates the blood and lymphatic circulation. It detoxifies the body through perspiration. Lack of exercise will cause toxemia, fluid stagnation and contribute to baldness.

The main cause of baldness, for men or women, will be a

combination of these factors. However, the most common cause not readily discussed is poor nutrition. If we are not eating and absorbing the nutrients we need for optimum health, including our hair, we will lose it.

The analogy I like to use is that of growing corn. Both hair and corn need a substance to grow from. The corn needs the earth and hair needs the scalp. Both have a bulb or root system. The hair is nourished by the blood vessels in the subcutaneous tissues just as corn draws its nourishment from the soil.

The average man has about 150,000 hairs on his head, each one of which grows up through the skin from its own follicle and lives from 3 to 6 years before falling out. A new hair should grow to take the place of the one that has "died," but if the follicle is not healthy and properly supplied with blood and nutrients, this does not occur, the hairs are not replaced and baldness is the result.

Applying creams and lotions, ointments and salves will do very little to get to the cause of the problem. I suppose if I really cared about my baldness, I would do something about it. I know I am under more stress than most, yet I handle it fairly well. I know I do not exercise enough and my diet could be better. I also have high testosterone, which I always thought was an Italian trait. Perhaps someday, I may write a book on how to re-grow hair. However, I will have to prove it can be done on me first.

Skin

The next body part to consider is the skin. The skin is the external manifestation of an internal balance, imbalance or condition. It is the largest detoxifying gland in the body. It can also be directly damaged by the sun if not taken care of properly, especially if you consume hydrogenated oils.

Our skin reflects the state of our physical, mental, emotional and even spiritual health. From nervousness, allergies, bacterial infections to dietary factors, if you consider The H.O.N.S.T.E.C. Syndrome, you will find the *cause*.

Growing up in southern California, I lived and live by the ocean. As a child and teenager, I spent a considerable amount of time in the sun at the beach. I loved to body and board surf. I never used sun screen and I always burned to the point of my skin becoming red, swollen, peeling and extremely painful. Sunburning is damaging enough at any age, but especially during our formative years.

At the same time I was destroying my skin, I had a terrible diet. Like my mother, I loved sugar. I ate candy and chocolate all day long. My mother never complained because she was the one supplying my habit. We would sit together and eat a whole box of See's chocolate covered cherries in one day. Suffice it to say, I ate a lot of hydrogenated fats and oils.

Although there are many contributing factors to healthy or unhealthy skin, diet plays the most important part. Because of my ignorance, I have unhealthy skin. However, through attending to it, I should be able to improve it. Remember, love and attention is a key to health and longevity.

If you go out in the sun for a *reasonable* length of time, you will *not* need sun screen. You want the healing rays of the sun to touch your skin. Suntanning converts subdermal (below) cholesterol into vitamin D. Since our diets are low in vitamin D, we need the sun to supply it. However, DO NOT SUN BURN!

Do not eat hydrogenated fats and oils. Read the label on your packaged and processed food. Matter of fact, don't eat packaged or processed foods. Also don't eat at fast-food restaurants. They all use trans fats: hydrogenated fats and oils. Protect your skin and it will protect you.

In addition to eating healthy and being careful in the sun, we should avoid toxic chemicals. As discussed under **'T'** in The H.O.N.S.T.E.C. Syndrome, toxic chemicals can cause terrible, irreversible skin damage. Because these poisons usually take years to show signs of toxicity, our government allows them to be sold and used. See the last page in this chapter for what can happen in just a *few* months after exposure to the most dangerous toxin known: dioxin.

Eyes

It has been said, "The eyes are the windows to the soul." I'm not sure if that's true, but it sounds good to me.

About 2,500 years ago, The Nez Perse tribe of Native Americans developed a system to identify ailments by looking into the sclera or whites of the eyes. On the other side of the world, the Chinese were developing the same diagnostic approach at the same time. The modern form of this art was first called Sclerology, by Dr. Stuart Wheelwright.

Dr. Wheelwright spent 25 years studying with the Nez Perse, reading over 80,000 people and noting similarities among those exhibiting the same health problems. Before his death in 1990, he passed the torch to Dr. Jack Tips, the current president of the *International Sclerology Institute:* www.sclerologyinstitute.org.

Dr. Wheelwright's research revealed that every major organ and gland corresponds to a particular area of the eye. By observing the length and shape of the blood vessels, he could accurately determine the sources and types of stressors affecting each patient's health. He then recommended changes in lifestyle, diet and exercise and encouraged specific herbs to help the patient heal themselves.

Within the sclera is the iris, the colored portion of the eye. In 1904, Dr. Henry Lane published a book entitled, *The Diagnosis from the Eye* which established a correlation between patterns found in the iris and specific dis-eases or conditions. He literally mapped out a topography chart showing the entire body. He called this system of visual interpretation Iridology.

Studying Dr. Lane's work, in 1919, Dr. J. Haskel Kritzer, published his version of an iris chart or map enhancing even more referenced areas, including the brain.

Dr. Bernard Jensen, a mentor of mine, met Dr. Kritzer in the 1930s. Through his studies and experiences during his practice of Iridiology, Dr. Jensen developed his own iris topography chart. The first version was copyrighted in 1948. He eventually wrote a definitive textbook entitled, *Iridology - The Science and Practice in the Healing Arts*. It was published in 1982 and represents over 50 years of work in Iridology and natural healing.

Before his death in 2001 at 93, Dr. Jensen passed the torch to David J. Pesek, Ph.D. Dr. Pesek teaches Holistic Iridology courses worldwide and has furthered the research and art of Iridology to even a higher level of understanding and interpretation, especially in the brain areas of thought and emotion on conscious and subconscious levels. Dr. Pesek is not only the president of the *International Institute of Iridology*, he is the president of the *American College of Iridology.* He may be reached at 1-866-456-6100. Go to Chapter 8 to see a chart of the eyes as developed by Dr. Pesek and his story.

Ears

There are 28 million people *legally* deaf or severely hearing impaired in the United States. [I suppose that means there are others *illegally* deaf?] There are over 250 million people in the world that fall under this category, half of which are classified as *preventable*. The most effective nutrients to prevent deafness are vitamins A and B complex.

Heredity is often blamed for deafness of certain types. We call it genetic predisposition, however, our ancestors are only responsible for our *susceptibility*, not for the dis-ease itself.

As the spinal-neurological chart demonstrates on page 49 above, the first and second cervical vertebra and corresponding nerves have a direct and indirect influence on hearing. Historically, it was for this very reason, chiropractic was introduced to the world.

Sometime around 1895, Dr. D. D. Palmer made a spinal "adjustment" to a deaf man named Harvey Lillard. From that one treatment, Mr. Lillard regained his hearing and Dr. Palmer started the philosophy, science and art of what is called chiropractic.

From acupuncture, chiropractic, naturopathic to effective massage and diet, when your orthodox medical doctor says there isn't anything more that can be done about your deafness or hearing loss other than a hearing aide, think twice.

Teeth

There is a real dividing line in dentistry today. Some dentists believe that cavities are caused by bacteria eating away at the enamel while others believe it is because of poor nutrition. It could be both, however, something doesn't make sense to me. If bacteria can eat away at our dental enamel, why is it when we die and are buried, the body is literally decomposed by bacteria except for the bones and teeth? If bacteria were responsible for cavities, then a corpse would continue to get cavities.

Although bacteria are found in the mouth and serve a purpose, Dr. George Meinig in his book, *New Trition*, clearly demonstrates how teeth develop cavities from the inside out. If we eat processed junk "food" and a high sugar diet, our blood pH changes to acid. These acids de-mineralize our tooth enamel making it susceptible to oxidative damage and decay.

In his classic work, *Nutrition and Physical Degeneration* published in 1939, Weston A. Price, M.S., D.D.S., F.A.C.D. traveled all over the world studying the diets and teeth of primitive people. The net result was always the same. A good natural diet meant good teeth; processed and devitalized foods *always* produced a high incidence of dental caries.

Some of the elements needed for sound teeth are absorbable calcium, phosphorus, magnesium, iodine and vitamins A, C and D. That is not to say we need to take isolated nutrients. What we need to do is stop eating junk food and start eating good food. To ensure we have all the nutrients we require, we should only consume organic whole-food nutritional supplements.

Do not brush your teeth with any toothpaste containing fluoride. It is a toxic poison. Just because it doesn't kill you immediately, does *not* negate its long-term effects. See Index *E-Resources* for more information.

Nails

Our nails contain carbon, hydrogen, nitrogen, sulphur, cystine, histidine, lysine, arginine, fat, sodium, calcium, potassium, magnesium and iron. The last five minerals are in the form of chlorides, sulfates, phosphates and carbonates.

White spots, ridges, brittleness and other nail abnormalities are all indications of a nutritional or hormonal imbalance and/or toxins. Painting over your nails with colorful polish and/or applying acrylic "false" nails does nothing to get to the cause of one's problem, if fact, acrylic nails can cause a fungal infection that will permanently destroy them.

As with the hair and skin, topical applications cover up *signs* and *signals* of internal challenges. To find a *cure*, always get to the *cause*.

Summation and New Remedy Book

Whether you have one of the above "diseases" or another named condition, you should know by now, the body will always show a *sign* or *signal* before the symptom of a "disease" develops. We simply need to learn how to read the body's messages.

There are two distinctive approaches to health or the lack of it. Natural healing uses non-toxic methods, *Experimental* orthodox medical treatment does not. Natural healing works *with* the body, attempting to get to the *cause* of a problem. *Experimental* orthodox medicine treats *symptoms*, not seeking the *cause*. Natural healers teach people how to heal themselves. *Experimental* orthodox medicine creates dependency through drug addictions.

In my next book entitled, *The Chappell Remedy Handbook,* I will cover every significant condition, "disease" and dis-ease I know, including a natural healing remedy for each. From infected toenails, to malaria, if it's out there, I'll have it in my book.

For the "baby boomers," now in their late 50's and early 60's, I will devote an entire chapter on how to *slow down* the aging process. **There is no such thing as anti-aging,** it's a slogan made up by public relation firms to sell products. Aging is part of life. Even if we live 4,000 years, we still age. However, we may be able to *slow down* this process, thereby looking and feeling in our twenties and thirties, when we are actually sixty and seventy years old.

[I wish my mother had experienced this kind of Love. I have always said, it is better to come *from* a broken home than to *live* in one. Seek Love and you will find it. It's worth the effort.]

Complete At Last

by

Eric C Wyndham

Before I was born, I remember being with the Source of all life, the Creator and Grand Architect of the Universe.

We sat for hours, playing and laughing the Great Mystery and I, loving and sharing, while I was learning, growing and understanding the importance of knowledge, wisdom, peace, justice, kindness, forgiveness and Love.

It wasn't too long before another guide, another angel, came to spend time in the presence of Enlightenment. Soon, my angel and I became one with and in Love. In time, God asked us what we wanted to do. In unison, we said, "To teach others the way of Truth like the Masters before us." We told God, we wanted to be humans.

She warned us that in so doing, we would temporarily forget our origin, our divinity and our true relationship with Him and each other. She said He would never leave us, for He would always be there to guide us back. After much thought, we held a final embrace and slowly transformed from our translucent blue figures to that which could be seen in this place called Earth.

As cautioned we lost our memory. We lived as humans experiencing pain and suffering, disappointment and ridicule. We went from dysfunctional families to relationships that became toxic, almost destroying our will, our life. Yet all the while, we still believed in a Sustainer we couldn't quite remember.

After years of service to humanity, teaching Love by example, I finally re-discovered my Heavenly partner, my beloved angel and that angel is you. I now remember what once was and what should be for I have re-discovered my own divinity.

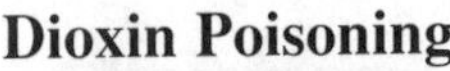

Dioxin Poisoning

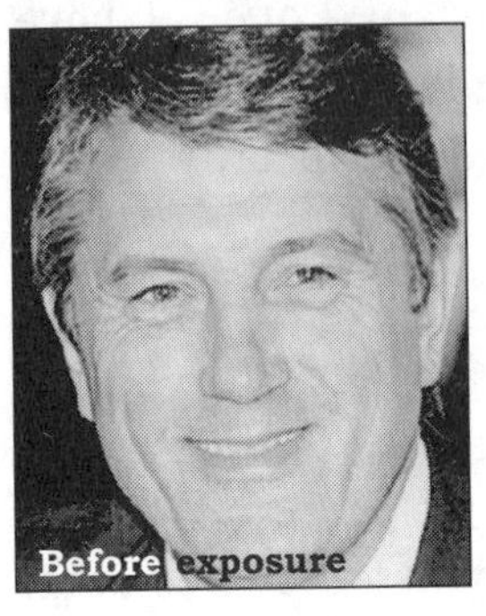

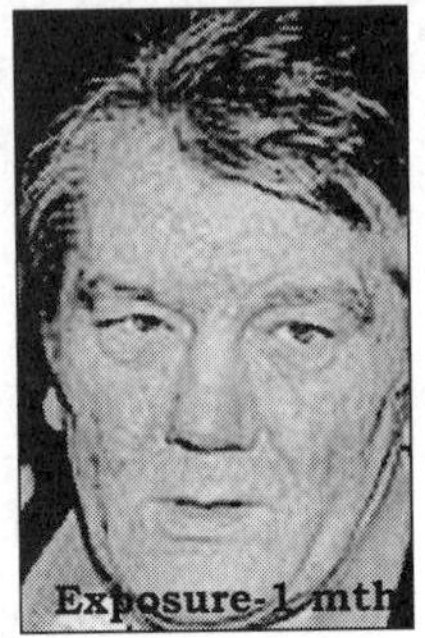

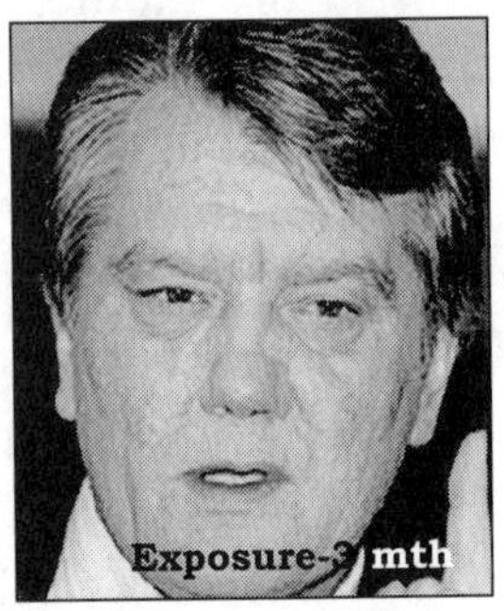

Viktor Yushchenko, the newly elected president of Ukraine, was *poisoned* during his campaign. He went from looking healthy on the left, to his current condition on the right within three months of ingesting dioxin at a dinner party.

Dioxin, T-2 or "Yellow Rain" is similar to Agent Orange, the toxin the United States sprayed on the Vietnamese people in the Viet Nam conflict back in the 1960s. The first sign of dioxin poisoning is skin damage.

According to our EPA, **"There is no safe level of dioxin."** It is found throughout the United States population at levels causing a variety of unacceptable adverse health effects.

Hundreds of chemical compounds can be denigrated to a dioxin or furan. The most toxic of all is TCDD and PCBs. Both are by-products of chlorine waste and PVC pipe incineration, pesticide manufacturing, pulp and paper bleaching.

Dioxins damage the immune system, skin and hormonal systems. They cause cancer, diabetes and lung dis-eases. They are fat-soluble and are mainly found in beef, diary, milk, chicken, pork, fish and eggs. Dioxins are bio-accumulative; they climb up the food chain in higher and higher concentrations.

Is it possible that "normal" aging with puffy eyes, rough skin and a bulbous nose is merely a *sign* or *signal* of subtle, toxic chemical poisoning or accumulation? It does *not* have to be dioxin. We have over 100,000 toxic chemicals currently *approved* for use in the United States. Take your pick.

Dis-ease is defined as lack of ease or harmony, it is NOT the same as "disease," a medical term for illness treated by medicine. *NEVER* attempt to stop or reduce your medication without the supervision of your medical doctor.

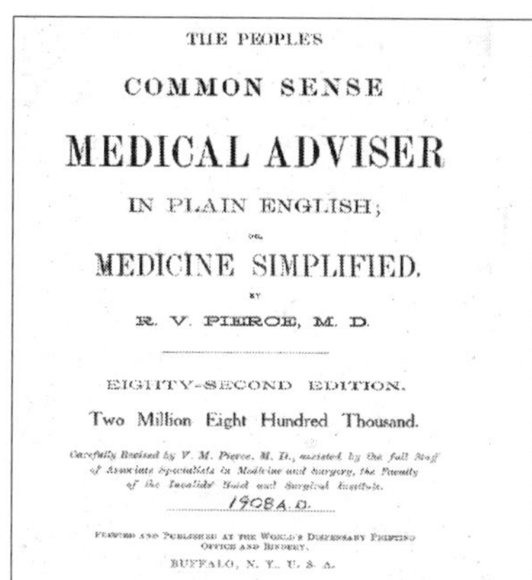

THE PEOPLE'S

COMMON SENSE

MEDICAL ADVISER

IN PLAIN ENGLISH;

OR,

MEDICINE SIMPLIFIED.

BY

R. V. PIERCE, M. D.

EIGHTY-SECOND EDITION.

Two Million Eight Hundred Thousand.

Carefully Revised by V. M. Pierce, M. D., assisted by the full Staff of Associate Specialists in Medicine and Surgery, the Faculty of the Invalids' Hotel and Surgical Institute.

1908 A.D.

Printed and Published at the World's Dispensary Printing Office and Bindery.

BUFFALO, N. Y., U. S. A.

CHAPTER 4 - *CURING* DIS-EASE WITH FOOD, HERBS, SUPPLEMENTS, EXERCISE, ELECTRONIC FREQUENCY DEVICES, THERAPY & MORE

"Every family needs a Common Sense Medical Advisor. It is in the interest and welfare of every person, not only to understand the means of preservation of health, but also to know what remedies should be employed for the alleviation of the common aliments of life." ***- Dr. R.V. Pierce, author of The People's Common Sense Medical Adviser (82nd edition-1908 A.D.).***

Dr. Pierce not only authored the above 82nd edition of his famous *Medical Advisor*, he was the medical director of *The Invalid's Hotel and Surgical Institute* and proprietor of the *World's Dispensary* in Buffalo, New York, both established in the mid 1800's. By 1908, he had sold the unheard of number of over *Two Million Eight Hundred Thousand* copies of his book. That's 2,800,000 copies! I am thankful to have one of the few remaining manuscripts of his most informative work.

I am consistently struck by the common sense and logic approach taken by pioneers of medicine. Seen today by our orthodox medical doctors as ridiculous, antiquated medical treatment, natural healers and even medical mavericks were *curing* dis-eases on a regular basis using detoxification, diet, herbs, rest, exercise, recreation, sun and water therapy.

Food

Let's start with food. Have you ever wondered why you eat? I mean, what is the real purpose of consuming food?

Fruits, vegetables, nuts, seeds, sprouts, legumes, dairy, grains, animal protein, oils, fats and everything in-between represent nutrients; water, light (chlorophyll), oxygen, vitamins, minerals, enzymes, amino and fatty acids, antioxidants, fiber and much, much more. It's simple. We normally eat to acquire nutrients as they are used to grow, heal and repair the body. We also convert these nutrients into energy to live and function optimally. Or do we?

We no longer eat to sustain life; we eat out of impulse driven by a suppressed appetite center and undernourishment.

Overfed and Undernourished

In addition to *normal* eating, one reason why Americans tend to eat beyond normal is because our food has become devitalized; the nutrients are not present in abundance and therefore our bodies keep signaling us to eat more.

Another reason we eat so much is because we are addicted to the drugs (chemicals) food processors put in the food to make it look, taste, smell or feel "better." In reality, chemical additives only serve to either extend the shelf life of the devitalized "Frankenfood" or excite one's numbed taste buds with salt, sugar or other harmful addictive substances such as MSG. After all, it's easier to sell and continue to sell a "food" item if the consumer is addicted to it.

We are also addicted to the oral gratification and satisfaction we receive by eating. It seems when things are not going the way we would like them to go, whether in our personal or business life, many find eating to be one way of forgetting their problems. Simply, stress can cause one to eat more. The more stress, the more we eat.

Still another reason we eat is to socialize and entertain. Every other commercial on television seems to wet our appetite and seduce us into eating more. We are compelled to live to eat, instead of eating to live.

Soil

Long ago before the industrial revolution in which modern civilization started using toxic chemicals and burning fossil fuels, oil and kerosene our air, water and food was pristine. The 'People of the Earth' knew how to live off the land. They knew what wild plants, roots and berries to eat and how to grow them. They knew how to rotate their crops and when to allow the land to rest. They only ate foods in season for they had no other choice. They knew how to combine their foods that ensured their health and survival.

The topsoil was alive and well. That is to say, it was full of nutrients, micro organisms and minerals. Food grown in this soil was equally alive and well. It was truly nutritious. 'People of the Earth' lived comparatively long and healthy lives. At least until modern civilization came to "help."

The Key

The healthiest people on the planet today all have one thing in common: they eat all natural, whole, live, organic and mostly raw food. They drink water that is not contaminated with chlorine, fluoride and other chemicals, yet is full of complex minerals. They have no *experimental* orthodox medical treatment: modern drugs, doctors or their procedures. Because they don't have automobiles and a "modern" industry that fills the air with hydro-carbonic acid, being out in the air everyday is healthy. They also feel the rays of the sun energizing their cells, knowing that it is healing.

It doesn't matter if these people eat mostly dairy, vegetables, fruit or animal, they do NOT live to eat. They eat to live. They eat only small amounts of food and only a few items at a time. They wear only natural fiber clothes and live in non-toxic shelters. From the jungle, desert, plains or mountains, these people have virtually NO stress as we know it. They have no bills, taxes or an oppressive government. There is no television, radio, newspapers or any vested interest media. They have a reverence for life and God or The Great Mystery. They live with nature, not against it. They love their family and friends and know their divine purpose. What an antithesis we are.

Devitalized Soil

Where once we tilled the land with wooden blades behind an ox or horse, we switched to steel and diesel-powered machines. Not knowing steel causes a different electrical charge to the earth and the food planted therein, we ignorantly continued. Instead of turning under the spent crops, we burned them, not realizing the value in the fiber and remaining nutrients and minerals, notwithstanding the mineralized ash. Instead of rotating the crops, giving the land a chance to recover from the last harvest or better yet, not planting at all in the seventh year, we kept and keep working the land without reprieve, further depleting it of nutrients and life force energy.

It is not just the rain and weather causing a run off of our top soil and subsequent minerals that have devitalized our food, but poor farming practices and management, in addition to our food-destroying preparation habits. Regardless, if our genetically engineered seeds, preservative, pesticides, insecticides and "Round Up Ready" crops are not toxic enough, even organically grown food eaten whole, raw and fresh, is now devitalized because of the soil, and therefore we simply don't have the nutrients in our food anymore. If it is not in the soil, it will not be in the food and will not nurture us.

So what is the answer? We need to either fully re-mineralize our soil and/or supplement our diet with whole-food nutrition. But not just any "formulae" will do, for there is a difference between isolated, chemist-formulated nutrients and natural whole-food nutrition. I am not talking about synthetic, dead, man-made nutrients verses natural living products. I am talking about formulated verses non-formulated. Perhaps we should learn those differences before gobbling up handfuls of so-called "supplements."

Isolated Vs Whole-Food Supplements

All naturally found nutrients have balancing, adaptogenic capabilities. All nutrients co-exist synergistic and antagonistically. Not unlike the plants and animals in a rainforest, desert or ocean, everything in nature finds a way to harmonize in relationship. Except of course if you work against nature, as with taking synthetic nutrients or so-called "natural" nutrients in an allopathic (symptom-treating) isolated application.

Let's say you are tired more than not and you have been told you have a B-12 or cyanocobalamin deficiency. If you go to a medical doctor and they "believe" in natural medicine, they may want to give you a B-12 shot. If you go to a naturopathic or chiropractic doctor, they most likely will give you a B-12 pill. So what's the difference? Unfortunately, taking an isolated nutrient like B-12, even a natural one, will eventually cause the other B Complex nutrients to lose their harmonizing balance with each other. In other words, too much B-12 can cause deficiencies in the other B's. And so it is with all nutrients, including vitamins, minerals, enzymes, amino and fatty acids.

The key to optimum health and longevity is not taking a basket full of food supplements. The answer is intelligently supplementing your modern-day nutrient deficient diet with whole-food nutritional supplementation; nutraceuticals. However, before you spend another penny, perhaps you should know what constitutes a nutrient.

Nutrients

By definition, a vitamin is an organic food substance. They exist in foods in minute quantities and are absolutely necessary for proper growth and the maintenance of health. They regulate metabolism and assist in the biochemical processes that release energy from digested food. Vitamins are either water-soluble or oil-soluble. Water-soluble vitamins must be consumed daily, as they cannot be stored and are excreted within four to twenty-four hours. These include vitamin C and the B-complex vitamins. Oil-soluble vitamins can be stored for longer periods of time in the body's fatty tissue and the liver. These include vitamins A, D, E and K. Both types of vitamins are needed by the body for proper functioning. Of all the vitamins, vitamin C seems to be the most easily destroyed nutrient and according to Drs. Linus Pauling and

Ewan Cameron, must be specifically added to the diet at doses large enough to be of value.

There are 18 major vitamins. For sake of space, the following will give you a basic understanding of at least 9 of them. Remember, isolated vitamins are typically used as drugs for a specific effect. They are primarily manufactured by a formulating chemist using hydrocarbon intermediates. They can technically be called "natural," since they can be said to be derived from "natural sources." But their isolated state is not at all the same as their "natural form" as found in real food. Do not take an isolated nutrient unless you are under the care of a knowledgeable whole food nutritionist, healer, doctor - or you know what you are doing.

As reported by LifeStar research, "Nutrients in food are never in a free-form." This means they do not exist in food as isolates. They are in a relationship. Food contains water and/or fat-soluble nutrients bound into a matrix of highly complex interlocking systems of proteins, carbohydrates, lipids, enzymes, co-enzymes, nucleic acids and countless other naturally occurring elements.

Scientific evidence strongly suggests that *proteins* are the transport mechanisms for nutrients in all known living systems. Plants only contain nutrients molecularly bound into relationships. Nature designed the human body to use vitamins and minerals the way they exist in plants. In that design, vitamins and minerals are always bound to soluble proteins, found or associated with carbohydrates, lipids and other naturally occurring constituents. This is not just a blend of isolates; it is a holistic relationship using whole food complexes. This delicate integration is usually compromised or destroyed in food processing.

Although oxygen and water are vital nutrients, light is often overlooked. Without the sun, most everything dies. Assuming one has plenty of all three, the following are considered essential nutrients:

Herbs

As we know, the Father of Medicine, Hippocrates, never used a toxic chemical or drug. He was an herbalist. He was the one credited with saying physicians should "first, do no harm." The only primary care *physicians* currently adhering to the dictates of Hippocrates are the natural healers such as chiropractors and *traditional* naturopaths. The others have forgotten their roots.

Herbal healing was the first system of healing in the world. It dates back to the beginning of time. From the Bible to ancient Chinese texts, herbs have always been used as remedies.

When I started my natural healing career, most of the herbs available were organic or wild harvested. They were picked at the proper times, dried or used fresh in compounds or tinctures (liquid extracts). Today, we have commercial growers and even pharmaceutical companies in the herb business. They are not concerned with quality, rather production and profit. Their herbs are no longer empowered with nutrients, alkaloids and healing properties. They may look like an herb, taste like one and smell like one, but that is as far as it goes.

To make an herbal tincture you need to let it brew for at least 30 days before pressing it, like a fine wine, herbs must be "cured," turned and attended to, before bottling. Commercial manufactures often do a *quick* brew of three to four days. This does not allow the herb enough time to be effective. It may look like an herb in a bottle and the label may say it is, but it is useless. You can take this colored water all you want, but it has little to no value.

In the 1800s, most pioneer families knew about herbs and their healing properties. After all, they lived in the plains and mountains far away from civilization. They learned about herbology from their parents, grandparents or the local natives. If they didn't know how to heal themselves, they died.

Living off the land meant they had to learn about the land, water, weather and techniques of proper sustainable farming. There were no magic chemicals to fool nature. You either knew what you were doing or you perished. Period.

Learning from Cuba and Castro

When the United States placed an embargo on Cuba in 1961, including sanctions against sending food or medicines, President Fidel Castro simply instructed Cuban doctors to learn alternative methods of medicine. Prevention became the only affordable means of keeping its population healthy. This is an interesting paradox. What was intended to be a punishment by the United States government, has turn out to be a blessing in the long run. I am not saying the Cuban people are not suffering, however, they are learning how to be *independent* of drug and sickness-based medicine. We should be so lucky.

In 1961, President Castro and the Cuban government decreed that all healthcare would be paid for by the government. Cuba, despite the ongoing U.S. embargo, which negatively affected Cuba's economy, has one of the best healthcare systems in the world. All Cubans receive free medical care. All areas of Cuba, whether urban or rural, have doctors. The government built clinics in rural areas that previously had none, and requires graduates of medical schools to provide a minimum of two years of healthcare service in these areas.

Healthcare for every citizen has been a top priority of President Castro, second only to education. The system emphasizes prevention, health education and community medicine.

Cuba's national public health system has gained an international reputation as a long-standing model for scientific research, development and health improvement. It has high health indicators such as a 6.3% infant mortality per 1,000 as compared to a 7.0% in the United States and a 32.0% in Latin America.

Medical grade ozone therapy is used in every hospital along with what the Cubans call traditional green medicine. Organic gardens are near every hospital providing food for the patients, doctors and staff. Synthetic, toxic fertilizers cost money the Cuban people can't afford. We should have such a problem.

Cuba is currently heavily investing in organic agriculture and in alternative medicine. Recently, Cuba bought two million bicycles, which are now a primary form of personal and business transportation. This was necessary due to the blockade, which decreases the petroleum and other raw materials getting to Cuba.

This may be one reason why the United States is really putting on the pressure. Cuba is showing the world, we do not have to depend on oil, gasoline, pesticides, insecticides, drugs and expensive medical procedures to function and live healthy.

Because animal protein and processed junk food is scarce, Cuba's cancer rate has dropped and so has their obesity and other degenerative dis-eases. People eat primarily beans, rice, potatoes, bread, eggs and occasionally chicken. They also love their herbs.

What are herbs and how do they work?

There are four basic classifications of herbs. For purposes of nutritional and herbal healing, only the first three categories are used.

1. Pot herbs - Also known as vegetables, have low toxicity at 1% with .5% buffers and low therapeutic effects. Pot herbs have 2% tonic nutrients, 1.5% fiber and 95% food nutrient activity.

2. Tonic herbs - From Iris moss, dandelion, parsley, kelp and many herbal teas, they have 8% toxic properties with 7% buffers. Tonic herbs have 24% tonic nutrients, 1% fiber and 60% food nutrient activity.

3. Therapeutic herbs - As the body adapts to the toxic properties of therapeutic herbs, it heals itself in the process. Golden seal, echinacea, chamomile, burdock, Oregon grape root and comfrey are just a few of the hundreds of therapeutic herbs available. The have 50% toxic property activities with 4% buffers. They have 15% tonic nutrients, 1% fiber and 30% food nutrient activity.

4. Drastic herbs - Drastic herbs are the poisonous plants. They cause drastic side effects. From poison ivy, hemlock, belladonna to Ipecac, there are hundreds of others. They have 86% toxic properties with 2% buffers. They have 2% tonic nutrients, 2% fiber and 8% food nutrients activity.

Herbology is not a science *easily* mastered. I have been studying and applying my knowledge of herbs for over 34 years. I am still learning. Caution is required not only when incorporating herbs for healing, but you should not use them in an allopathic application for symptomatic relief. In other words, it is easy to use herbs to mask symptoms the way medics use drugs, never getting to the cause of why you need an herb or drug in the first place.

The best advise I can suggest to anyone interested in using herbs for medicinal purposes, is to acquire a copy of Dr. John Christopher's *School of Natural Healing* book on herbology and Jethro Kloss' *Back to Eden*. Once you feel proficient enough to include herbology in your life, start with *one* herb and verify that it works as indicated. Always use organic herbs that have not been fumigated, irradiated or genetically engineered.

Next time you are anxious, irritable, agitated or can't sleep, have a cup of valerian root tea. You can buy valerian root already in a tea bag or loose. You can also buy the whole root and prepare it for brewing. If you really want to be an herbalist, you can grow it yourself. Camomile, hops and passionflower all have similar effects. They are very relaxing and soothing. Try one at a time or compound (mix) them into a concoction.

For every (drinking) cup of hot water (only use distilled), pour a teaspoon of one or mixed herbs in and let steep for a few minutes. Some herbs need more time; some need less. This is where a good herbal book comes in to explain the differences.

Once you have expressed enough of the herb into the hot water, strain into another cup and drink. Over time you will learn how long to let steep and how much of each herb you want to mix.

Red clover is an herb used for most conditions, illnesses and dis-eases. It is an excellent blood purifier. Whether you have a "cold" or cancer, this herb makes a delicious tea.

Basic Vitamins

[Note: Although all following nutrients are contained in kamut, spirulina, chlorella, barley, alfalfa, rice germ/bran and purple dulse, the additional food sources may also be helpful.]

1. Vitamin A (Retinal) - also known as beta carotene, is found in milk, butter, eggs, carrots and leafy green and yellow vegetables and in beef liver (not recommended). Vitamin A provides for the first line of defense against invading toxins since it establishes healthy skin and mucous membranes. Vitamin A is part of the powerful antioxidant group of nutrients and has been known to actually destroy carcinogens - cancer producing substances.

Functions within the Body-Vitamin A

Immune System - helps the body resist infections, virus and cancer.

Skin and Mucous Membranes - helps skin elasticity and cell growth.

Eyes - including visual purple production (essential for night vision).

Cell growth and elasticity - promotes growth and vitality, repairs and maintains body tissue, helps prevent premature aging (skin elasticity) and senility (nervecells).

Deficiency Symptoms - Allergies, appetite loss, soft tooth enamel, skin blemishes, dry hair, rough dry skin, loss of smell, sinus trouble, fatigue, susceptibility to infections.

Therapeutic Uses -Acne, heart disease, diabetes, allergies, arthritis, asthma, hyperthyroidism, recurring infection, athletes foot, sinusitis, tooth and gum disease, cystitis, bronchitis,"cold," psoriasis, peptitis, migraine headaches, vision deterioration.

2. Vitamin B1 (Thiamin) - is found in wheat germ, dulse, black strap molasses, Brewer's yeast, okra, sunflower seeds, egg yolk, Brazil nuts and in beef liver (not recommended). B1 is a water-soluble vitamin as are all the B-complex. Enters and leaves the body each day and for optimum health you should consume it daily. Thiamin helps burn carbohydrates for energy, so having optimal body uptake is important in a weight-management program.

Functions within the Body-Vitamin B1

Carbohydrate Metabolism - energy, growth, learning capacity, circulation.

Organ Muscles and Body Muscles - aids digestion, circulation, prevents liquid retention, prevents constipation, muscle-tone maintenance (intestine, stomach, heart).

Deficiency Symptoms - Muscular weakness, digestive disturbances, numb hands and feet, fatigue, irritability, nervousness, mental depression, shortness of breath, pains around heart, beriberi (a neurological disease often causing numbness and tingling in the toes and feet, stiffness in ankles, pains in legs and finally paralysis of leg muscles).

Therapeutic Uses - Alzheimer's, diarrhea, constipation, diabetes, indigestion, heart disease, congestive heart failure, stress, mental illness, nausea.

3. Vitamin B2 (Riboflavin) - is found in Brussels sprouts, almonds, wheat germ, prunes, cheese, apples, carrots, lemons, grapefruit, kelp, coconut, milk, eggs, cereals, yeast, leafy green vegetables and in beef liver (not recommended). It helps the mitochondria (fat-burning furnace within the cell) of muscle cells to produce energy. It is important in weight management because you always want to maximize the optimal performance of those "fat-burning" furnaces. Food processing destroys up to 80% of natural riboflavin. A study done at Cornell University revealed that just moderate levels of exercise increase riboflavin needs of healthy women.

Functions within the Body-Vitamin B2

Metabolism - digest carbohydrates, fats and proteins, produces energy.

Eyes - reduces chances of cataract formation.

Skin, nails and hair - promotes growth and strength.

Deficiency Symptoms - Bloodshot and burning eyes, cataracts, corner of mouth cracks and sores, dizziness, poor digestion, premature wrinkles, slow growth, red sore tongue.

Therapeutic Uses - Arteriosclerosis, baldness, high cholesterol, cystitis, oily skin, hypoglycemia, light sensitivity, mental retardation, muscular disorders, nausea, weight control, premature wrinkles and stress.

4. Vitamin B3 (Niacin) - is found in rice, almonds, wheat germ, whole bran, rhubarb, whole barley, buttermilk, lobster, haddock, chicken and in beef liver (not recommended). It is a water-soluble vitamin that works in the glycogen stage of the energy cycle, in the fatty acid oxidation for energy process and in tissue respiration. Excess niacin above 30 mgs may cause vascular dilation accompanied with flushing, burning and itching. This is commonly called a "niacin flush." This is uncomfortable, but not toxic and is sometimes a strategy for breaking through a migraine headache.

Functions within the Body-Vitamin B3

Metabolism - digests carbohydrates, fats and proteins.

Organ Muscles - improves circulation, lowers cholesterol, dilates blood vessels, increases blood flow, produces sex hormones, aids in the production of hydrochloric acid.

Brain - aids in the functioning of the nervous system.

Deficiency Symptoms - Appetite loss, canker sores, cold hands/feet, depression, fatigue, halitosis, headaches, indigestion, insomnia, muscular weakness, nausea, nervous disorders, pellagra (a painful skin disorder with inflammation of the tongue and lining of the mouth. Also a serious digestive disorder causing diarrhea as well as mental depression), skin eruptions.

Therapeutic Uses - Acne, baldness, canker sores, diarrhea, halitosis, cardiovascular disease, leg cramps, migraine headaches, arthritis, schizophrenia, poor circulation, stress.

5. Vitamin B5 (Pantothenic Acid) - is found in nearly all plants, royal jelly honey, egg yolk, wheat bran, molasses and in beef liver (not recommended). It is a crucial nutrient for energy metabolism. It also makes brain neurotransmitters and natural body steroid hormones. Deficiency of Vitamin B5 in rats causes highly notable failure of cartilage growth and lesions like the lesions in osteoarthritis.

Functions within the Body-Vitamin B5

Metabolism - used for conversion of fats, carbohydrates and proteins into energy.

Organ Muscles - used for production of neurotransmitters, adrenal hormones, and antibodies, enhances stamina.

Adrenal gland - vital for the production of steroids in the adrenal gland.

Deficiency Symptoms - Fatigue, appetite loss, nausea, headache, tingling in hands, depression, anxiety.

Therapeutic Uses - Stress, fatigue, arthritis, depression, migraine headache.

6. Vitamin B6 (Pyridoxine) - is found in whole grain cereals, Brewers yeast, brown rice, green leafy vegetables, honey, prunes, cabbage and egg yolk. It functions in the formation of body proteins and amino acid metabolism, chemical transmitters in the nervous system, red blood cells, and prostaglandins. Because this B vitamin is involved with the multiplication of cells, it plays a vital role in pregnancy and in proper function of the immune system, mucous membrane, skin, red blood cells and brain chemistry.

Functions within the Body-Vitamin B6

Digestive system - hydrochloric acid production, fat and protein utilization (weight control), alleviates nausea.

Blood - promotes red blood cell formation.

Organ Muscles and Body Muscles - antibody formation, maintains sodium/potassium balance (nerves).

Skin - promotes healthy skin, reduces swelling in tissues.

Deficiency Symptoms - Acne, anemia, arthritis, convulsions in babies, depression, dizziness, nervous disorders, hair loss, irritability, learning disabilities, muscle spasms, urination problems weakness.

Therapeutic Uses - Alcoholism, arthritis, allergies, bursitis, hypoglycemia, insomnia, bronchial asthma, cardiovascular disease, premenstrual edema, weight control, anemia, epilepsy, fatigue, seborrhea, neuritis, shingles, stress.

7. Vitamin B9 (Folic Acid) - is found in raw milk, Brewers yeast, whole grains, dates, spinach, green leafy vegetables, tuna, oysters, organ meats, salmon and in beef liver (all animal sources are not recommended). It is an essential part of cellular division and DNA synthesis (the genetic code for the replication of every new cell). Of critical importance is with women taking birth control pills. A side effect of birth control pills is the depletion of folic acid.

Most birth defects from folic acid deficiency will occur within the first few weeks of pregnancy when most women don't even realize they are pregnant. Infant neural tube birth defects like spina bifida, if related to Vitamin B9 deficiency, are totally preventable if women would practice good nutrition, prevention and take whole-food nutritional supplements.

Functions within the Body-Vitamin B9

Organ Muscles and Body Muscles - Analgesic for pain, body growth and reproduction, hydrochloric acid production, formation of cells, aids in digestion, production of myelin, protein metabolism.

Blood - red blood cell formation.

Glands - improves lactation.

Nervous System - makes a protective coating surrounding the nerves, prevents nerve damage.

Deficiency Symptoms - Anemia, canker sores, digestive disturbances, graying hair, growth problems, impaired circulation, fatigue, mental depression.

Therapeutic Uses - Anemia, arteriosclerosis, baldness, high cholesterol, constipation, heart disease, loss of libido, overweight, macro-cystic anemia.

8. Vitamin B 12 (CyanoCobalamin) - is found in raw milk, kelp, cheese, eggs and salt-water fish, oysters and liver (all animal sources are not recommended). It helps prevent pernicious anemia, a deadly type of anemia characterized by large, immature red blood cells. The fastest way to nutritionally short circuit your body is a Vitamin B12 deficiency. B12 keeps the electrical nerve impulses moving through your body. Two of the most common nutrient deficiencies in the elderly are folic acid (B9) and vitamin B12. These deficiencies lead to motor-skill disturbances, confusion, delusion, fatigue, memory loss, numbness and ringing in the ears.

Functions within the Body-Vitamin B12

Blood - regulates red blood cell formation, utilization of iron.

Organ and Muscles - increases energy, cell longevity, metabolism (carbohydrates, fat, protein), promotes growth, needed for proper digestion.

Nervous System - prevents nerve damage and helps with nerve impulses.

Deficiency Symptoms - Chronic fatigue, general weakness, confusion, delusion, nervousness, pernicious anemia, memory loss, numbness, poor appetite, walking/speaking difficulties, ringing in the ears.

Therapeutic Uses - Alzheimer's disease, baldness, brain damage, cardiovascular disease, arrhythmia, dermatitis, eczema, depression, leg cramps, pernicious anemia.

9. Vitamin B15 (Pangamic Acid) - is a derivative of the amino acid glycine and is found in brown rice, sesame seeds, Brewer's yeast, sunflower and pumpkin seeds and organ meats (not recommended). It is one of those substances that the "nutritional authorities" at the Food and Drug Administration (FDA) consider of no value in human nutrition, because their education on nutrition is limited, yet they like to think they know all there is to know and all that will ever be known!

Pangamic acid (B15) increases general and myocardial resistance to hypoxia - insufficient supply of oxygen to living tissue usually caused by air pollution or carbon monoxide poisoning. It also lowers blood cholesterol levels and aids in protein synthesis.

Protein and Vitamins

Protein from the Greek word 'protos' means the first - an essential part of the human diet. Vitamin from Latin 'vita' means life and 'amine' meaning salts - the salt of life. When it comes to protein and vitamins, there is nothing more complete than the ingredients in Super Kamut. From kamut, spirulina, chlorella, alfalfa, barley, rice germ and bran and purple dulse, this is a maximum super green food.

Super Kamut® (Part of the LifePack System)

It's a fact: Mainstream medicine focuses on treating the symptoms of disease with drugs. The only real difference between drugs and poisons are dosages and intent. The human body runs on nutrients, not drugs. Researchers have figured out that the human body requires over 100 different nutritional building blocks, yet it is becoming increasingly difficult to acquire these nutrients from our food. Why?

Study after study has shown that anyone who doesn't consume 5-10 servings of vegetables per day is missing out on nature's ultimate insurance policy. Vegetables provide the body with a multitude of compounds including enzymes, minerals, antioxidants, chlorophyll and especially protein and vitamins. However, if the soil in which the vegetables have been grown is de-mineralized, the food will be equally as de-mineralized, hence the need for whole food supplementation.

Fruits, vegetables, grasses and other plants are primary sources of protein. Animal protein is secondary. Of all the primary sources of protein, Egyptian Kamut® is the most nutritious.

What Is Kamut®?

Over four thousand years ago the Egyptians grew a specialized wheat grass. Reportedly consumed by only pharaohs, kings, queens and other royalty, it was called Kamut® (kuh-moot). Long having disappeared, allegedly in 1945 an American soldier stationed in Egypt, broke into an ancient burial crypt and discovered a stone urn containing hundreds of Kamut® kernels. He sent these kernels to a relative in the United States whereby they were soon sprouted. With no interest in a Super Kamut® kernel the remaining dried kernels laid in a glass jar until 1980. Rediscovered and because the kernel is twice the size of common wheat with 20 to 40% more protein and nutrients than American wheat with a rich, buttery flavor, it is now seen as the best source for whole food protein nutrition.

Kamut® is known for its intense cleansing properties and is unsurpassed in its ability to balance the immune system and promote healing. Kamut® contains many of the essential amino and fatty acids, vitamins, minerals, enzymes and other co-factors. It is one of the most nutrient dense/rich whole foods we can consume. Kamut® is an heirloom, non-hybrid ancient grain from the Nile region of Egypt and has never been crossbred. Its recent cultivation in the U.S. encourages agricultural biodiversity and limits the reliance on mono-agriculture. Kamut® contains 20 to 40% more protein, 27% more lipids and measures higher in 8 of the 9 minerals found in common wheat. It also contains numerous trace minerals which it draws from the rich soil where it is grown.

Kamut® as opposed to regular wheat, is significantly higher in magnesium (23% higher) and zinc (25% higher). In terms of vitamins, Kamut® contains more riboflavin, thiamine and niacin than common wheat, and is significantly higher in vitamin E.

Kamut® has many of the properties of common wheat with far less of its allergenic component: two-thirds of those tested with wheat allergy will have less or no allergy to Kamut®. Like all wheat, it is glutinous, yet the majority of gluten-sensitive individuals can eat it without adverse side effects. Those with celiac and other gluten intolerance conditions should first test for reactions with very small portions.

Medallion Laboratory in Minneapolis, MN, did a complete nutritional analysis of the ancient grain QK-77 which is currently sold under the brand name of Kamut®. These results were compared with figures compiled by the USDA for hard red spring wheat, hard red winter wheat, soft red wheat, soft white wheat, hard white wheat and durum. These grains are normally referred to as common wheat. Since Kamut® may be used as a substitute for any of these wheats, an average number for all the wheats in the USDA report was used.

As an overall summary, it can be said that Kamut® has higher nutritional value than the common wheats. The most striking superiority is found in the protein level of this grain.

Kamut® wheat is also significantly higher in total lipids. Since lipids are higher in energy than carbohydrates and proteins, Kamut® wheat can be described as a high-energy grain. The vast majority of the nutrition in this grain, however, is in the form of complex carbohydrates whose value in the diet is well documented.

Because Kamut® is made up of such a large seed (about 2-3 times the size of a normal wheat kernel); the ratio of the seed coat to the seed volume is less than other wheats. The proportionately less seed coat area explains why the percent of fiber which is found in the bran located in the seed coat is a little less than in the smaller kernels of the other wheats.

When vitamins are compared, there is no trend. Of the seven vitamins normally found in wheat, Kamut® has higher concentrations of four and lower concentrations of three. Again, it is of interest to note, however, that there is 30 percent more vitamin E in Kamut®.

Kamut® has significantly higher levels of all the major fatty acids usually found in wheat. Of course like all wheat, Kamut® has no cholesterol. Kamut® also has higher levels of sixteen out of the eighteen amino acids usually found in wheat. The concentrations of six amino acids are 34 to 65 percent higher in the Kamut® than in the average wheat. These amino acids are threonine, cystine, arginine, histidine, aspartic acid and serine.

There is one other significant difference between Kamut® and average grains in the USDA report. That difference is the moisture content. Low moisture is characteristic of grain grown under dry land conditions of the western end of the northern great plains; (Montana, western Dakotas, southern Alberta and Saskatchewan). This low moisture helps to naturally protect the grain from insects and spoilage. It also slows the oxidation of natural products once the flour is ground. That means there is less nutritional loss between grinding and processing. The result is a more nutritious and wholesome product for the consumer.

Kamut® wheat grass is my first choice for a nutrient rich,

whole food protein complex and is why I call my whole food nutrient dense protein/vitamin powder Super Kamut®. (Kamut® is a registered trademark of Kamut International, Inc.).

Spirulina

Spirulina is an amazing source of complete, highly digestible vegetarian protein, proportionately higher than meat and fish and has the greatest source of B-12 analogue in nature.

There are family species of microalgae such as blue-green algae, spirulina and aphanizomenon, and green algae chlorella and dunaliella. Spirulina's scientific name is arthrospira platensis. This edible algae has a long history of safe human consumption and over 30 years of safety testing. Special farms where spirulina is cultivated under controlled conditions, do not allow the growth of other contaminant blue-green algae, as found in lakes and waterways.

These tiny green spiral coils harvest the energy of the sun, growing a treasure of bio-available nutrients. Allegedly, this first photosynthetic life form was designed by nature 3.6 billion years ago. Blue-green algae produced the oxygen in our atmosphere allowing all higher life forms to evolve. It contains everything life needed to evolve into its rich diversity today. This immortal life form has renewed itself for billions of years. In the past 20 years it has reintroduced itself to humanity. Spirulina contains billions of years of successful evolutionary wisdom coded in its DNA.

More Nutrition Per Acre Than Any Other Food

Spirulina can produce 20 times more protein per acre than soybeans. If we can use unusable resources to grow the most powerful food on earth, we can help stop cutting the last of the primordial forests to grow food. By bringing spirulina into our personal lives, we become part of the solution to improve the health of our planet.

Spirulina contains compounds like phycocyanin, polysaccharides and sulfolipids that enhance the immune system. Spirulina contains the most remarkable concentration of functional nutrients ever discovered in any food, plant, grain or herb and no other algae, blue-green or chlorella, has been the subject of such intense research over the past 30 years.

Several years ago, the National Cancer Institute announced sulfolipids from blue-green algae like spirulina were remarkably active in test tube experiments against the AIDS virus. In 1993-95, research showed natural polysaccharides in spirulina increased T-cell counts, strengthened the immune system and raised disease resistance in chickens, fish and mice. The animal feed industry is embracing spirulina as a new probiotic to replace overused anti-biotic drugs in animal feed. In 1994, a Russian patent was awarded for spirulina as a medicine for reducing allergic reactions from radiation in the children of the Chernobyl disaster.

The Healthiest Whole-Food Is Your Best Defense

The foods we eat are the first line of defense from the negative effects of lifestyle stress, pollution, radiation and toxic chemicals. Yet so many processed foods are nutritionally empty. They leave us vulnerable to poor health and low energy.

The good news is many essential nutrients recommended by experts to help protect our bodies are concentrated in spirulina. This amazing algae from the sea contains the most powerful combination of nutrients ever known in any grain, herb or food.

World's Highest Beta-Carotene Food Reduces Long-Term Health Risks

Spirulina beta carotene is ten times more concentrated than carrots. So even if you don't eat the recommended 4 to 9 servings of fruits and vegetables every day (most people eat only 1-2), ensure yourself of the highest source of beta carotene by taking spirulina to help support your body's defense. It is 60% easy-to-digest vegetable protein without the fat and cholesterol of meat.

People are eating less meat and dairy protein because they want to lower fat, cholesterol, and chemicals in their diet. Spirulina is the highest protein food with all the essential amino acids and has only a few calories to keep your waistline where you want it.

A rare essential fatty acid is a key to health.
Gamma-linolenic acid (GLA) in mother's milk helps develop

healthy babies. Studies show nutritional deficiencies can block GLA production in your body, so a good dietary source of GLA can be important. Spirulina is the only other whole food with GLA.

Iron for women and children's health .

Iron is essential to build a strong system, yet is the most common mineral deficiency. Spirulina is rich in iron, magnesium and trace minerals and is easier to absorb than iron supplements.

High in Vitamin B-12 and B Complex.

Spirulina is the highest source of B-12, essential for healthy nerves and tissue, especially for vegetarians.

Unusual phytonutrients for health and cleansing.

Scientists are discovering the benefits of polysaccharides, sulfolipids and glycolipids, and the rainbow of natural pigments that give spirulina a deep green color. Green (chlorophyll), blue (phycocyanin) and orange (carotenoids) colors collect the sun's energy and power. Chlorophyll is a natural cleanser and is often referred to as nature's green magic.

Scientists at the Osaka Center for Cancer and Cardiovascular Diseases have confirmed in human studies that taking an extract of spirulina can have positive effects on the production of cancer-fighting immune cells in the body. Results of this study have been published in the journal *International Immunopharmacology* Vol.2, No. 4.

This latest study, performed on 12 adult males, found that the oral administration of a hot water extract of spirulina (outdoor grown and spray dried) helped the immune system to produce cancer-fighting immune cells called natural killer (NK) cells. By analyzing the blood cells of volunteers, the group showed a significant increase in NK cell production and an increase of the killing ability of these NK cells.

Moreover, in vitro stimulation of blood cells with BCG cell-wall skeleton (a bacterial cell-wall material) resulted in a significant increase in IL-12 production in cells from volunteers given spirulina than in cells without pre-exposure to spirulina. IL-12 is a cytokine that stimulates natural killer cells. It facilitates cell-killing activity of NK cells.

While more research is needed to confirm and expand upon these results, this study shows that spirulina has the potential to mitigate cancer. It also suggests that taking spirulina helps arm the body with defensive natural killer cells that can act on cancer cells as soon as they develop, thereby preventing cancer's onset.

There was still an increase in natural killer cell activity that continued to be observed up to five weeks after stopping administration of spirulina.

The researchers studied natural killer-cell activity using IL12/IL18 mediated interferon gamma production. This is the first time that the molecular mechanism of the human immune enhancing effects of spirulina has been explained. The study also confirms results from earlier animal studies by the same group and results from an in vitro study using human peripheral blood mononuclear cells by a group of researchers at the University of California, Davis.

Containing a wide variety of nutrients and with an unmatched digestibility coefficient of 95%, spirulina is an extraordinary whole food. Its visible color is a deep blue green; however, it contains other intense colors including red and orange pigments. These pigments represent life enhancing substances such as phycocyanin, polysaccharides, chlorophyll, gamma linolenic acid and mixed carotenoids. Spirulina provides excellent nutrients for the eyes, skin, nervous system and assists in purifying one's blood.

Chlorella Plankton

Chlorella belongs to the eucaryotic cell category of algae and lives in fresh water as a single-celled plant. Its size is about that of a human erythrocyte; i.e. between 2-8 microns in diameter. The name chlorella derives from two Latin words meaning 'leaf' (green) and 'small', referring to the unusually high content of chlorophyll that gives chlorella its characteristic deep emerald-green color. Chlorella is also rich in protein, vitamins, minerals, "C.G.F." (Chlorella Growth Factor) and other beneficial substances.

Under favorable growth conditions; strong sunlight, pure water and clean air, chlorella multiplies at an incredible rate. The process of reproduction can generally be divided into several steps: growth, ripening, maturity and division. At the division stage, a "mother" cell divides into four 'daughter' cells. This complete reproduction cycle can take less than 24 hours.

As a source of bio-available essential nutrients, chlorella compares well with any whole food on earth. It is a complete protein containing 19 amino acids in excellent ratios as well as the highest quantities of chlorophyll and RNA / DNA ever discovered within a natural source. It is, also, an abundant source of vitamins and minerals plus essential fatty acids.

Extensive research has and is being conducted on chlorella. Probably its most outstanding feature is its ability to help a person's body detoxify harmful air, water, food-borne heavy metals and chemical pollutants; precursors to many of today's degenerative disease conditions.

Chlorella's unique phytochemical known as CGF, or Chlorella Growth Factor, is believed to be responsible for many of the therapeutic effects that have been reported in scientific journals throughout the world. In Japan, chlorella is by far the most popular nutritional supplement today with over five million people taking it on a daily basis. The Japanese are among the longest living people of all the industrialized nations.

An individual chlorella cell is barely larger than a human red blood cell which allows for micro fine filtering. This filtering process excludes any potentially toxic strain of algae or inorganic matter from entering the harvest. The chlorella in QCI's Super Kamut® is chlorella pyrenoidosa which is a fresh-water micro-algae cultured in pure water containing over 70 minerals and trace minerals. It is also grown in natural sunlight so that it remains a wholesome natural food, as nature intended. This is the premium grade of chlorella.

Rapid, low-temperature spray drying is used to crack the individual chlorella cell walls. This process preserves the phytonutrients and RNA / DNA values thus providing maximum absorbability. If the cell wall is not broken, the nutrients in chlorella are almost entirely unavailable as they are protected by a tough cellulose shell.

One of its main functions is as a superior detoxifier, and is especially good before and after having silver / mercury amalgams removed from one's teeth. It helps to chelate with and draw heavy metals out of the body.

In tests, chlorella was added to the diet of mice with fatty livers. After administration of this diet over an extended period, there was a marked reduction in this fatty condition. Mice that were injected with cancer cells showed a higher resistance to this challenge if they had been fed with chlorella. Another test showed that Chlorella Growth Factor will improve their resistance to abdominal tumors and increase the number of immune cells in the abdominal cavity.

Chlorella can promote cell reproduction, reduce cholesterol and increase hemoglobin levels. Since chlorella is such a broad-spectrum product, it can help to support and repair organs and tissues that have been injured by a variety of causes.

Numerous research projects in the USA and Europe have indicated that chlorella can also aid the body in the breakdown of persistent hydrocarbon and metallic toxins such as DDT, PCB, mercury, cadmium and lead as well as strengthening the immune system response. The fibrous materials in chlorella will also improve digestion and promote the growth of beneficial aerobic bacteria in the gut. Other research programs have indicated that regular use of chlorella can help to guard against heart disease, reduce high blood pressure and lower serum cholesterol levels.

It could be said that there is no other green plant from under the sea that is more beneficial to the human body than chlorella. With the many positive findings of scientific researchers around the world, this food should become an indispensable part of our daily diet so that we can enjoy the many health benefits that it has to offer. As a perfect food, chlorella has no peers.

Dis-ease is defined as lack of ease or harmony, it is NOT the same as "disease," a medical term for illness treated by medicine. *NEVER* attempt to stop or reduce your medication without the supervision of your medical doctor.

Alfalfa

Alfalfa was first discovered by the Arabs, who named it the father of all foods as it is one of the most complete foods there is. It is more nutritious than almost any other herb, contains many important enzymes, proteins, minerals and vitamins and has been used for food and medicine for thousands of years. Alfalfa cleans, builds and strengthens the body and rebuilds decayed teeth. The alkaloid in the leaves strengthens the central nervous system, helps prevent cholesterol accumulation in the veins, helps chemical imbalance and neutralizes uric acid, just to mention a few of its many attributes. It has been found helpful for numerous conditions, including arthritis, ulcers, high blood pressure, constipation, infections, asthma, allergies, anemia and many others.

Alfalfa has very deep roots, commonly growing to 60 or 80 feet deep, some alfalfa roots have been found more than 150 feet deep! This is why it is so rich in minerals. Much of our soil has been seriously depleted by using agricultural chemicals. The surface of the soil is now depleted of rich minerals because of improper use of the land, thus it is then difficult to get the minerals we need in our food. Trace mineral deficiency can act to impair hereditary transmission, as shown by the abnormalities that are becoming more common. Nature has been making normal birds, butterflies and animals for millions of years. If wild animals can do it, why can't we? It is because they, by their instinct, select the right foods and do not meddle with nature's food by changing it. The condition of any civilization's soil is crucial to their health and their very existence.

Rich in Many Vitamins and Minerals

Alfalfa was brought to America around 1850 and today is the largest crop grown in this country. By nature alfalfa is very alkaline, which helps to eliminate excess uric acid, it is also extremely rich in chlorophyll. Chlorophyll promotes healing more than other substances and is similar to our blood pH. Alfalfa also contains several different compounds of calcium. It is rich in potassium, magnesium, vitamins A, E, K, D, B6 and protein. It has high amounts of phosphorus, iron, potassium, chlorine, sodium, silicon, magnesium, B1, B2 and B12. Alfalfa is such a good all around herb that many different animals thrive on it alone.

A surprising fact about alfalfa is that it is higher in protein than beef. Alfalfa is 18.9 percent protein, while beef is 16.5, eggs are 13.1 and milk is 3.3 percent. Alfalfa contains all seven essential enzymes: lipase to break down fat; amylase for carbohydrates; sucrase which converts cane sugar into dextrose; peroxidase, which is an oxidizing aid for blood; pectinase to digest starches; coagulase to coagulate milk and help to clot blood emulsion to act on sugars which helps digestion; and protease which digests proteins.

Herbalists have used alfalfa for many different purposes. The one word that keeps appearing is "tonic." The plant is a kidney tonic, prostate tonic, reproductive tonic, musculoskeletal tonic, glandular tonic and so forth. Alfalfa has traditionally been one of the best herbal treatments for arthritis, gout and rheumatism.

Alfalfa has a proven cholesterol-lowering effect. Steroidal anti-inflammatory action is suggested by its content of plant steroids, and by some research that found an estrogenic effect on ruminants (grazing animals). Alfalfa has also been shown to possess antibacterial action against gram-negative bacteria and contains at least one protein with known anti-tumor activity.

According to leading authorities, alfalfa alkalizes and detoxifies the body, especially the liver. It is good for all colon disorders, anemia, hemorrhaging, diabetes, ulcers and arthritis. It promotes pituitary gland function and contains an anti-fungus agent.

Alfalfa's blood-purifying properties have been attributed to its high chlorophyll content. In fact, it is probably due not only to chlorophyll but also several other components contained therein. It appears that alfalfa works on inflammation (arthritis, rheumatism) and as a general tonic by removing toxins from the blood, including high molecular weight alcohol (triacontanol, octacosanol). It also reduces cholesterol and serum lipids while the flavonoids relax the smooth muscles. The alkaloids help reduce blood sugar levels and the saponins support the digestive system by helping to balance the intestinal flora.

The high amount of beta carotene in alfalfa acts to help strengthen epithelial cells of the mucous membranes of the stomach, and could be the source for its beneficial effect on ulcers. You can't have a real "super food" without organic alfalfa.

Barley

Scientific research has shown that the juice from young barley leaves is rich in vitamins (especially beta carotene, B complex vitamins and vitamin C), minerals (including potassium, calcium, iron, phosphorous and magnesium), chlorophyll and muco-polysaccharides, which play a major role in the structural integrity of body tissue. Of the 3000 enzymes known and identified, barley grass contains up to 1000, including the potent antioxidants super oxide dismutase (S.O.D.), catalase, peroxides, cytochrome oxidase and dehydrogenase.

Cytochrome oxidase is an enzyme essential for cell metabolism. In the body there are two forms of fat: brown fat contains cytochrome oxidase and is metabolically active, white fat contains nothing harmful and is not metabolically active. Regular consumption of barley juice may stimulate weight loss, probably due to barley's enhancement of the cytochrome oxidase enzyme system.

Barley is also an important source of the superoxide dismutase enzyme (SOD), a potent antioxidant. Normal metabolic activity produces dangerous superoxide free radicals which can damage cell walls and are linked to premature aging and many diseases, including cancer and heart disease. In mice inoculated with cancer, barley juice had a surprising curative effect, probably due to the juice's high level of SOD.

Continuing research has revealed numerous other benefits of barley juice. Barley juice is very alkaline and can contribute to maintaining the body's acid-alkaline balance. Isolated compounds from barley juice are found to have hypercholesteromic, anti-inflammatory and anti-ulcer properties. A new antioxidant, 2-O-GIV, has been isolated and reported to have antioxidant activity equal to or superior to vitamin E.

Finally, studies have shown that when barley juice is added to injured cells, the cell's DNA repairs itself rapidly. This may contribute to preventing abnormal changes in the cell structure, which could lead to cancer and rapid aging.

Barley grass is one of the green grasses, the green vegetation that can supply sole nutritional support from birth to old age. Barley has served as a food staple in most cultures. The use of barley for food and medicinal purposes dates to antiquity. Agronomists place this ancient cereal grass as being cultivated as early as 7000 B.C.. Roman gladiators ate barley for strength and stamina. In the West, it was first known for the barley grain it produces.

Astounding amounts of vitamins and minerals are found in green barley leaves. The leaves have an ability to absorb nutrients from the soil, if therein. These are easily assimilated throughout the digestive tract, giving our body instant access to vital nutrients. These include potassium, calcium, magnesium, iron, copper, phosphorus, manganese, zinc, beta carotene, B1, B2, B6, C, folic acid, and pantothenic acid. Indeed, green barley juice contains 11 times the calcium in cows' milk, nearly 5 times the iron in spinach, 7 times the vitamin C in oranges and 80 mg of vitamin B12 per hundred grams.

Barley also contains glucan, a fiber also found in oat bran and reported to reduce cholesterol levels. The root contains the alkaloid hordenine that stimulates peripheral blood circulation and has been used as a bronchodilator for bronchitis. Barley bran, like wheat bran may be effective in protecting against the risk of cancer.

Drinking barley green juice is often recommended by people who study and practice natural healing techniques. In recent years it has become popular among those seeking a potent source of the antioxidant and phytochemical properties attributed to deep green leafy vegetables.

In today's world, "eating right" is becoming more and more difficult. Barley provides more chlorophyll, protein, enzymes, trace minerals and phytochemicals at a very reasonable price. Easy to use and wonderfully palatable, barley is a beautiful rich green powder.

Stabilized Rice Germ and Bran

Brown rice germ and bran are excellent sources of Gamma-oryzanol (esters of ferulic acid), a potent antioxidant within plant cells. Gamma-oryzanol has been found effective in lowering blood cholesterol and triglyceride levels. Brown rice germ and bran are also excellent sources of both soluble and insoluble dietary fibers. Dietary fibers help to bind bile acids, lower blood cholesterol, increase satiety after eating, increase fecal weight and volume, decrease transit time of food through the colon, and decrease insulin response after a carbohydrate meal. Adequate daily fiber consumption helps prevent constipation, carbohydrate disorders and hypercholesterolemia.

Rice bran is the outer coating of the rice kernel. Worldwide it is removed from the white portion of rice in a process known as polishing. Polishing breaks up the coating into smaller particles, which begin to oxidize almost immediately. Attached to and also a part of the rice bran in a portion called the rice germ, which can be likened to an egg and contains the reproductive system of the rice kernel.

During the polishing process the oil portion of the bran is damaged and starts to degrade in several ways, one of which is by enzymatically induced rancidity. In other words, a naturally occurring enzyme in the oil that helped make the oil now starts to take it back. Within about 12 hours there is enough damage to effectively reduce the nutritional advantages of the rice bran and make it unfit for human consumption. Or so we thought.

It is estimated that between 50 and 60 million metric tons of rice bran is discarded worldwide every year because of the degradation induced by the milling process. This most valuable nutrient source is typically thrown away.

Various attempts at stabilizing rice bran have been attempted since the early 1900s and it wasn't until 1978 that the results of a successful stabilization process were scientifically published. By the early 1980s a process had been developed by the United States Department of Agriculture that effectively deactivated the enzyme in the rice bran oil that contributed the most to the degradation of the rice bran.

As of 2001, there are two plants in the United States that effectively stabilize rice bran using a non-chemical process. Except for certain export purposes, the product of these two plants is licensed to only one company, which is the sole source of stabilized rice bran in the United States. Virtually all stabilized rice bran on the American market being used in any product originates from this single source. As a raw material, this stabilized rice bran is sold through distribution channels to eventually become various forms of finished products. Various manufacturers can then modify stabilized rice bran to fit their individual markets and retail channels.

Rice, like other grains, consists of three parts: the outer bran, the starchy endosperm that makes up the bulk of the grain, and the germ or heart. The bran and germ are the parts of the grain that provide the nutrition and these are the parts that are removed in the process of refining the brown rice to white rice. White rice has an advantage over brown rice as it is resistant to insect infestation. It has so little nutrition even bugs aren't interested. There is nothing much in white rice or in any refined grain such as white wheat flour that interest our cells either.

Rice germ and bran contain many nutrients that work together. In particular, rice germ and bran contain nutrients not readily found in other foods or supplements. Rice germ and bran are one of the most potent food sources of phytochemicals, also called phytonutrients, which are plant compounds. These food sources or plant compounds work synergistically with other nutrients to enhance absorption and utilization.

One of the phytonutrients as mentioned is gamma-oryzanol,

which can be effective in the treatment of elevated cholesterol and triglyceride levels. It has a positive effect on fat metabolism and blood lipids. Lipolytic effect means that it helps burn fat in order to provide energy, which is then used to build lean body mass. This is no small matter when the majority of Americans would like to lose weight and/or increase their energy. It also contains essential oils as well as inositol and choline for optimal fat digestion.

Another phytonutrient is lipoic acid, which helps produce energy in muscles and protects the liver - which is an important system for detoxifying poisons. Lipoic acid also stabilizes blood sugar to calm down sugar cravings and energy swings and is an important antioxidant. In addition, it helps recycle vitamins E and C so the body can get more antioxidant protection from them.

Stabilized rice germ and bran contain antioxidants to help protect against free-radical damage and the de-generative disease processes that often result: cancer, heart disease, arthritis and diabetes. There are over 74 know antioxidant compounds in rice germ and bran. It has a number of forms of vitamin E, including tocopherols and tocotrienols. Tocotrienol isomers and compounds are 40 to 1,000 times more potent than alpha-tocopherol as antioxidants. Tocotrienols promote T-cell development and thus enhance the immune system.

Stabilized rice germ and bran are one of the richest sources of B vitamins found in nature. From B1 to B15, it has it all. Rice germ also contains most of the essential amino acids required to maintain a healthy life.

Purple Dulse

Purple dulse seaweed is one of the richest sources of bio-available minerals on the planet. It contains all the minerals and trace minerals that are found in the oceans and the earth's crust. For QCI's Super Kamut®, I chose purple Scandinavian dulse because it not only has the highest mineral concentration, it also tastes mild. Many seaweeds smell and taste fishy and are offensive to most people.

Dulse (dillisk/ sea grass/ Palmaria palmata) is a sea

vegetable that grows in the inter-tidal zone, the region of shoreline found between high and low tides, along North Atlantic and Northwest Pacific coastlines. Dulse is found attached to rocks by means of a holdfast, it grows between 25 and 45 cm in length and is characterized by red or purple translucent fronds.

Dulse is harvested by hand during the spring and summer months, then spread thinly on netting, cured in open fields by the wind and sun. During frequent turning, any adhering shells or other debris are removed. Dulse is deemed cured when the outer surface of the frond is covered with sea salt, which has moved to the outer surface of the frond from within as a result of capillary action. In this cured state, dulse has a shelf life of several years, if kept dry and out of strong direct sunlight, therefore, dulse may be consumed at leisure.

Dulse is a low-calorie food stuff, containing high levels of roughage, important in sustaining proper bowel and intestine function and is an excellent dieting health food, eaten on its own or used as an ingredient when accompanying salads and other dishes.

Biochemical Benefits of Dulse

Dulse is a rich source of potassium, an essential cellular ion and low in sodium salts. A recent study suggested that the majority of Westerners exhibit potassium deficiency, due to the methods commonly employed to cook vegetables, such as boiling which leaches this essential ion out of the vegetable and is thrown away with the cooking medium. Consuming dulse is an excellent way of obtaining potassium, vitamins and minerals in the diet. Including the following:

1. As previously noted, zinc is an important ion required for the proper function of an enzyme called DNA polymerase. Zinc is also essential for maintaining normal levels of vitamin A in the blood.

2. Manganese is required for a surprising number of essential enzymes, such as pyruvate carboxylase, a key enzyme involved in energy production from sugars and therefore, this ion has cardinal importance. Magnesium is found bound to adenosine

triphosphate (ATP), the energy currency of the cell and this important energy molecule is involved in the majority of the biochemical process the cell undergoes.

3. Iron is recognized for its important role as a central component of hemoglobin. In the red blood cells, these cells transport oxygen around the body through the blood stream. Eating dulse can prevent or alleviate anemia.

4. Iodine prevents gout and must be ingested by people who obtain nutrition from food-stuffs grown in iodine poor soils. This ion plays a role in controlling thyroxine concentration, a body hormone that regulates energy levels within the body. People who are run down or are affected by lethargy often find that reduced thyroxine levels are at fault.

5. As stated above, Vitamin A or retinol aids vision especially at night. This vitamin can prevent and alleviate night blindness, it also helps to prevent dry skin and hair.

6. Vitamin B1 plays an important role in keeping nerve cells functioning properly, it also has a metabolic coenzyme role (as do the other B vitamins). It is also associated with pyruvate decarboxylase, important for energy production in the cell.

7. Vitamin B2 or riboflavin, is another coenzyme found in the mitochondria, the power house of the cell. It is here the majority of the energy of the cell is produced from sugar, therefore, involved in that capacity, demonstrates this vitamins vital metabolic role.

8. Vitamin B6 or pyridoxine, another important metabolic molecule, functions as a coenzyme that assists the reactions of many enzymes involving amino acids and it is essential for the metabolism and conversion of these amino acids.

Vitamin E or tocopherol protects cellular membranes against attack from free radicals, thus, this vitamin protects the cell against damage and potential cancer-causing agents, keeping the cell functioning properly.

Nature's Minerals

"If it weren't for minerals, after cremation, there would be nothing to urn."

- Phaelae

The Miracle Elements: Fossilized Stony Coral Minerals

In all the years I have been investigating natural healing, nutrition and working with degenerative dis-eases, I believe the most *effective* whole food mineral supplement complex available today is fossilized stony coral.

Stony corals are sea animals, which includes the hydroids, jellyfish and sea anemones. By secreting a highly mineralized limestone, the stony corals build a housing of protective cups into which the soft polyp animals can retreat when disturbed. The limestone housing is made of all the minerals available in the ocean.

The stony corals are inhabitants of the reefs of Okinawa, the Caribbean and other islands, where the fossilized stony corals of several excellent products come from. In addition to supplementing much-needed minerals, research over many decades has proven the presence of an amazing number of antibiotic, anti-viral and anticancer substances in some of the different corals.

Only fossilized stony coral is collected from above the seashore and is over 20,000 years old and older, buried in the earth when the oceans were free of all chemical debris and contamination. Okinawian and Caribbean fossilized stony coral is also free of radiation contamination by atomic weapon experimentation and destruction. Other island corals are possibly not.

Stony coral minerals are so easily accepted by our body that surgeons can use pieces of coral in bone transplants without rejection. It is almost impossible to overdose on coral. Fossilized stony coral has never been known to cause any adverse side effects such as constipation or gas.

Elements contained within fossilized stony coral:

Major Minerals (10) found in large quantities.

Calcium (Ca)	Strontium (Sr)
Magnesium (Mg)	Chlorine (Cl)

Sulfur (S)	Aluminum (Al)
Hydrogen (H)	Silicon (Si)

(Deuterium - stable mineral isotope of hydrogen)

Sodium (Na)	Iron (Fe)

Trace Minerals (32 elements) that are present in amounts less than .01 percent of the body.

Antimony (Sb)	Manganese (Mn)
Arsenic (As)	Mercury (Hg)
Barium (Ba)	Molybdenum (Mo)
Beryllium (Be)	Nickel (Ni)
Bismuth (Bi)	Osmium (Os)
Boron (B)	Palladium (Pd)
Cadmium (Cd)	Phosphorus (P)
Cesium (Cs)	Zinc (Zn)
Chromium ((Cr)	Potassium (K)
Cobalt (Co)	Rhodium (Rh)
Copper (Cu)	Rubidium (Rb)
Fluorine (F)	Selenium (Se)
Germanium (Ge)	Silver (Ag)
Iodine (I)	Tin (Sn
Lead (Pb)	Tungsten (W)
Lithium (Li)	Vanadium (V)

Use Unknown Minerals (31)

Bromine (Br)	Dysprosium (Dy)	Scandium (Sc)
Tantalum (Ta)	Erbium (Er)	Europrium (Eu)
Tellurium (Te)	Terbium (Tb)	Gadolinium (Gd)
Gallium (Ga)	Thallium (Tl)	Thorium (Th)
Gold (Au)	Hafnium (Hf)	Thulium ™
Titanium(Ti)	Holmium (Ho)	Indium (In)
Ytterbium (Yb)	Yttrium (Y)	Zirconium (Zr)
Iridium (Ir)	Lanthanum (La)	
Lutetium (Lu)	Neodymium (Nd)	
Niobium (Nb)	Platinum (Pt)	
Praseodymium (Pr)	Rhenium (Re)	
Ruthenium (Ru)	Samarium (Sm)	

Compatible Enhancing Agents/Nutrients

Bicarbonate buffers are key minerals. The more we become acidic the more our buffer reserves are depleted. Poor eating habits and medications cause acidosis. The body will take minerals from bone, teeth, fluids, and other tissues, all to keep the pH of the blood 7.35 to 7.45 or slightly alkaline.

Calcium (Ca) - The great alkalizer is a major essential element/mineral. 99% of all calcium is located in the bones and teeth. 60% of the calcium in blood serum is the ionic (bio-available) form. Ionized calcium is of great importance in blood coagulation, function of the heart, muscles and nerves. Any substance that releases calcium from the cells causes the cells to divide. Calcium deficiency may be one cause of cancer. It also brings about increased excretion of lead in lead poisoning. Calcium has a major role in the function of the brain, heart, kidney, liver, muscles, skin and spleen. Sugar, salt and other chemicals drive calcium out of the body. Calcium must be ionized prior to being absorbed and needs adequate gastric acidity and hydrochloric acid for uptake.

Magnesium (Mg) - is the seventh most abundant element present in the body following calcium. Magnesium plays a major role in maintaining the electrical potential across muscle and nerve membranes. Muscle spasms can be the result of a deficiency of magnesium and so can heart attacks. When magnesium is absent from cells, the structure of ribosomes, which contains the vital nucleic acids, is destroyed. Mitochondria control the enzymes that break down glucose into energy. Without magnesium the enzymes cannot be activated and the mitochondria disintegrate.

Potassium (K) - is necessary for the proper working of the digestive tract. Deficiency leads to constipation. Potassium affects eight separate body enzymes that can function ONLY when potassium is present in sufficient quantity. From the heart to nerves and blood cells carrying carbon dioxide out through the lungs, potassium is essential. Excessive heat can cause so much potassium loss one can die from heat prostration. Early symptoms of potassium deficiency are weakness, impairment of neuro-muscular function, absent reflexes, mental confusion, soft and sagging muscles and dry skin. In teenagers, acne is a sign of potassium deficiency.

Vitamin D - Vitamin D comes from the ultraviolet rays of the sun, egg yolk, butter, fish oils, shitake mushrooms and yeast, to name a few. By adding Vitamin D3 it allows calcium and other minerals to be more readily absorbed in the intestine.

Vitamin D is converted in the liver to calcidiol, which is the major circulating form of vitamin D3. Parathyroid hormone is transported to the kidney where it stimulates the production of the hormonal form of vitamin D3 called calcitriol from the calcidiol. Calcitriol is the active hormone that by itself stimulates the intestinal absorption of calcium. Calcitriol, in the presence of the parathyroid hormone, stimulates the mobilization of calcium from bone and the re-absorption of calcium in the kidney. Without Vitamin D3, this does not happen.

Betaine HCL - is a precursor to hydrochloric acid in the stomach which helps digest the mineral complex. It is an excellent addition.

Malic Acid - is an extract from apples and is used to keep calcium from clumping in the stomach.

Marine verses Fossilized Stony Coral

In light of the television infomercials by Robert Barefoot and *The Calcium Factor* promoting his marine coral product, I thought I would explain the significant difference between marine coral and fossilized stony coral.

Barefoot acquires his coral from either Marine Bio or a similar company from Okinawa. The process used to remove what he is calling dead stony coral from a marine bed, is through dredging and vacuuming. A large ship hovers over a coral reef while dredging and vacuuming up what is called sea floor coral rubble. Contained within this "rubble" are coral larvae which have settled to the ocean floor along with a litany of other organisms vital to the health of the nearby coral reef. From this process, the free floating particles (sediment) of sea life and rubble cause a tremendous turbidity in the water. This sediment covers the living coral reef choking off life-giving oxygen and light.

Because all marine coral, including Mr. Barefoot's, is from our current polluted oceans, it may contain high levels of mercury, lead and other heavy metals in addition to all the toxic chemicals currently being dumped in our oceans including DDT. In order to remove these contaminant's, marine coral is usually heated to over 1,200 degrees Fahrenheit. This process has been known to change the crystalline structure of minerals, thereby causing a loss in their effectiveness.

Barefoot claims his marine coral has a calcium-to-magnesium ratio of 2 to 1. What he is NOT telling us is the magnesium is most likely either added into his product at the processing plant or is mixed with Dolomite. Since the human body has a calcium-to-magnesium ratio of 48 to 1 and fossilized stony coral minerals have a ratio of 43 to 48 to 1, I question why anyone would want to synthetically add a known calcium antagonist at a level that circumvents and supercedes nature? And yet many companies are adding magnesium to their isolated calcium supplements at a 2:1 ratio. Why? Because they have been told it's "ideal." What they don't know is how this "ideal' ratio came to be.

In 1945 or thereabouts, vitamin companies were trying to get people to take more of their isolated limestone-derived calcium. Fortunately, when you take an isolated calcium, the body will reach a level where it can't take any more. At a certain saturation point, the consumer of this isolated calcium will become constipated. In order to remedy this natural occurrence, the formulators, at the time, added magnesium, a known antagonist to calcium. This stopped the constipating side effect of taking an overdose of isolated synthetic calcium. Once they reached a calcium-to -magnesium ratio of 2:1, constipation stopped. Recommending a calcium-to-magnesium ratio of 2:1 is only for the benefit of the company selling their "junk" product and is ludicrous, to say the least.

Therefore, there are three major reasons not to consume or buy marine coral:

1. Extracting marine coral destroys our delicate marine eco-system.

2. Commercial marine coral must be heated to be purified of toxic chemicals and heavy ocean metals. This process alters the structure of minerals contained therein.

3. Changing the balance of calcium to magnesium, as found in nature, is not wise and is unhealthy.

To the contrary, fossilized stony coral is harvested from land quarries. This coral has been out of the ocean for thousands, if not, millions of years. It is the water that has passed through fossilized stony coral that the Okinawans drink on a regular basis. This has contributed to the people of Okinawa living a long and healthy life, not marine coral.

Please don't just take my word for it. Here are a few quotes from other experts on marine coral minerals:

"Clearing large areas of coral rubble would certainly impact reef ecosystems, not only because coral larvae settle on rubble, but also because there are countless organisms that inhabit spaces within corals and rubble. Removing coral rubble from areas where the underlying sediment is unsuitable for larval settlement would certainly inhibit new corals from attaching and growing. I can't conceive that this practice would not negatively affect the long-term integrity of most coral reef ecosystems."

Michael Dowgiallo, Ph.D.
Coral Reef Program Coordinator
National Oceanic and Atmospheric Administration

"This activity (dredging and vacuuming) can harm the corals and the organisms that live in and on them in two ways: First, the dredging and vacuuming activity lessens and stirs up large amounts of sediment in the water. This sediment smothers and kills corals and other organisms in the ecosystem. An additional adverse effect of stirring up the sediment with dredging

and vacuuming activities is that the turbidity of the water prevents light from reaching the corals and the corals need light in order to survive and grow. Secondly, reefs are formed (and grow) by a process of bioaccretion (cementing together) of carbonate particles that have been removed from the living coral by bioerosion. If all the sediment that has accumulated around a reef (especially that which has already begun to solidify and hence does not risk smothering the reef) is scraped away, the reef loses its capacity to grow and keep up with the sea-level rise. Failure to grow and keep pace with sea-level rise would mean the demise of the reef because the corals need light and thus must be near the surface in order to live."

Marjorie L. Reaka-Kudla, Ph.D.
Professor, Department of Biology
The University of Maryland

"I would have an extremely hard time believing anyone who suggests that this activity (dredging and vacuuming) would be benign. Dead corals may act as a substrate for new colonizers, so vacuuming up even dead corals or coral fragments might hinder the ability of reefs to recover in the future. Even if dredging & vacuuming is occurring where there are no (or few) corals, there are certainly other organisms being directly affected, such as sea whips and anemones, many of which also provide structure to benthic habitats and thus provide essential ecosystem functions (such as hiding places for juvenile fish and substrate for various life stages of benthic invertebrates)."

Clark Field, Ph.D.
School of Aquatic and Fisheries Sciences

There seems to be much confusion relative to the many different forms of calcium, their bioavailability and bio-efficiency. Chemists, "doctors" and so-called "nutritionists" are frantically being employed to validate and legitimize any and all calcium products claiming to be the "best" form and healthiest available.

Perhaps a brief lesson in calcium chemistry and history will clear up any ambiguities one may have concerning this subject.

Chemistry

Calcium is a major essential mineral and the most abundant mineral in the body. It has an atomic mass or molecular weight of 40.08. Although above-the-sea fossilized stony coral minerals are NOT just calcium, but part of a whole food mineral complex, the calcium contained therein is in a carbonate form chemically known as CaCO3. Above-the-sea fossilized stony coral calcium differs from all other calcium carbonate forms because it was created by an invertebrate making it organic and it becomes 98 to 100% ionic when dissolved in solution. Ionic means the dissociation of a substance in solution into its constituent ions, and ions are positively or negatively charged particles. Since all minerals must be ionized in order to be absorbed, above-the-sea fossilized stony coral calcium is actually ionic calcium carbonate, not just carbonate and is therefore much more bio-available and bio-efficient than all other forms of calcium.

Let's just look at a few of the other "popular" forms of calcium and their percentage of calcium per 100 milligrams of compound:

1. Calcium Gluconate is 9% calcium and is commonly found in corn sugar extracted calcium.
2. Calcium Lactate is 13% calcium and is commonly found in dairy products.
3. Calcium Citrate is 21% calcium and is commonly made by heating and mixing limestone with citric acid.
4. Calcium Chloride is 27% calcium and is commonly found in sea brine and made by Dow chemical.
5. Calcium Phosphate is 31% calcium and is commonly found in cow and pig bone.
6. Calcium Carbonate is 40% calcium and is commonly found in inorganic limestone, organic fossilized stony coral and oyster shell.

The total molecular weight of calcium carbonate compound

which has other elements in it, is approximately 100 milligrams (mg), of which 40% is pure elemental calcium. This means for every 1,000 mg of calcium carbonate 40% or 400 mg is pure calcium. Scientists tell us that only 10% of calcium is absorbed from calcium carbonate. Therefore, of the 400 mg of pure elemental calcium from 1,000 mg of calcium carbonate, only 40 mg (10%) becomes absorbable calcium. However, this is not the case with calcium carbonate found in above-the-sea fossilized stony coral minerals. Why? Because above-the-sea fossilized stony coral calcium becomes ionic in solution.

Ionic Calcium (Ca++) is commonly found in above-the-sea fossilized stony coral and has a molecular weight of 40.08. Remember, for every 1,000 mg of calcium carbonate 40% or 400 mg is pure elemental calcium. However, scientists tell us that 98 to 100% of ionic calcium is absorbable as opposed to calcium citrate, which has the next highest absorbability at 50%. Because the 400 mg of pure elemental calcium from 1000 mg of calcium carbonate as found in above-the-sea fossilized stony coral is organic and IONIC, a minimum of 392 mg (98%) becomes absorbable calcium. That's 392 milligrams per 1,000!

Regardless of what the hypesters are telling you, it is clearly obvious, of all the calcium available on the market today, calcium carbonate has the greatest percentage of pure elemental calcium (40%). And of all the calcium carbonates available, above the sea fossilized stony coral minerals, being organic and ionic, has the greatest absorbability (98% min.). I have formulated a whole-food mineral complex from above the sea, fossilized stony coral. I call it **Coral Blend**. It is part of my LifePack System®. See QCI Products® Index E- *Resources*.

History

Finally, as a matter of history, one of the healthiest societies on earth is the Okinawans from Japan. They also have one of the largest populations of centurions in the world. It is a known fact they consume vast amounts of above-the-sea fossilized stony coral minerals in their water. They also till these minerals into their soil and feed them to their livestock. The Okinawans do not consume supplemental calcium gluconate, calcium lactate, calcium citrate, calcium chloride, calcium phosphate or calcium carbonate from inorganic ground-up limestone or oyster shell. They simply drink a highly fossilized stony coral mineral water from above the sea and eat foods they have been mineralized with the same. The Okinawans do not take isolated processed minerals. Therefore, for optimum health and longevity neither should we. The answer is quite clear: Above-the-sea fossilized stony coral minerals provide a whole-food mineral complex along with pure ionic 98% bio-available calcium. There is no better mineral complex, period.

Stable 'O' (Part of the LifePack System)

Stable 'O' is a liquid concentrate of electrolytes of oxygen, which become available to the body in molecular form when ingested. Electrolytes are any substances that dissolve in water and conduct electricity. The unique sodium chlorite formulation in Stable 'O' stabilizes millions of oxygen molecules in solution with electrons. The molecular oxygen is released upon contact with stomach acid. **Stable 'O'** helps to provide molecular oxygen to the bloodstream. Secondly, it may kill anaerobic bacteria, viruses and parasites on contact, without harming other tissues or friendly aerobic bacteria.

The key to how **Stable 'O'** works so effectively is the specific "enzyme-enhancing" qualities of the chlorite ion. Chemically speaking, the chlorite ion is a molecule of chlorine and oxygen with a strong negative charge. The same molecule with a neutral charge is chlorine dioxide, an even more potent oxidizer and super-effective killer of microbes.

When you dilute Stable 'O' in water, the highly alkaline pH of the Stable 'O' is rapidly lowered from a pH of 12 to about a pH of 8. This lowering of the pH in water causes the separation of chlorite ions and stabilized oxygen molecules (02) from the sodium atoms. Tiny amounts of chlorine dioxide are also released. When Stable 'O' is swallowed with water, it typically encounters stomach acid with a normal pH of 3 to 4. The reaction created in the stomach environment is even stronger and generates more molecular oxygen and more chlorite and chlorine dioxide destroying viruses, bacteria and protozoa.

The amount of sodium in the end product is negligible. Cells, particularly leukocytes, use the chlorite to increase the efficiency of peroxidase enzymes. When used as directed **Stable 'O'** combines with the natural body functions and immune responses to become an effective nutrient with virtually no toxic side effects.

The reason **Stable 'O'** works so well is our bodies are mostly water and bodily fluids account for most of our body weight. Human blood plasma closely resembles primeval sea-water. (If you have ever tasted your own tears, they are "salty" like the sea). The red blood cell carries 99% of our oxygen needs, while the plasma feeds both food and a very important 1% of oxygen needs to the cells. If the red blood cells are oxygen deficient, it is possible for them to pick up the oxygen from the plasma. Cells always get their oxygen from the plasma. Oxygen goes from the lungs to the red blood cells, into the plasma, then into the cells.

With **Stable 'O'** it is possible to raise the plasma oxygen level, thus increase the cellular oxygenation level and provide the red cell a buffer against carbon monoxide. Our bodies should be 75% water, 40% of that inside the cell walls. Ideally, our body water should be saturated with dissolved oxygen. By drinking *charged distilled water with **Stable 'O'** it helps reverse dehydration, fight free-radical damage, reverse tissue hypoxia, increase nutrient absorption and cleanse and remove toxins.

What Is Medical Grade Ozone? - Oxygen 03

Ozone is an elemental form of oxygen (02) occurring naturally in the Earth's atmosphere. Ozone (03) is created in nature when ultraviolet rays from the sun pass through oxygen atoms in the atmosphere causing the oxygen atoms to temporarily recombine in groups of three, hence the chemical designation 03. After lightning or a thunderstorm, the air usually has a fresh clean smell due to the small amounts of ozone created by the storm. Ozone is also produced commercially in ozone generators, which send an electrical discharge through specially designed condensers containing oxygen.

In 1924, Otto Warburg, M.D., discovered that cancer cells could not survive in an oxygen-rich environment, in fact, he won the Nobel Prize for his work in this field. Since that time, we have learned that most anaerobic pathogens, bacteria and viruses die in an oxygen-rich environment.

In wasn't until 1932, however, that the medical use of ozone was seriously studied by the scientific community. Ozonated water was used as a disinfectant by Dr. E.A. Fisch, a German dentist. One of his patients was the surgeon Erwin Payr, M.D., who immediately saw the possibilities of ozone in medical therapy. Dr. Payr, along with the French physician Paul Abort, was the first medical doctor to apply ozone gas through rectal insufflation to treat mucous colitis and fistulae. In 1945, Dr. Payr pioneered the method of injecting ozone intravenously for treatment of circulatory disturbances. Additionally, it is used by most of Europe to kill all bacteria in public drinking water.

The first physicians to treat cancer with ozone were Drs. PG Seeger, A. Varro and H. Werkmeister. During the next twenty years, hundreds of German physicians began using ozone in their practices to treat a wide variety of dis-eases through a number of applications. Horst Keif, M.D. is believed to have been the first doctor to use ozone therapy to successfully treat patients infected with the human immuno-deficiency virus (HIV).

Today, some eight thousand health practitioners, including chiropractors, naturopaths, homeopaths and medics in Germany use ozone in their practices. It is estimated that over twenty million ozone treatments have been given to over two million patients in Germany alone over the last forty years. While considered by our AMA-controlled and FDA enforced health care system to be experimental and therefore illegal, except for water purification, the medical uses of ozone are well known, well established and well documented outside of the restrictive confines of the United

States. The reason for this restriction is quiet obvious: Ozone is inexpensive and very effective. On the other hand, drugs are a billion dollar a year enterprise sanctioned by the financially vested AMA and FDA.

Ozone is gaining momentum as a preferred treatment and has proven effective in treating thirty-five or more dis-eases with a great degree of success. Ozone is totally non-toxic when used appropriately and has proven very effective against life-threatening challenges such as cancer, AIDS and AIDS-related infections. The list of treatable dis-eases using medical grade ozone continues to grow. In countries where socialized medicine is the norm and because it is inexpensive, ozone is openly used as a tool in the battle against dis-ease.

Personally, I prefer not to accept students for my wellness educational classes, unless they incorporate oxygen therapies, especially ozone. Although ozone can be legally only used for water purification in the United States and for medical conditions in certain states, Nevada being one, it's nice to have a machine in case you are outside the United States where ozone is used to cure dis-ease. I not only recommend an ozone machine for most conditions, I recommend it for everyone as one way to prevent illness and acquire optimum health.

In spite of our prejudicial and restrictive health laws, many individuals today are purchasing ozone equipment to self-treat in the privacy of their own homes. The use of ozone equipment for self-treatment is relatively simple, where almost anyone can perform the easy, low-cost treatment at home.

Ozone is made up of three atoms of oxygen, which is highly unstable and is quick to react with other substances. Ozone has a very short life and returns quickly to its two-atom state, (02 - oxygen). In commercial and medical applications ozone has to be generated on-site and used immediately for its full effect.

Medical grade ozone or oxygen therapy is truly a major key to one's health success, as it purifies the blood; gets rid of bacteria, viral infections, pathogens and pyrogens, boosts the immune response of the body and oxygenates at the cellular level.

I predict ozone will prove to be one of the most important modalities used to eliminate dis-ease in the next generation. That is of course if we are free to make our own health choices. The only machine I currently recommend is the **Oxy-Charge® Water Purification System**. (See Index E-*Resources* at the back of the book.)

ProDigestives: (Part of the LifePack System®)

There is convincing evidence derived from the works of Drs. John Beard, Francis Pottinger, Jr., Weston Price, Edward Howell and William Donald Kelly that the destruction of enzymes in the cooking and processing of food is, perhaps, the most significant factor in chronic and degenerative diseases in both humans and animals.

It begins with a phenomenon known as digestive leukocytosis. "Leukocytosis" is a pathological condition defined in Dorlands Illustrated Medical Dictionary as "a transient increase in the number of leukocytes in the blood, resulting from various causes, such as hemorrhage, fever, infection, inflammation, etc."

Leukocytosis was first discovered in 1846. At first, it was considered normal because everyone who was tested had it. Paul Kautchakoff, M.D. later found that leukocytosis was not normal. In fact, the major cause of leukocytosis was discovered to be the eating of cooked food. An entire category of leukocytosis was classified as "digestive leukocytosis," that is, the elevation of the white blood cell level in response to the lack of enzymes in cooked food in the intestine. It is pathological because the pancreas was never intended to provide 100% of the digestive enzymes needed as is the case when eating cooked food.

Dr. Kautchakoff divided his findings into four accepted classifications according to the severity of the pathological reaction in the blood:

1. Raw food produced no increase in the white blood cells.
2. Commonly cooked food caused leukocytosis.
3. Pressure cooked food caused even greater leukocytosis.

4. Man-made, processed and refined foods, such as carbonated beverages, alcohol, vinegar, white sugar, flour, and other foods, caused severe leukocytosis. Cooked, smoked and salted animal flesh brought on violent leukocytosis consistent with ingesting poison. However, microwaving any food or liquid (especially baby formulae) causes extreme and violent molecular damage and leukocytosis, consistent with ingesting a highly toxic poison.

This phenomenon occurs after eating cooked food, since prolonged heat above 118 degrees Fahrenheit destroys enzymes in food. Three minutes in boiling water destroys the enzymes; pasteurization destroys 80% to 95%; and baking, frying, broiling, stewing and canning destroys 100%. Nature designed food with sufficient enzymes within it to digest that food when it is ingested. When enzymes are destroyed by cooking or other processing, ingesting that food triggers the body's immune system, and it responds with leukocytosis.

Many health professionals are coming to the conclusion that this syndrome is an abusive scenario that puts significant stress on the pancreas, accounting for the enlarged pancreases of people in industrialized societies, and contributing to blood sugar problems such as diabetes and hypoglycemia, as well as the proliferation of obesity, cancer and other chronic degenerative disease.

What Is An Enzyme?

The medical dictionary defines an enzyme as "a protein produced in a cell capable of greatly accelerating, by its catalytic action, the chemical reaction of a substance (the substrate) for which it is specific."

This is the standard definition taught in medical school. But more significantly, enzymes are the body's workers. Enzymes operate on a biological and chemical level, perhaps even the energetic level, and although vitamins, minerals, hormones, proteins and other substances are essential to life, it is enzymes that perform the work and utilize these substances in restoring, repairing and maintaining health and life. Enzymes are the closest thing to what can be described as a "life force." Without them, life would not exist. In fact, when enzyme levels fall below a given level in any living system, life ceases.

Attempts to produce synthetic enzymes have failed. Science has identified over 80,000 different enzyme systems, and it is suspected that there may be hundreds of thousands, even millions of different types of enzymes. Yet although science endeavors to know what certain types of enzymes are made of, no one has yet been able to directly measure or take a picture of one.

What Do Enzymes Do?

Enzymes build, orchestrate and unify the physical expression we call "life." They seem to know precisely what to do and when to do it. They "assemble" molecules during their formative growth and they take molecules apart when individual cells are fractured. Enzymes create and modulate every system in the body. Enzymes help assemble a human body from a one-cell organism into a 50 to 70 trillion-cell life form. Enzymes are involved in repairing the body when it is damaged; they transport, use, and transform oxygen molecules and every other nutrient the body needs; they break down metabolic waste and the by-products of cells; they quench free radicals, and they split off unwanted molecules from nutrients, adding necessary ones. The physical existence of every human being and the existence of all other living organisms are totally dependent upon the ability of enzymes to do their job.

Cells can even create "customized" enzymes for specific purposes. For example, prior to 1947 cyanocobalamin, the commercial form of vitamin B-12, did not exist, yet the body is usually able to custom manufacture an enzyme to split off the cyanide molecule from the cobalamin which was added in the manufacturing process to stabilize the product and increase shelf life.

Unless the appropriate enzyme is created and removes the cyanide, cyanocobalamin is biologically inert in the body. There have been documented cases where infants have been harmed or worse from receiving B-12 (cyanocobalamin) shots because the infant's body lacked the ability to make the appropriate enzyme to split the cyanide molecule off. The result was cyanide poisoning.

Enzymes do things that in a laboratory require up to 2,000 degrees Fahrenheit to duplicate. Enzymes are present in raw food in direct proportion to the proteins, complex carbohydrates, lipids and other food constituents that exist there. Food enzymes break food down so its constituents are small enough to pass into the blood or lymph system, enabling the body to effectively utilize them.

Eating cooked or manufactured food forces the body to call upon the immune system to donate enzymes in the digestive process, a process nature did not intend the immune system to participate in habitually. It was meant to function as a back up. But when it is chronically called upon to fulfill this role, it creates a stress upon the body that contributes to premature aging and a pathological enlargement of the pancreas, with chronic depletion of metabolic enzymes from white blood cells. The immune system's primary defense mechanism in the blood is the secretion of appropriate enzymes by specialized blood cells that disassemble foreign substances that threaten the local ecology. When food is eaten that does not have sufficient enzyme levels within it to accomplish digestion, the condition such an insufficiency creates and triggers the immune response.

The sleepy, lethargic feeling many people get after eating is a symptom of the depletion the body suffers in this process. There are simply not enough metabolic enzymes left in the blood after eating to run the body at pre-meal levels. The depletion results in a loss of energy taken from operating the body to digest what was ingested.

How Does the Body Get Its Enzymes?

We are born with the ability to produce our own metabolic enzymes, an ability that appears to be limited. Dr. Edward Howell, a famous enzyme researcher, equated it to being born with an enzyme bank account that is finite. We have an enzyme capability designed to last our entire lifetime. How often we make withdrawals and how big they are determines our enzyme "balance," and that balance affects the level of health we enjoy. It may also affect the length of our life span. When we constantly write checks out of our enzyme account without making deposits, we end up running our body on deficits. These deficits inevitably show up as problems in the body. Those who write lots of checks and make few deposits, sooner or later are likely to end up with degenerative and other disease.

Of course, we also get enzymes from outside sources other than food, such as those made by a variety of intestinal bacteria. An example of this is lactose. Lactose intolerance is a deficiency in ß-galactosidase, a lactose-digesting enzyme made by certain strains of acidophilus bacteria living in the intestine. If the bacteria in the intestine does not exist in sufficient numbers to produce enough ß-galactosidase, an intolerance to dairy products may result.

Due to modern food processing, packaging and preparations that make longer shelf life possible, prepared food is essentially dead relative to human and animal nutritional needs. Over 80% of the average American diet today is comprised of processed and fast food. Food is even irradiated, without being labeled to give consumers an informed choice, thereby destroying enzymes without cooking - and without us knowing it.

Studies Show

Enzyme-rich raw food diets and their positive effect on various diseased conditions in both humans and animals have been well documented throughout the world. The first major scientific paper on enzymes was published by Dr. John Beard in the early 1900s. Dr. Beard was an embryologist who successfully treated cancer using a pancreatic extract, which he described in his book, *The Enzyme Treatment of Cancer and Its Scientific Basis.*

In the early 1930s, and over the following 25 years, Francis M. Pottinger, Jr., M.D. and Weston Price, D.D.S. conducted studies on cats using two diets. One diet consisted of two-thirds raw meat, one-third raw milk and cod liver oil. The second diet consisted of two-thirds cooked meat, one-third raw milk and cod liver oil. Studies revealed the following:

Multiple generations of cats on the *raw* meat diet were healthy. They had adequate nasal cavities, excellent tissue tone, good fur with little shedding, and no facial deformities. The calcium and phosphorous content of their bones was consistent. Their internal organs developed and functioned normally. Throughout their lifespan they were resistant to infections, fleas and other parasites. They were free of allergies and miscarriages were rare. Litters averaged five kittens, with mothers experiencing no difficulty nursing.

Multiple generations of cats on the *cooked* meat diet were not so healthy. They had many variations in facial bone and dental structure. Their long bones tended to be increased in length and smaller in diameter, showing less calcium.

In the third generation, some of the bones were as soft as rubber. Other indications were heart problems; nearsightedness and farsightedness; under activity or inflammation of the thyroid gland; infections of the kidney, liver, testes, ovaries and the bladder, arthritis and inflammation of the joints and inflammation of the nervous system with paralysis and meningitis. Infections of the bone showed up regularly, often appearing to be the cause of death. By the time the third generation was born, the cats were so physiologically bankrupt that none survived more than six months.

Cats on the cooked meat diet were more irritable. There was evidence of role reversal, with female cats becoming the aggressors and male cats becoming docile and passive, either acting perverted or showing no interest in sex. Some females were dangerous to handle. Increasingly abnormal activities occurred between the same sexes. Vermin and intestinal parasites were rampant. Skin lesions and allergies were frequent and progressively worse from one generation to the next. Pneumonia and empyema (accumulation of pus) were principal causes of death in adults, with diarrhea, followed by pneumonia, the cause of death in kittens.

Females frequently had ovarian atrophy and uterine congestion. Males often failed to have active sperm development. Spontaneous abortion in pregnant females was about 25% in the first deficient generation, increasing to about 70% in the second generation. Deliveries were difficult, and many females died in labor. The mortality rate of kittens was high. Some mothers failed to lactate. Many failed to become pregnant, and those that did had difficulties. The average weight of kittens was 16% less than those born to mothers raised on a raw meat diet.

When cats of the cooked meat-fed first and second generation groups were returned to a raw meat diet, it took about four generations to recover a state of normal health. Improvement in resistance to disease was noted in the second generation, with allergic manifestations persisting into the third generation. By the fourth generation, most of the severe deficiency symptoms disappeared, but seldom completely. Once a female cat was subjected to a deficient diet for a period of 12 to 18 months, her reproductive efficiency was so reduced that she was *never* able to give birth to normal kittens. Only when the kittens were put on an optimum diet did a gradual reversal and regeneration take place.

Also in the 1930s, Drs. Ernst Freund and Max Wolf identified in the blood, a "normal substance" as an enzyme that decomposes fatty materials and proteins. Later Dr. Wolf discovered enzymes could in fact, destroy cancer cells and tumors.

Although it was Dr. John Beard in 1910 who contributed to our knowledge of enzymes, on April 15, 1940, in the *Journal of the American Association for Medico-Physical Research*, Dr. Edward Howell was formally recognized as the discoverer of the vital role of enzymes in human nutrition.

Dr. Howell pioneered more than 50 years of research and scientific experimentation with overwhelming evidence indicating that the primary cause of degenerative disease in humans is enzyme deficiencies exacerbated by enzyme-deficient mothers passing on genetic deficiencies to their offspring. Numerous studies have documented that when captive or domesticated animals are fed diets similar to human diets common to industrialized nations, they develop diseases similar or identical to human beings.

In 1965, independent of Dr. Beard's work, William Donald Kelly, D.D.S., discovered a link in cancer and pancreatic enzyme deficiency. Dr. Kelly is a metabolic researcher and creator of four holistic medical concepts considered the most advanced in their field: *Non Specific Metabolic Therapy, The Science of Optimum Health and Metabolic Ecology and Metabolic Typing*. He not only has treated over 33,000 patients, he started his career by healing himself of pancreatic and liver cancer using natural healing and pancreatic enzymes. His booklet *One Answer to Cancer* and book *Cancer: Curing the Incurable* are best sellers and priceless.

Dr. Kelly proved that the presence of a malignant tumor in an individual indicates that he has a *deficiency* of active pancreatic enzymes. In addition to detoxification and optimum nutrition, Dr. Kelly helped develop effective proteolytic (protein digesting) enzymes, specifically pancreatin, to help the body destroy cancer cells. Dr. Kelly believes the direct cause of cancer is the changing of an ectopic germ cell into an ectopic trophoblastic cell from not having enough pancreatic enzymes. In light of what we know happens to our pancreatic enzymes, due to cooked food, poor nutrition and environmental pollution, Dr. Kelly's theory is quite plausible.

Digestion Starts in the Mouth

Teeth break up food and mix it with saliva. Saliva in turn helps to form a bolus and protects the pharyngeal and esophageal mucosa, primarily with secretory IgA antibodies. Saliva also helps to re-mineralize the teeth with calcium salts. (This is one reason why I recommend brushing your teeth at night, just before bed, with CoralWhite® tooth treatment). The enzymes lingual lipase, salivary amylase and ptyalin, initiate fat and starch digestion.

Stomach

From the mouth, our food travels to the stomach. The stomach mechanically churns food, breaks up and emulsifies fats and exposes molecules to additional enzymes. In doing this, it produces 1 to 2 liters of gastric juices per day.

Gastric juice has several components:

1. Hydrochloric acid is secreted by the parietal cells. It activates pepsinogen to convert to pepsin and renders some minerals, such as calcium and iron, more absorbable. Stomach acid prevents bacterial overgrowth by creating an essentially sterile environment. One exception is Helicobacter pylori which have been linked to stomach ulcers.

2. Mucus forms an acid and pepsin-resistant coating of the stomach lining.

3. Gastric lipase begins the hydrolysis of fats.

Small Intestine

Most digestion and absorption takes place in the small intestine and is mediated by pancreatic enzymes and bile. The process involves several steps:

1. Secretion of pancreatic juices which is controlled by the vagus nerve and the duodenal hormones secretin and cholecystokinin. Hormone production, in turn, is simulated by the presence of fat, protein and acid chyme.

2. Amylase splits starch to maltose.

3. Secretion of bicarbonate which neutralizes stomach acid.

4. The proteases typsinogen, chymotrypsinogen and procarboxypeptidase are activated to trypsin, chymotrypsin and carboxypeptidase. These enzymes digest proteins to oligopeptides and amino acids.

5. Lipase hydrolyzes diglycerides and triglycerides, producing long-chain fatty acids.

6. Bile secreted by the liver is stored in the gall bladder. Bile salts solubilize and emulsify fats, enabling enzymatic hydrolysis.

The crypts of Lieberkuhn of the intestinal mucosa also produce immunoglobulins, which protect the gastric mucosa from microbes and small amounts of digestive enzymes such as peptidase and disaccharidases.

Large Intestine

A primary role of the large intestine is the absorption of water and electrolytes. The large intestine also provides an environment for microbial fermentation of soluble fiber, starch and undigested carbohydrates.

Anaerobic colonic fermentation results in the production of short-chain fatty acids (SCFAs), the main energy source for colonic epithelial cells. It is these SCFAs, in combination with amines derived from protein degradation, that provide buffering and create the slightly acidic pH of fecal matter.

More Food For Thought!

The benefits of a raw food diet are evidenced by the classic Arctic Eskimo diet of 80% saturated fat consisting primarily of raw fat and raw meat. Essentially, these people were disease-free. Their sled dogs ate the same diet and were also disease-free. A study of over 3,000 of these people revealed that none of them had high cholesterol, heart disease, arteriosclerosis or high blood pressure. Only one out of 3,000 was slightly overweight. This 80% saturated fat diet is almost twice that of the average American diet, and more than three times what the American Heart Association says is safe, calling into question the presumptions made by traditional science as to the causes and source of these diseases.

In the wild, animals on their natural diets are relatively free of degenerative disease. When animals are put on human diets, two things consistently occur: The animal's life span is cut by as much as 85%, and their weight increases by as much as 64%. Animals on human-style diets have lower brain weights than their wild counterparts.

Animals in captivity, such as laboratory mice, have a brain weight almost half that of their wild counterparts. Brain weight between animals on enzyme-deficient diets and the same species on natural diets consistently differs. Dr. Howell noted that after assessing more than 50 reports in published scientific literature, when rats are given a "factory diet," body weight goes up and brain weight goes down. These deficient laboratory animals on "factory food" are considered healthy by the scientific community using them, and results deduced from their experiments form the backbone of the laboratory development of pharmaceutical drugs and medicine for human use.

How Can You Reduce Your Body's Enzyme Depletion?

More people are eating raw food today and buying organic produce, while aware of the hazards of chemical and other tampering with the food chain. But modern life, worldly schedules and restaurant patronage do not always support a raw food diet. Fortunately, and largely through the research of the aforementioned doctors, plant and animal digestive and proteolytic (protein digesting) enzymes are now available to help compensate for the lack of food enzymes in cooked food.

Those enzymes that breakdown starches, proteins, fats and cellulose are amylase, protease, lipase and cellulase. The enzymes that breakdown protein and cancer cells are proteolytic.

Proteolytic enzymes are found in plant food such as pineapple and papaya as bromelain and papain, animal stomach extract as pepsin and pancreatic extract such as pancreatin, trypsinogen and chymotrypsinogen. Taking these enzymes when you eat cooked or processed food not only provides support for your body's natural digestion of starches, proteins, fats and cellulose, but they help in the routine digestion of cancer cells. They supplement what your body would normally obtain through eating enzyme-rich raw food.

Plant digestive enzymes work in both the stomach and the intestine. In addition to helping alleviate the effects of an enzyme-deficient diet, plant digestive enzymes have the ability to operate through a broad pH range within the temperature range of the digestive system, and they are not harmed by stomach acid. They help prevent your enzyme reserves from being depleted when these reserves are called upon to do digestive work that nature's design never intended.

In contrast, animal digestive and proteolytic (protein

digesting) enzymes are composed of pepsin, pancreatin, trypsinogen and chymotrpsinogen. Although at one time, they were thought to be destroyed in the stomach due to an acid pH, in a recent Russian study, it was found that pancreatic enzymes are not destroyed by stomach acid. Therefore, enteric coating of enzymes is not necessary, especially because on their unreliable absorption.

All instances of dis-ease, ill health, aging and injury involve tissue damage at the cellular level. These cellular events may be in progress for months or years before they actually manifest as a problem, but they always reflect a breach of cellular integrity that ends up as a physical problem. The common cause of this cellular damage is oxidative stress known as free-radical pathology.

Free radical damage is involved with every degenerative dis-ease known. Over 6,000 studies reveal free-radical induced tissue damage as the common link. Unabsorbed oxygen is the most common source of free radicals in the body. Antioxidant enzymes are the body's defense system with no other purpose but to protect the body against the effects of free radical damage. Antioxidant enzymes are complex molecules made up of protein chains called peptides and trace minerals.

What is in QCI's ProDigestives?

Because of accepted industry standards, based on *misinformation*, there has never been a proteolytic and digestive enzyme in one capsule or tablet. Not until now.

I have revolutionized the nutrition industry by being the *first* manufacturer to produce an all-inclusive digestive enzyme.

After 30 years of trial and error, I have developed the *only* proteolytic and digestive enzyme on the market today. It contains the following ingredients:

1. Papain
2. Pancreatin
3. Bromelain
4. Lipase
5. Chymotrypsin
6. Amylase
7. Protease
8. Trypsin
9. Invertase
10. Glucoamylase
11. Nattokinase
12. Cellulase
13. Serrapeptase

Remember, the healthiest people in the world eat mostly

raw food. This allows their body to produce more metabolic enzymes for healing and repairing. Americans eat mostly cooked food. This depletes their metabolic enzymes to make more digestive enzymes. By taking proteolytic and digestive enzymes, we allow our body to make the metabolic ones. We must take enzymes that combine digestive and proteolytic.

Essential Fatty Acids: The Scientific Basis for Essential Fatty Acid Supplementation Using Organic Flaxseed Oil. *"The red blood cells in the lungs give up carbon dioxide and take on oxygen. They are then transported to the cell site via the blood vessels, where they release their oxygen into the plasma. This released oxygen is attracted to the cells by the resonance of the pi-electron oxidation-enhancing fatty acids. Otherwise, oxygen cannot work its way into the cell. Electron rich fatty acids play the decisive role in respiratory enzymes, which are the basis of cell oxidation."* **- Ed McCabe, Oxygen Therapies**

In spite of the wisdom of Ed McCabe, for whatever reason, fats and oils have developed a *bad* reputation. Perhaps it is because we don't know the difference between natural, healthy fats and oils as opposed to unhealthy, man-made, unnatural, toxic fats and oils? Again, we are being mislead into believing intentional corporate misinformation on fats and oils, the latest being so-called, "Heart-Healthy Oil" from our fast "food" restaurants. (See discussion under Trans Fatty Acids below).

Lipids

Fats and oils belong to a group of biological substances called lipids. Lipids are biological chemicals that do not dissolve in water. Just pour some vinegar in a glass and then some olive oil over it. If you don't aggressively shake it, the oil and vinegar won't temporarily mix. However, once you have mixed the two, if you let it stand for a minute or so, the vinegar and oil will again separate. Without the addition of a surfactant, the oil will not dissolve in a water-base solution. All lipids act the same way.

Fats and Oils Are the Same

Oil is simply fat in liquid form and fat is simply oil, which is solid at room temperature. As affirmed by Ed McCabe, nutritional dietary fat plays a very important role in our health, vitality and longevity. Fats are vital for all growth processing, renewal of cells, brain and nerve functions, even for the sensory organs - eyes and ears, and for the body's adjustment to heat, cold and quick temperature changes.

Although vegetarian diets typically provide 10% of the calories from fat, many health organizations recommend we consume 20% of our calories from fat. In fact, restricting one's caloric intake to 10% fat may have a beneficial therapeutic effect, but it is too deficient to be an optimum preventive diet, a diet that can build and maintain health and prevent disease. Even though some people need more dietary fat than others do and at certain times of the year, the typical American diet provides 30 to 40% of its calories from fat, and it shows.

If you doubt me, just look at our pre-teen and teenage children. Girls develop breasts at 7 years old and boys have a beer belly before they know what beer is. (In all fairness, estrogen, zeno-estrogens and estrogen mimickers also play a part in pre-puberty breast development). Treating obesity in children and adults is a billion-dollar industry and growing. In addition, an unhealthy high-fat diet, bad fats or not, promotes tumors, cancers, heart disease, auto immune diseases like multiple sclerosis and rheumatoid arthritis, many skin diseases, gall bladder and liver disorders and especially diabetes and other degenerative conditions.

Fats, as an energy/fuel, digest more slowly than other foods and help the body to produce body fat for insulation, for protecting the vital organs and holding them in place. Of particular importance, fats and oils are necessary for the assimilation of the fat-soluble vitamins A, D, E and K. They also serve as regulatory messengers (hormones) and structural components of cell membranes and prostaglandins. However, since the energy released in the body from fat combustion is more than twice that of other foods, (proteins and carbohydrates yield four calories per gram and fats provide nine calories per gram), it is easy to see, if we don't metabolize or "burn off" excess fats, we can easily acquire health concerns like the above, including obesity, especially when consuming animal and diary fat and mutated, toxic, hydrogenated oils.

The typical diet for overweight people is processed, junk and fast foods with heavy meat and diary intake. Don't forget the *diet* soda illusion. Just because you consume an aspartame-laden soft drink called "diet" (synthetic sweeteners like aspartame are known neuro and excito-toxins and have been linked to Parkinson's) with your cheese (fat) hamburger (fat) and french fries (fat), doesn't mean you have converted your fat meal to something healthy. You are only fooling yourself all the way to the morgue.

Metabolizing Fats and Oils

Since chewing begins to separate fats in the mouth it is imperative that we chew our food properly. With eating fast food, comes fast eating. In other words, most Americans don't chew their food properly and therefore start their health problems accordingly. As a matter of fact, most people don't really eat their food, they consume it similar to a vacuum cleaner.

The next stage in metabolizing fats and oils is in the stomach with hydrochloric acid breaking down fats and separating the lipids from foods so that the enzyme, pancreatic lipase, can begin splitting the fats. Bile from the gall bladder emulsifies fats, breaking them down further so that the above lipase and other enzymes can act on individual triglycerides (fats) to release diglycerides, monoglycerides and fatty acids. In the small intestine, fatty acids are absorbed directly through the intestinal wall. The diglycerides and monoglycerides are reconverted into triglycerides to be transported through the intestines, to the blood stream and to the liver.

Saturated, Polyunsaturated, Monounsaturated and Trans Fatty Acids

Fats or lipids are composed of building blocks called fatty acids. A fatty acid molecule consists of a long chain of carbon atoms in a carbon-carbon double bond with hydrogen atoms "attached." Healthy fat is made of three fatty acids bonded together with glycerol to form a triglyceride. Triglycerides comprise about 95 percent of the lipids in food and in our bodies. The other 5% is from phospholipids and sterols (with the exception of toxic, brown fat from hydrogenated oils or trans fats). All triglycerides have a similar structure: being composed of three fatty acids attached to a glycerol molecule.

There are three major categories of fatty acids: saturated (dense), polyunsaturated and monounsaturated (less dense). These classifications are based on the number of hydrogen atoms in the chemical structure of a given molecule of fatty acid. Although all oils contain all three types of lipids, they are usually classified according to which type predominates. As an example, peanuts are 60% monounsaturated, 22% polyunsaturated and 18% saturated. Therefore, peanut oil is classified under monounsaturated fatty acids. However, with the advent of molecular manipulation and genetic engineering, nothing is safe from cross breeding and mutation, leading to a future with intentionally confusing and changed classifications.

Saturated Fatty Acids (solid at room temperature)

Saturated fatty acids have all the hydrogen the carbon atoms can hold. Saturated fats are considered "heavy" and are usually solid at room temperature. They are more stable than the other fats, that is; they don't combine readily with oxygen and turn rancid. Saturated fatty acids raise blood cholesterol and the risk of coronary heart disease rises as blood cholesterol levels increase. Although saturated fats usually come from animal fat: fat meats, beef, veal, lamb and pork and their byproducts including milk, butter, lard etc., coconut and palm oil are two saturated vegetable oils.

The liver uses saturated fats to manufacture our cholesterol. However, excessive dietary intake of saturated fats can significantly raise the blood cholesterol level, especially the level of low-density lipoproteins (LDLs) or "bad cholesterol." The reason LDLs have been called "bad cholesterol" is because they are supposedly responsible for plaque formation in the arteries. Research has shown acid pH and inflammation has more to do with the *cause* rather than the consequence.

Palmitic, stearic and arachidonic acids (omega 6) are found primarily in saturated animal fats. If we eat too much animal fat/protein, we risk consuming too many saturated fats and omega 6 fatty acids. The key here, as in nature, is balance. Unless you have the genetic make-up from generations of eating mostly animal protein and fat, as the Eskimos of Alaska and others similar to them do, it is best to eat less saturated fat and more unsaturated.

Unsaturated Fatty Acids

Unsaturated fatty acids have at least one *unsaturated* bond - a place where hydrogen or oxygen can attach to the molecule. There are two common types of unsaturates both are discussed in detail:

Polyunsaturated Fatty Acids (liquid even at refrigerator temperatures)

Polyunsaturated fatty acids have more than one unsaturated bond. Polyunsaturated oils, which contain mostly polyunsaturated fatty acids, are liquid at room temperature and in the refrigerator. Unfortunately, they easily combine with oxygen in the air becoming rancid and therefore must be refrigerated after opening. This particular fatty acid is found primarily in flax and hemp seed, sunflower, safflower, corn, soybean and certain vegetable oils. (Note: I do NOT recommend soybean oil because the beans are all genetically engineered and the oil is highly processed). Certain fish oils are also high in polyunsaturates. Unlike the saturated fats, polyunsaturated fats contain no cholesterol and actually lower your total blood cholesterol level. However, because they do become rancid very easily, they should be refrigerated upon opening. In addition, taking large amounts of polyunsaturates may lower one's high-density lipoproteins (HDLs) or "good cholesterol." HDL cholesterol is called good because it picks up LDL from the arterial walls and transports it to the liver where it is broken down into bile acids and flushed from the body. As always, moderation and balance is the key.

Alpha-linolenic acid (omega 3 and the most important) and linoleic acid (omega 6) presence determines the sub-classification of polyunsaturates. These fatty acids are classified as essential since our body cannot manufacture them.

Monounsaturated Fatty Acids (liquid at room temperatures and solid in the refrigerator)

Monounsaturated fatty acids have only one unsaturated double bond. These fatty acids are mostly found in vegetable and nut oils such as olive, peanut, walnut, almond and canola. However, I do NOT recommend canola oil because it comes from the rapeseed plant and is used in Canada as an industrial oil. It is also genetically engineered to keep from going rancid which makes it difficult, if not impossible, to breakdown in the human body.

Monounsaturated fatty acids appear to reduce blood levels of low-density lipoproteins (LDLs) without affecting high-density lipoproteins (HDLs) or "good cholesterol."

If your olive oil does NOT become solid in the refrigerator, it may be because it was blended with irradiated, hydrogenated, corn or some other polyunsaturated oil. I suggest you take it back where you bought it and *demand* your money back. Simply buy another brand.

As cooking oils, monounsaturated fatty acids strike a balance between saturated and polyunsaturated fatty acids. They do not cause cholesterol to accumulate as do saturated fats and they do not easily become rancid, as do polyunsaturates. The degree to which oils are monounsaturated is determined by the amount of oleic acid (omega 9) present.

Trans-Fatty Acids

A trans-fatty acid is a polyunsaturate that has been transconfigured, transformed or transmutated into a synthetic fat called trans-fat through heating with temperatures reaching 450 degrees Fahrenheit. In nature, most unsaturated fatty acids are cis fatty acids. Cis means that the hydrogen atoms are on the same side of the double carbon bond. In trans fatty acids the two hydrogen atoms are on opposite sides of the double bond.

Hydrogenation is a process used to harden liquid oils into solid food "stuffs" like margarine and shortening. Hydrogenation is also used to increase shelf life of food "stuffs" from bread to cookies, ice cream to crackers. To hydrogenate an oil, it must be heated while adding pressurized hydrogen gas and either nickel, zinc, copper or another reactive metal catalyst. This process breaks the carbon double bonds and attaches the hydrogen to the molecule. This chemical hardening is done to achieve increased plasticity (stiffness) of the liquid oils at room temperature. However, this process creates a fat that interferes with metabolic absorption efficiencies and tends to congregate at adipose tissue sites.

Hydrogenated, trans fats or "brown" fats are very difficult to excrete from the body and are extremely harmful and toxic. It is the fat fast food restaurants and others use to fry their chicken, fish and french fries. Make no mistake, hydrogenated trans-fats are a mutation and are extremely unhealthy. It is NOT "Heart Healthy" as the fast "food" restaurants claim. It is still a toxic oil.

Essential Fatty Acids (EFAs)

Again, two polyunsaturated fatty acids are linoleic (LA or omega 6) and alpha-linolenic (ALA or omega 3) acids or what has been called vitamin F. They are classified as essential fatty acids because the human body is unable to manufacture them, therefore we must consume them in our diet. (Fish require only one fatty acid and plants require neither since they make their own.) LA and ALA also meet the definition of essential to wit:

1. We must have them to live and to be healthy;
2. Our bodies cannot make them from other substances;
3. Deficiency results with gradual deterioration of cells and tissues and ultimately in premature death; and
4. Increasing the intake to adequate levels reverses the signs brought about by deficiency.

Linoleic acid (LA or omega 6) is abundant in safflower (80%), sunflower (?) and corn oils (59%) in hemp (60%) and somewhat in flax seed/oil (14%). If linoleic acid (LA) is provided by foods, our cells can make other fatty acids: GLA or gamma-linoleic acid, DGLA or dihomogamma-linoleic acid and AA or arachidonic acid. However, bad fats; margarine, shortening, trans-fatty acids, hard "saturated" fats, sugar, lack of minerals; magnesium, selenium, zinc, lack of vitamins B3, B6, C, E, viruses, obesity, diabetes, aging and rare genetic mutations can all inhibit omega 6 conversion. Note: Although gamma-linoleic acid (GLA or omega 6) is present in evening primrose (9%), borage (22%) and black currant (17%) seed, these substances have predominately linoleic acid (LA).

Alpha-linoleic acid (ALA or omega 3) is abundant in flax (58%) and hemp (20%) seed. However, flax seed and oil also have oleic (OA or omega 9 at 19%) and linoleic acid (LA or omega 6 at 14%) in it. This makes flax the best oil to not only provide an abundance of omega 3, but also the balance of omega 6 and 9. If alpha-linoleic acid (ALA) is provided by foods, our cells make other fatty acids: SDA or stearidonic acid, EPA or eicospaentaenoic acid and DHA or factors that affect LA above, taking either flax or hemp seed/oil or DHA from black currant seed oil or EPA and DHA from fish oils, especially krill and northern ocean algae should be considered.

Essential Fatty Acid (EFA) molecules carry slight negative charges that cause them to repel each other. This allows them to carry oil-soluble positive charged toxins from deep within the body to the skin surface for elimination. This is also one reason why those with impure diets have dermatological conditions. Have you ever wondered why some people get skin cancer and others do not?

Those individuals who are healthy to begin with can stay out in the sun all day. Those individuals that are clinically or pre-clinically *unhealthy* end up acquiring skin cancer with minimum exposure to the sun. It is our choice of oils that make the difference in skin cancer, NOT the sun. In addition, EFAs store electric charges that produce bio-electric currents important for nerve, muscle, cell membrane functions and the transmission of messages.

EFAs help form a barrier that keeps foreign molecules, viruses, yeasts, bacteria and fungi outside the cells and keeps the cell's proteins, enzymes, genetic material and organelles inside. EFAs play many roles, they: 1. regulate oxygen use, electron transport and energy production; 2. help form red blood pigment (hemoglobin) from other substances; 3. keep fluid producing (exocrine) and hormonal producing (endocrine) glands active; 4. help make joint lubricants; 5. are precursors of derivatives like DHA, which are needed by the most active tissues - brain, retina, adrenal and testes; 6. help generate electrical currents that make our heart beat in an orderly sequence; 7. are precursors of prostaglandin's (PGs), which are hormone like substances that regulate blood pressure, platelet stickiness and kidney function; and 8. are help our immune system fight infections by enhancing peroxide production. In short, essential fatty acids are paramount to optimum health.

Although the amount needed varies with levels of one's activity and stress, nutritional state, the season and individual differences, linoleic acid (LA omega 6) has the highest daily requirement. One to two percent of our calories or 1 teaspoon (3 to 6 grams per day), will prevent signs of deficiency in most healthy adults. LA optimums are around 3 to 6 percent of calories or 1 tablespoon per day. However, vegetarians carry up to 25 percent of their body fat as linoleic acid (LA), while meat eaters carry around 10 percent. People with degenerative diseases average only about 8 percent of their body fat as linoleic acid.

Alpha-linolenic acid (ALA omega 3) optimums range between 1 to 2 teaspoons per day. By taking organic flax seed oil and using butter or extra virgin olive oil instead of margarine and substituting extra virgin olive oil for processed oils such as canola, corn, safflower, sunflower and soybean, the optimum amounts of both LA (omega 6) and ALA (omega 3) are realized at the ideal ratio of 4 to 1 respectively. (Try making a salad dressing with 3 parts olive oil and 1 part flaxseed oil for the ideal ratio.)

These two essential fatty acids form two separate lines of chemical derivatives that act as competitive regulators of our metabolism. When the two are consumed in the correct ratio, metabolic balance can be better realized with optimum health the end result. When one consistently and ignorantly consumes heavy amounts of just one of the fatty acids, essential or not, they often develop dis-eases that reflect this imbalance. By consuming trans and hydrogenated fats, it expedites the ultimate outcome of accelerated aging, sickness and finally premature death.

Flax Seeds and Oil

Flaxseed oil has been keeping civilizations of the world healthy for thousands of years. It contains the above essential fatty acids and each 100 grams contain 26 grams of protein, 14 grams of fiber, 12 grams of mucilage, 14 grams of minerals; potassium, phosphorus, magnesium, calcium, sulphur, sodium, chlorine, iron, zinc, manganese, silicon, copper, fluorine, nickel, cobalt, iodine, molybdenum, chromium and 9 grams of water.

Flaxseed oil is a highly mucilaginous food (12 g/100g) and is very beneficial for the healthy workings of the alimentary canal and elimination system. Flaxseed oil is an excellent food to prevent and remedy constipation. It also supplies complete high-quality protein. However, it contains 45 to 50% fat, so do not overeat! One to two tablespoons of oil per day for the average active adult will not cause weight gain.

If you want to consume flaxseed, be aware, chewing will not typically break the husk of the seed, therefore you should use a small grinder. (see *Source* page). Ground flax seeds will turn rancid within a few days, therefore it is better to grind them fresh and eat them at once.

Health Benefits of Omega 3, 6 & 9
Fatty Acids in Flaxseed

As stated, the two essential fatty acids (LA & ALA) form the membranes of every cell in the body. They control the way cholesterol works in the body and the way glucose is absorbed in the cell. They make up a very large part of the brains active tissues and are the only fats that become prostaglandins, which play key roles in regulating the cardiovascular, immune, digestive and reproductive functions. They also control inflammation and healing, body heat and calorie burning (weight loss).

Although not essential, oleic fatty acid (OA omega 9) is another fatty acid contained in flaxseed and oil (19%) and even more abundant in olive oil. Oleic acid is present in all foods that contain fat and is easily produced in the body from stearic acid.

Atherosclerosis involves the accumulation of foam cells along the arterial wall. Lipids provided by oxidized low-density lipoproteins (LDLs), transform macrophages into these foam cells. Oleic acid is the principal lipid of a class that makes LDLs resistant to oxidation, and therefore a diet rich in oleic acid reduces foam cell accumulation rates and lowers the chances of atherosclerosis.

From heart disease, arthritis, psoriasis, cancer, hypertension and stroke to symptoms of fatigue, dry skin, indigestion, immune weakness, sore joints, and allergies, imbalances or deficiencies of essential fatty acids are one cause that must be addressed and corrected.

Health Benefits of Lignans in Flaxseed

Lignans are steroid-like compounds found in many plants, with one of the richest known sources being Golden Yellow & Brown flaxseed. They contain 100 to 800 times more lignans than 66 other plant foods. Lignans are found in the outer shell of the flaxseed and have anti-viral, anti-fungal, anti-bacterial and anti-cancer properties. With the elements in flaxseed and oil, including lignans, flax not only has value in treating cancer in general, but particularly colon and breast cancers. The cells of these cancers, which have estrogen receptors, can be inhibited by the anti-estrogenic compounds in lignans, specifically enterodiol and enterolactone. Lillian Thompson, Ph.D. and Paul Gross, M.D. of Toronto, Canada, have shown in numerous animal studies, that lignans can reduce the growth of breast cancer by more than 50%.

Health Benefits of Fiber in Flaxseed

The rich fiber in flaxseed produces short chain fatty acids including butyrate, acetate, and propionate. Butyrate in particular

Dis-ease is defined as lack of ease or harmony, it is NOT the same as "disease," a medical term for illness treated by medicine. _NEVER_ attempt to stop or reduce your medication without the supervision of your medical doctor.

has been shown to suppress the growth of cancer in the colon of humans and cancer in general in animals.

Flaxseed contains both soluble and insoluble fiber. Fiber has the ability to reduce LDL cholesterol and triglycerides and has a very low glycemic index, which is important to anyone who needs to keep blood sugar and insulin levels down.

The National Cancer Institute (NCI) officially recognizes the value of fiber in the prevention of cancer, specifically colon cancer. Flaxseed with its healing fiber maintains bowel regularity and health.

How to Make the Budwig Flax Seed and Oil Diet

The Flaxseed and Oil Diet was originally proposed by Dr. Johanna Budwig in 1951, a German biochemist and expert on fats, oils and cancer. Dr. Budwig discovered that the absence of linol-acids (linoleic and linolenic) in the average American diet, is responsible for the production of oxydase, which induces cancer growth and is the cause of many other chronic disorders. The beneficial ferments of oxydase are destroyed by heating or boiling oils in foods and by nitrates used for preserving meat, etc. This is the exact diet most Americans and others of modern societies consume.

The use of oxygen in the human body can be *stimulated* by protein compounds of sulphuric content, which make oils water-soluble and are present in cheese, nuts, onion, leek, chive, garlic, and especially *cottage cheese*. Use only unrefined, cold-pressed oils with linoleic and alpha-linolenic acids, such as flaxseed. Such oil should be consumed with foods containing the right proteins. The best combination is low-fat organic cottage cheese and finely ground flaxseed with fresh flaxseed oil.

The flaxseed should be freshly ground and of the Golden Yellow & Brown variety. Not all flaxseed and oils are the same. After years of clinical application, I only use **H.C. Golden Yellow & Brown** varieties with **Omega 369** flaxseed oil. **Omega 369** flaxseed oil is the best, purest, most carefully prepared flax oil in the world today. I should know. I have it made under my exact specifications. **H.C. Golden Yellow & Brown** flaxseed are organically grown with the utmost of care in HSO (homeostatic soil organisms) saturated soil, bringing to life every plant and seed.

Recap

Our body energy resources are based on lipid metabolism. To function efficiently, cells require true polyunsaturated, live, electron-rich lipids, present in abundance. By consuming **H.C. Golden Yellow & Brown** flaxseed with **Omega 369** flax oil, we satisfy all the fatty acid nutritional requirements the body needs for optimum health and vitality.

Oils are essential for the biological and physiological function of the cells. Oils have been highly underestimated in the importance of health and longevity. In over 34 years of helping people overcome all types of degenerative dis-eases, I can unequivocally state, the "right oils" are one of the golden rules you must follow if you are searching for the so-called "secret" to optimum health.

The right oils are *not* genetically engineered or irradiated and are pesticide-free, organic and cold/first-pressed. These oils are either stored in dark bottles found in the refrigerated section of your health food store, as flax or hemp oil or found in glass bottles such as peanut, sesame and extra virgin olive oil.

The wrong oils are Round-Up Ready™ soy, corn, canola or any other genetically engineered "Frankenfood" sprayed with pesticides or bombarded with radiation, hydrogenated or transmutated. The main purpose of processing oils is to extend shelf life, not yours. To the contrary, trans-fats and oils, including hydrogenated, are near impossible to digest and therefore accumulate in the body in atherosclerotic plaque formation, sealing glucose/insulin cellular receptor sites, fatty degenerative deposits especially the heart and liver and in uncontrollable obesity .

Never consume any packaged foods having hydrogenated oils in them. Do NOT assume because something is sold in a health food store, that it is truly healthy. Read *every* label. If you need a degree in chemistry to understand the ingredients contained in a so-called "food" item, put it back on the shelf.

Never use margarine or any substitute for real butter. No matter what the media tells you, organic unsalted butter is healthier for you than all substitutes. Remember, you can't fool Mother Nature. At least not for very long, that is. The key here is balance and moderation. A little real, unsalted butter is an excellent food, however, over-doing anything, including water, is unhealthy. Practice using common sense and logic.

Vitamin C Deficiency, Scurvy and Collagen

As long ago as 1500 B.C., physicians knew about scurvy, even though they didn't call it that. It was first fully described by Aristotle in 450 B.C. as a syndrome characterized by lack of energy, gum inflammation, tooth decay and bleeding problems. Since that time, we have learned much more.

With scurvy, the body literally falls apart as collagen is broken down and not replaced. The joints begin to wear down as tendons shrivel and weaken. The blood vessels disintegrate leading to bruising and bleeding as vessels rupture throughout the body. Teeth loosen and fall out as the gums and the connective tissues holding teeth also begin to erode. Organs once held firmly together by connective tissues also lose structural strength and begin to fail. In time, the various body tissues weaken and the immune system and heart give out, leading to death. It's not a pretty picture.

History

As the sailing explorers of Great Britain traveled throughout the seas, many of these brave new-world champions never made it to their destination. On one occasion, sailors too sick to travel were left on the shore of a New England coast. The aboriginals, finding this dying lot, gave them a tea made from evergreen (spruce) needles. The men soon recovered. At some date in history, someone decided that scurvy must by caused be something people ate or didn't eat. Even the famous Captain Cook knew of certain foods to prevent this dreaded curse and gave his men barley tea.

By the nineteenth century it was well known that lemon juice protected against scurvy and thus became a mandatory daily drink for all British seamen. Lemons were replaced with limes and thereafter, British sailors and the English in general were called "Limeys." We now know, scurvy is a disease caused by vitamin C deficiency, which adversely affects the collagen in the body and multiple organs and tissues.

Examples

As a chiropractic student, I participated in dissecting several cadavers. Anytime an unknown transient dies in Los Angeles or someone simply wills their body to science, chiropractic and allopathic medical schools may receive their remains, in whole or in part. On one particular day, I was the dissecting team leader overseeing a new cadaver. In reading their case history and viewing the body, I determined that a heart attack diagnosed as the cause of death was in fact, undiagnosed scurvy. It wasn't too difficult. The body had multiple lesions, hemoraggic bruising and paper-thin skin. To prove my point to my professor and other students, I simply made a full longitudinal incision in the anterior thigh area and removed the femur as if pulling a bone out of an overcooked chicken. To the amazement of those witnessing such a spectacle, I proved what scurvy really looked like. Lack of vitamin C not only can predispose one to frequent so-called "colds," but by affecting collagen, it can cause a litany of health problems, sub-clinical scurvy being one.

A couple of years ago, I went to visit a dear friend of mine in the hospital. This gentlemen was one of the most knowledgeable individuals I have ever met. As a medical doctor, he has written dozens of books, over 300 scientific articles and has over 75 pages in his biography. He spent 25 years as a scientific researcher for the C.I.A. and was the inspiration for the movie "Medicine Man" with actor Sean Connery. He knows more about the healing effects of laetrile than anyone else in the world - having written the definitive book on it.

Relative to botanicals, natural healing, oceanic plants and animals, healing and toxic chemicals, he is absolutely brilliant. There is only one criticism I have for my hero and dear friend; he did not practice what he knows to be optimum health. Because he eats junk food including hydrogenated oils, drinks soda and gets little to no exercise, he had a stroke or Cerebral Vascular Accident (CVA). With a CVA, the mid-cerebral artery usually weakens and eventually ruptures, causing hemorrhaging into the brain. Many people die within days. Many more are left with paralysis or permanent memory loss. One look and I could tell his stroke was caused by a vitamin C deficiency. His skin was thin, pale and scaly. He had multiple bruises running down both arms with so-called "age" or "liver" spots on his hands. He just had the "look."

When you don't have enough vitamin C, you won't have enough collagen. If you don't have enough collagen, your arterial blood vessel walls will be weak. Once weak, they are predisposed to rupture plain and simple.

Several days after I last saw my friend, he had another stroke and died. I believe it could have been prevented.

Looking Younger

Collagen is the protein that forms connective fibers in tissues such as teeth, ligaments, bones, skin and cartilage. Collagen fibers keep bones and blood vessels strong and help to anchor our teeth to our gums. Collagen also acts as a matrix that gives support, shape and bulk to blood vessels, bones and organs such as the heart, kidneys and liver. Collagen is required for the repair of blood vessels, bruises and broken bones. As the most abundant protein in the body, collagen accounts for more mass than all other proteins put together.

The loss of collagen is one reason why we age, why our skin loses its "tone" and our muscles lose their shape. It is why some bruise so easily and others have bleeding gums and even blood in the stool. So many of our so-called "diseases" are actually just signs of imbalance, deficiencies and toxicities. In this case, what our body is begging for is more vitamin C, more collagen.

In order for the body to make protein matrix collagen, actually procollagen, the body requires vitamin C and two amino acids, proline and lysine. Procollagen is then used to manufacture one of several types of collagen found in different tissues throughout the body. To this date, science has discovered at least fourteen different types of collagen, the top four being:

Type 1 makes up the fibers found in connective tissues of the skin, bones, teeth, tendons and ligaments.

Type 2 is made up of round fibers found in cartilage.

Type 3 forms connective tissue that gives shape and strength to organs, such as the liver, heart and kidneys.

Type 4 forms sheets that lie between layers of cells in the blood vessels, muscles and eye.

Vitamin C

Of all the vitamins known, vitamin C supplements are the most widely taken. From the so-called "common cold" to cancer, vitamin C has purportedly been the vitamin of choice with hundreds of thousands of testimonials proclaiming the efficacy of this famous nutrient.

"Vitamin C is the most potent anti-toxin known. It can effectively neutralize or minimize the damaging effect of most chemical carcinogens in food and the environment and thus be of great value in cancer-prevention programs. It will also help prevent the formation of free radicals which are causatively connected with breast cancer." **- Paavo Airola, N.D., Ph.D.**

"Supplemental vitamin C has value for the prevention of all forms of cancer...and in every stage of the disease."

- Linus Pauling, Ph.D.

Although Drs. Paavo Airola and Linus Pauling thoroughly understood the significance of vitamin C, it was Dr. Albert Szent-Gyorgi that actually discovered it.

Albert Szent-Gyorgyi Ph.D. (1893-1986), one of the most respected and honored biochemists of the 20th century and recipient of the Nobel Prize in 1937 for his research in bio-chemistry, discovered what is called vitamin C or ascorbic acid from lemons in 1932. However, what was thought to be a simple compound, is in fact, a complex similar to the B vitamins. Although not widely accepted at this time, I predict, in the not too distant future, we will thoroughly discover complexes within vitamin C and they will be known as C1, C2, C3 etc. This is important because of the difference between whole-food nutrition and isolated nutrients.

If one takes pure ascorbic acid (vitamin C) without the supporting C complex, bioflavonoids, rutin, hesperidin (a.k.a. vitamin P) and other whole-food nutrients, the net result relative to health, not only is incomplete nutrition, it is a forced nutritional imbalance.

An orange is not simply ascorbic acid. It is a complex of nutrients, including the C complexes, bioflavonoids, water, amino acids (protein), fat, minerals; calcium, iron, magnesium, phosphorus, potassium, sodium, zinc, copper, manganese, selenium, B complex vitamins, folic acid, vitamin A, vitamin E, saturated, monounsaturated and polyunsaturated fatty acids and other UNKNOWN nutrients.

It is the UNKNOWN nutrients that make whole-food nutritional supplementation far superior to isolated, man-made supplements. The UNKNOWN nutrients found in whole food nutrition, may be what really makes vitamin C so important and so affective. Under UNKNOWN nutrients, I also include the life force or energy field or that which is seen and not seen. However, only time will tell as science discovers what nature has known since the beginning of creation.

Uses

Vitamin C obviously has a wide range of clinical applications. It produces a positive immunological response to help fight bacteria and viruses. It enhances the production and activity of interferon, an antiviral substance produced by our bodies. It has also been helpful for relief of back pain and pain from inflamed vertebral discs, as well as the inflammatory pain that is associated with general sprains and strains.

In gouty arthritis, vitamin C improves the elimination of uric acid, (a protein metabolic waste product (irritant)), through the kidneys. In asthma, vitamin C relieves bronchiospasms caused by chemical toxins and subsequent histamine production. It is also used for problems of rapid aging, burns, fracture healing, bedsores and other skin ulcers and to speed wound healing after an injury or surgery. Peptic and other stomach ulcers seem to heal more rapidly with vitamin C therapy. As an antioxidant, vitamin C is effective in preventing the formation of free radicals, which play a major role in the origin of disease.

Stress Relief

Vitamin C is also known as the stress vitamin. It has a propensity or affinity for the adrenal glands, which are the stress glands. Its support of adrenal function and role in the production of adrenal hormones, epinephrine and norepinephrine, helps the body handle infections and stresses of all kinds. The more stress one is under, the more vitamin C is drawn up by the adrenal glands. If the adrenals consume most of the available vitamin C there will be little left for all the aforementioned tissues. The end result will be one if not more of the vitamin C deficiency diseases.

Vitamin C also supports the thyroid by stimulating production of thyroxine (T4) hormone, helping with problems of fatigue and slow metabolism. It also aids in cholesterol metabolism, increasing its elimination and thereby assisting in maintaining healthy cholesterol.

Tryptophan, an amino acid, is converted in the presence of vitamin C to 5-hydroxytryptophan, which forms serotonin, an important brain chemical. Vitamin C also helps folic acid convert to its active form, tetrahydrofolic acid and helps tyrosine to form the neurotransmitter substances, dopamine and epinephrine.

Known Depletors of Vitamin C

If stress isn't enough, to make things worse, vitamin C is a water soluble nutrient and is easily oxidized within hours. Even under ideal conditions, vitamin C does not stay in the body longer than four hours. It is not stored in the liver as with the oil-soluble nutrients: vitamins A, D, E or K. Therefore, it is paramount that we consume or supplement our diet with a truly bio-available whole food vitamin C at least three times per day. In addition to the stresses of life, the following are known to deplete vitamin C:

1. Cortisone or prednisolone used for any inflammation, especially arthritis.
2. Sulfa drugs stimulate the urinary excretion of vitamin C two to three times the normal amount.
3. Antibiotics not only destroy vitamin C, but the B complex, as well.
4. Deficiencies of vitamin A lead to depletion of vitamin C resources.
5. Smoking, drinking alcohol and caffeine, coffee, tea and cola beverages can destroy vitamin C within minutes.
6. Baking soda and other food additives, preservative, colorings etc.
7. Heat and light; cooked food and foods like citrus that have been cut or juiced and left out in the air or light.
8. Aluminum and copper cookware destroy vitamin C.
9. Infections, fevers, aspirin and other pain medications, environmental toxins, petroleum products, carbon monoxide (car exhaust), heavy-metal exposure; and lead, mercury and cadmium all destroy vitamin C.

Best Whole-Food Sources of Vitamin C

The best-known whole food sources of vitamin C are the citrus fruits; oranges, lemons, limes, tangerines, grapefruits and *rainforest fruits*. However, rose hips, acerola cherries, sago palm, papayas, cantaloupes and strawberries all have an abundance of vitamin C. Good vegetable sources are red and green peppers, broccoli, Brussels sprouts, tomatoes, asparagus, parsley, dark leafy greens, cabbage and sauerkraut.

Requirements

One of the easiest tests for vitamin C deficiency is a capillary fragility test. In my clinic I used a Petechiometer®, which actually tests the integrity of one's capillaries. Whether you have an instrument or not, if you bruise easily, you are demonstrating a vitamin C deficiency and possibly other imbalances. Although it only takes 20 to 30 milligrams of absorbable vitamin C on a daily basis to keep one from developing pre-clinical scurvy, when seeking optimum health, we need to take more vitamin C than just the minimum to keep us from getting sick.

Although the Recommended Daily Allowance (RDA) set up by the United States government is a mere 60 mg per day, this amount is absurdly insufficient for optimum health. If you want to know what it is like to take a nutrient at the minimal level, try holding your breath for as long as you can just before you pass out. Then take another breath. What you are doing is breathing the minimal amount of air/oxygen to just barely survive. You won't be able to function very well; run, play, work or think, but you will survive. This is what we do when we take supplements according to the governments RDAs.

According to natural healers, doctors, researchers and clinicians in the field, the recommended dose of a whole-food vitamin C complex for the average non-smoking, non-alcohol-drinking adult, is 3,000 milligrams (mgs) per day. That is 1,000 mgs, three times per day. If you are ill from allergies, infections to cancer, this dose can go all the way up to 10,000 mgs per day or more. Some practitioners are recommending up to 50,000 mgs per day, however, at this dose you should be under the care of a natural healing doctor that is highly experienced in natural healing.

There are virtually no side effects to taking vitamin C with the exception of a loose stool. Sometimes when a dose is higher than one can absorb, the ascorbic acid will stimulate the bowels thereby causing diarrhea. Simply cut down the dose until your bowels are back to normal. Then you can slowly increase the dose over time thus avoiding a bowel problem.

Ultra C

After years of clinical application, research and experimentation, I have developed the finest, whole-food vitamin C complex ever created. From rose hips, acerola berries, pineapple-extracts, rutin, hesperidin and rainforest fruits, **Ultra C** is the ultimate, whole food vitamin C.

Adults need 1,000 mgs three times per day. If ill, increase accordingly.

Remember, for a more youthful appearance and vibrant health, we must have significant amounts of healing, repairing nutrients. Vitamin C is part of the LifePack System®. If your arms, legs, hands, face or any part of your body is sagging, in addition to exercise, you need nutritionally support. If you bruise easily or have varicosities (swollen veins), you are simply demonstrating nutritional deficiencies. If you have bone or teeth problems, start taking vitamin C today and plenty of it.

Staying Health and Looking Good

There is no mystery as to why we get sick. We basically and ignorantly create our own illnesses. It is therefore our responsibility to create our own cures. With the exception of genetically engineered organisms that have circumvented nature and are designed to kill, all cures are found in nature. We must become familiar with these remedies and thereafter incorporate nature into our lives.

First and foremost, my LifePack System® is designed to enhance, through whole-food nutraceutical supplementation, a good nutritional foundation based on eating organic, healthy food, breathing non-contaminated air/oxygen (if that is even possible) and drinking pristine water. Assuming one is at least doing that, and knowing our soil has been and is currently de-mineralized, it is imperative we supplement our mineral-and nutrient-depleted food, organic or not. It is for that reason my LifePack System® was developed.

Recap

To recapitulate, my LifePack System® supplies every known vitamin, mineral, amino and fatty acid, enzyme, antioxidant and even stabilized oxygen. It is one of the most comprehensive and complete nutritional programs ever formulated. It consists of the following highly concentrated nutrients:

1. **Super Kamut®: Full Complex Protein & Vitamin Powder** -

A whole food protein/vitamin powder made of Egyptian kamut, spirulina and chlorella plankton, alfalfa and barely grass, rice germ/bran and purple dulse. Each morning mix one to two tablespoons of Super Kamut in almond or rice milk, vegetable or fruit juice. Use a blender and put fresh fruit, berries or a banana in it when using the milks or fruit juice, thereby making it a smoothie, however, don't use any fruit if you have Cancure® and you are on Dr. Chappell's intensive or extreme diet plan.

2. **Coral Blend: Fossilized Stony Coral Mineral Complex -**

Made from fossilized stony coral minerals, with vitamin D3, malic acid, vitamin C & K and betaine HCL. Take one capsule three times per day with or without meals. For the most comprehensive information on this product, read my book, *The Miracle Elements: Fossilized Stony Coral Minerals.*

3. **Stable 'O': Stabilized Oxygen -**

A liquid concentrate of electrolytes of oxygen to compensate for air pollution and oxygen deprivation. Squirt 10 to 20 drops of Stable 'O' in the above 8 oz. glass of Ultra C and charged distilled water each time you have a glass. Take three times per day minimum.

4. **ProDigestives: Proteolytic & Digestive Enzymes** -

This is the only proteolytic and digestive enzyme on the market today. ProDigestives contains pancreatin, chymotrypsin, trypsin, papain, bromelain, amylase, invertase, lactase, lipase, cellulose, glucoamylase, nattokinase and serapeptinase. Take one capsule three times per day with or without meals.

5. **Omega 369: Organic Flaxseed Oil -**

Contains all the essential fatty acids required by the body for optimum nutrition. Each morning mix one tablespoon of Omega 369 Flaxseed oil and one tablespoon of freshly ground HC Flaxseed in with your Super Kamut® smoothie, in your favorite salad dressing (if eating salad) or low-fat cottage cheese.

6. **Ultra C: Whole-Food Vitamin C -**

A combination of whole-food vitamin C from citrus, rose

hips, acerola berries and proprietary rainforest fruits. Mix one scoop (1 gram) of Ultra C in an 8 oz. glass of charged distilled water and take three times per day away from meals

7. **Acai Plus -**

For a complete description of this amazing berry from Brazil, see Index E-*Resources.* Take one capsule three times per day with or without meals.

This System® is not a one-a-day, synthetic, isolated, vitamin pill program. This is serious whole-food nutritional supplementation. This is the 'crème de la crème' of all current nutraceuticals on the market today. Nothing is more comprehensive. Nothing can compare to the all-natural and organic ingredients used in my System®.

If we want optimum health, we must nourish ourselves with optimum nutrition. As stated, even organic food if grown on devitalized soil will not provide the nutrients we need to prevent illness. We must supplement our diet with all the nutrients the body needs to be healthy. My System® is designed to do just that and more.

Exercise

This is the easy part. Never work out. That's right. Never go to a gym, run, jog or do anything you call "working out." Why? Because right from the start, you have defeated yourself.

Would you rather play and have fun or work? Do musicians work music or play music? See the difference? Now that I have your attention, let me explain.

You may go to a gym, run, jog or do any exercise you want, just don't call it "working out." As long as you are making it fun, you will be encouraged to continue.

When I want an overweight child to lose weight, I don't tell them they need to exercise or work out. I simply give them a ball and tell them to play. As a consequence of having a good time playing, they lose weight.

The first exercise you should learn to do is breathing. That's right, breathing. Most people have *never* learn to breathe from their entire lung(s). Lying down on your back, take a deep breath through your nose, expanding your rib cage as far as possible, but leave some room for the second and third steps.

In the second phase, continue breathing in, but this time fill the lower lung by pushing your lower abdomen out and dropping your diaphragm. To help do this visualize that you are pregnant.

In the third and final phase, continue to breathe in and raise your shoulders up towards your ears. This raises the clavicles off the apex of the lungs, filling the upper portion.

Do this exercise every morning before you get out of bed, breathing in through the nose and out through the mouth at least ten times. While you're doing this technique, silently say, "I am young. I am strong. I am healthy." Repeat this affirmation during your whole breathing exercise. This sets your intention for the day.

Electronic Frequency Devices:

Arizona Sauna of California

The above will be briefly covered in Index E-*Resources* in the back of the book.

Therapies: Healing Modalities

Chiropractic

The roots of chiropractic care can be traced all the way back to the beginning of recorded time. Writings from China and Greece from 2700 B.C. and 1500 B.C. mention spinal manipulation and the maneuvering of the lower extremities to ease low-back pain. Hippocrates, the Greek physician, who lived from 460 to 357 B.C., also published texts detailing the importance of chiropractic care. In one of his writings he declares, "Get knowledge of the spine, for this is the requisite for many diseases."

In the United States, the practice of spinal manipulation began gaining momentum in the late nineteenth century. In 1895, Daniel David Palmer founded the chiropractic profession in Davenport, Iowa. Palmer was an avid reader of the medical journals of his day and had great knowledge of the developments that were occurring throughout the world regarding anatomy and physiology.

In 1897, Daniel David Palmer opened the Palmer School of Chiropractic, which has continued to be one of the most prominent chiropractic colleges in the nation.

Throughout the twentieth century, doctors of chiropractic gained legal recognition in all fifty states. A continuing recognition and respect for the chiropractic profession in the United States has led to growing support for chiropractic care all over the world. The research that has emerged from "around the world" has yielded incredibly influential results, which have changed, shaped and molded perceptions of chiropractic care. The Chiropractic Health Report in New Zealand published in 1979, strongly supported the efficacy of chiropractic care. The 1993 Manga study published in Canada investigated the cost effectiveness of chiropractic care. The results of this study concluded that chiropractic care would save hundreds of millions of dollars annually with regard to work disability payments and direct health care costs.

Doctors of chiropractic have become pioneers in the field of non-invasive care promoting science-based approaches to a variety of ailments. A continuing dedication to chiropractic research could lead to even more discoveries in preventing and combating maladies in future years. (American Chiropractic Association)

Naturopathy

Hippocrates is thought to have been one of the first practitioners to use a combination of therapies such as diet, exercise, fresh air and rest to restore health in his patients. The "father of medicine" was well ahead of his peers (who blamed evil spirits for disease) when he theorized that illness occurred when the body's systems were out of balance. Hippocrates treated the body as a whole, rather than a series of parts, a principle still applied in naturopathy today.

The modern form of naturopathic medicine is said to have come out of the "natural cures" that were widely practiced in European spas and natural mineral springs in the 18th and 19th centuries. It spread to the United States where German-born doctor Benedict Lust set up the first school of naturopathy in 1896.

The term naturopathy is believed to have been coined from the words "nature" and "homeopathy." Benedict Lust was against any processed foods as he said that they destroyed the nutritional value and all the chemicals present within, our body is not designed to absorb them.

The above personnel had made a big difference in promoting and spreading the word on naturopathy, but there are still a few people who need to be credited for their work and dedication in this natural-healing method. They are: Louisa Lust, wife of Benedict Lust, Dr. Henry Lindlahr, Otis G. Carrol, Fredrick W. Collins, Linda Burfield Hazard and Bernarr Macfadden. These people helped spread the word on naturopathy unconditionally. With proven reports and journals, they tried their best to do what they could do to help people by giving them a choice of life without side effects, rather than living with side effects.

Though alternative medicine was met with fierce resistance from the AMA, the spirit to spread the word on natural care never faded. Where the word of cure spreads like a fire, soon, alternative medicine is carving its own niche among people. There are a few who never trusted natural medicine, but are seeking it now as a choice to live a longer and a healthier life. In a survey in 1998, it was shown that alternative medicine is very common with people aged from 29-49, which composes 38% of the total U.S. population.

Acupuncture

Acupuncture has been practiced for many centuries, and by many different nationalities and cultures. Records indicate acupuncture started in ancient China, possibly as long as 4,000 years ago. In ancient China, three legendary characters have been regarded as the founders of Chinese medicine. The earliest is Fu Xi, also called Bao Xi, a legendary tribe leader who was believed to have made many innovations, such as the production of nine kinds of needles. The second is Shen Nong, the Divine Husbandry Man, who was said to have taught the art of husbandry, and discovered the curative virtues of herbs by tasting a hundred different varieties. The third is Huang Di, the Yellow Emperor, who was said to have discussed medicine, including acupuncture, with his ministers and who, like Fu Xi, was credited with having made nine kinds of needles.

From the Third Century A.D. onwards, acupuncture became a more specialized discipline in China with many outstanding specialists, and numerous valuable books. The first book devoted exclusively to acupuncture is the Zhenjiu Jiayi Jing (*A Classic of Acupuncture and Moxibustion*) compiled by Huangfu Mi (214-282) between 259 and 260. In this book, the name and number of points of each channel and their exact locations are defined and systematized, and the properties and indications of each point and the methods of needling are presented in great detail. The acupoints of the four limbs are arranged according to the Three Yin and Three Yang Channels of the feet and hands. The number of acupoints has increased from the 295 listed in the Neijing to 349 A.D.

In the early 17th century, a trend appeared among quite a few scholarly doctors whereby acupuncture, together with surgery, was regarded as an insignificant and petty skill that was inferior to herbal medicine. In 1822 Emperor Dao Guang, in the second year after ascending his throne, issued an imperial edict stating that acupuncture and moxibustion were not suitable forms of treatment for a monarch, and should be banned forever from the Imperial Medical Academy. Although the ban was limited to the court, by the second half of the 18th century the general study and practice of acupuncture was at a low ebb. By this stage, however, acupuncture and moxibustion had already arrived in Europe and the West. It was first introduced through reports by Jesuits in the 17th century. In England, James Morris Churchill began to use acupuncture for pain control and Sir William Osler recommended the use of acupuncture in the treatment of lumbago.

Over the past 50 years in China, acupuncture, together with the whole system of traditional Chinese medicine, has been designated a national cultural heritage.

Since the 1950s Chinese official policy has been to encourage the study of traditional Chinese medicine and the integration of the two medical systems, traditional Chinese medicine and Western medicine.

Massage

Massage is a universal instinct. Humans have known that it helps to rub a sore limb and that to touch is beneficial. For that matter apes know this as well, and indeed so do most other mammals. Writing a history of massage is therefore a curious project, much like writing a history of breathing or of dancing or of mating; we know that it must have happened continuously throughout history, but it is almost impossible to get an accurate idea of precisely what was being done, where, and by whom. This essay should not be seen as a comprehensive or reliable chronicle; rather it flits through the past and settles momentarily upon those documented characters and periods that seem interesting.

Massage - China

New age practitioners will claim that massage extends back to 3000 B.C. in China, or that it is documented in ancient Chinese writings from 2000 B.C. These claims seem rather dubious. The earliest known writing - Cuneiform, used by the Sumerians, dates from shortly before 3000 B.C. and almost all remaining fragments from the period are only administrative and economic. Chinese writing dates from around 1400 B.C., near the start of the Shang dynasty, and it is from around this time that we can reliably date massage.

The first professional massage exam was instituted in China some fifteen hundred years later, with the introduction of Schools of Occult Studies to complement the more commonly accepted Confucian schools. These were devoted to such subjects as Buddhism and Taoism that transcended the practical ordered affairs of government. Students of medicine were tested in massage and acupuncture as well as treatment of general bodily "diseases."

The first level of qualification, the hsiu ts'ai (cultivated talent) was equivalent to the current British BA degree; the ming

Dis-ease is defined as lack of ease or harmony, it is NOT the same as "disease," a medical term for illness treated by medicine.
NEVER attempt to stop or reduce your medication without the supervision of your medical doctor.

ching (understanding the classics) and chin-shih (advanced scholar) corresponded to a Masters degree and a doctorate. Possession of these qualifications was very prestigious.

Massage - India

The history of massage is typically written by doctors and so, as seen in the previous section, we are left with a very medical perspective. Indian massage, however, provides a delightful counter example.

Most records of Indian massage focus not on its medical qualities but on its sensual. The erotic sculptures at Khajuraho and elsewhere, for instance, and the Kama Sutra, bear testament to a culture that understands and uses these properties to change peoples' moods, to arouse them and to delight and soothe.

It seems likely that the English word massage comes from the Portuguese word "amasser," to knead, which was used by the French colonists in India in the 18th century. But as mentioned above it is the current tradition to seek to give a subject dignity by ascribing to it improbable ancient roots; in this case, the Arabic massa, to touch, has been suggested as an alternate etymology.

Massage - Greece

While we could only guess that massage was widespread in other cultures, we have definite evidence that it was common in Ancient Greece. In the medical field, massage was a typical Hellenistic remedy along with poultices, occasional tonics, fresh air and a corrective diet. The top schools in Ancient Greece were those of gymnastics; the practice of athletic sports and the required nudity set apart the Greek way of life from that of barbarians. The schools were essentially open-shaped sports grounds with cloakrooms, washstands, training rooms, massage rooms and classrooms around the outside.

Although massage was common in Ancient Greece, we shall touch upon a few noteworthy individuals. Aesculapius worked in Thessalay (near Macedonia) in the 5th century B.C. He is reported to have treated patients with relaxation, diet, hydro therapy, herbs, massage, advice and tender loving care. Serpents were used at this stage as tools in curing patients; and it is the Staff of Aesculapius, with a serpent knotted around it, that has become the symbol of medicine.

Hippocrates used friction in the treatment of sprains and dislocations, and kneading to treat constipation. Hippocrates was also the first person to use the term aphorism in his eponymous book, "Life is short, Art long, Occasion sudden and dangerous, Experience deceitful, and Judgment difficult. A physician must be experienced in many things but assuredly also in rubbing." He held that all disease results from natural causes and should be treated using natural methods: rest, healthy food, exercise, proper diet, fresh air, massage, baths, music and visits to friends - to restore the body to a healthy state, and that it essentially had the power to heal itself. Hippocrates is often described as holistic but, paradoxically, he is also noted for his rational approach to anatomy, medicine, therapy and prognosis, and for separating medicine from philosophy and religion.

Asclepiades of Bithynia (in Asia Minor) lived from 124 B.C. to 44 B.C.. He went to Rome to teach oratory before taking up medicine. Good food, fresh air, enemas, hydrotherapy, local applications to cleanse wounds and massage were his principle treatments. He was known for his common 'horse' sense and perceptive knowledge of human nature, and for inventing the shower bath. He became friends with such dignitaries as Cicero, Crassus and Mark Anthony, and did much to win acceptance for Greek medicine in Rome.

Massage - Rome

The Romans too were keen on massage. Those who could afford it would start by bathing themselves or being bathed by attendants, and having any stiff muscles rubbed with warm vegetable oil. Then came a full body massage to awaken nerves, stimulate circulation and free the action of their joints. Finally their entire body was rubbed with very fine oil to keep their skin elastic and supple. This combination of bathing, cleaning and massage appeared in every country that the Romans conquered. Julius

Caesar himself was 'pinched' every day.

Massage - Persians

Medical knowledge, including that of massage, made its way from Rome to Persia in the Middle Ages. Manuscripts, for instance, were collected and translated by Hunayn Ishaq in the 9th century. Later in the 11th century copies were translated back into Latin, and again in the 15th and 16th centuries, when they helped enlighten European scholars as to the achievements of the Ancient Greeks. This renewal of the Galenic tradition during the Renaissance played a very important part in the rise of modern science.

Massage - Western Europe

An early record of massage in Western Europe comes from Ambroise Pare (1510-1590) who wrote about it in one of his publications, but was widely ridiculed. In 1780 Clement Joseph Tissot wrote the more successful *Gymnastique Medicinale et Churgicale* which covered occupational therapy as well as massage.

International Association of Infant Massage (IAIM) - was founded in the 1980's and is headquartered in Ventura, California. IAIM promotes nurturing touch and communication between newborns and their parents. Parents learn how to relax and soothe their baby, which deepens bonding, improves communication and contributes to development.

Classes consist of 4 weekly sessions of 1-1/2 hour each. It includes: 1. The theory and practice of infant massage. 2. Teaching a baby to relax. 3. Discussion of family bonding. 4. How to vary the massage as the child grows. 5. How to deal with special problems such as colic, intestional difficulties; excessive gas & constipation. 6. Individualized help with specific childcare needs.

Although there are many groups illegally using the IAIM name, only a certified IAIM practitioner knows the safest techniques concerning infant massage. To learn more about this extremely important process, call IAIM at 1-805-644-8524.

Rolfing

Rolfing was the invention of Dr. Ida P. Rolf, and has evolved over a 50-year period. Starting with an early family illness, Dr. Rolf began to study the work of the early osteopaths, and the pioneers who brought yoga from the East. She was a researcher at heart having graduated with a Ph.D. in Biochemistry in 1916, which lead to a career in organic chemistry at the Rockefeller Institute. It was this strong foundation, willingness to learn, and curiosity that led to some fundamental additions to the understanding of human movement potential.

Up until the 1950s the body of work was yet to be taught to others. After realizing what she had to offer, Dr. Rolf began teaching what was then known as "Structural Integration;" with her earliest students being osteopaths, chiropractors and pre-medical students. Looking for a group of people who would follow her method of understanding the body, Dr. Rolf created the Rolf Institute in 1971 and began a program that became known as Rolfing ("Structural Integration"). She looked for students who were willing to work within a window of understanding that would allow Rolfing to evolve as a discipline of its own, not an adjunct or a subject within another school of thought.

Yoga- (Sanskrit for "union")

Yoga originated in India some 5,000 years ago and yogis, ascetics and Hindus traditionally practiced it. Yoga was introduced to the West in the 19th century, the discipline having been translated from Hindu texts.

Scholars believe that yoga grew out of Stone Age Shamanism, because of the cultural similarities between Modern Hinduism and Mehrgarh, a neolithic settlement (in what is now Afghanistan). In fact, much of Hindu ideas, rituals and symbols of today appear to have their roots in this shamanistic culture of Mehrgahr. Early yoga and archaic shamanism had much in common as both sought to transcend the human condition. The primary goal of shamanism was to heal members of the community and act as religious mediators. Archaic yoga was also community-oriented, as it attempted to discern the cosmic order through inner vision, then to apply that order to daily living. Later, yoga evolved into a more inward experience, and yogis focused on their individual enlightenment and salvation. The first archaeological evidence of yoga's existence is found in stone seals excavated from the Indus Valley. The stone seals depict figures performing yoga postures. These artifacts officially put yoga on the history books circa 3000 B.C., and more importantly, link it to the great Indus-Sarasvati Civilization.

Hydrotherapy

From the beginning of time water has been used to heal, to hydrate, and to sustain life. The healing powers of mineral waters are mentioned in the Old Testament and by the time the ancient Greek civilization was established, the use of water as a healing resource was well known. This fact is evident in the number of tourists that, to this day, still travel to visit the early Roman baths.

The history of hydrotherapy probably goes as far back as human history. A form of self-prescribed and self-administered hydrotherapy that most small boys on hot days have experienced is a plunge or a swim in cold water. The invigorating effect of cold water is well known. The ancient Romans built and used public bathhouses for therapeutic purposes. Doctors Calvin and Agatha Thrash, in their book *Home Remedies* copyright 1981, mention in their chapter on the history of hydrotherapy that for years hydrotherapy has been a respected method of treatment in the United States. It was recognized that the "brand bath" (spraying and sponging with cold water accompanied by vigorous rubbing) was considered very useful in the treatment of typhoid fever in 1927. It was recognized as "powerfully stimulating to the nervous system, fortifying the patient to conquer the infection." It was felt that the benefits accrued through the circulatory system, the immune mechanisms and the neuromuscular system.

Colon Therapy

Colon hydrotherapy, a popular form of treatment among certain physicians in the 1930s and 40s is undergoing resurgence.

Colon lavage was first recorded 1500 B.C., in Ebers Papyrus, which dealt with the practice of medicine. These enemas were described as the infusion of aqueous substances into the large intestine through the anus. Hippocrates recorded using enemas for fever therapy. Galen (2nd century A.D.) also recognized and was proponent of the use of enemas. Pare in 1600 A.D. offered the first distinction between colon irrigation and the popular enema therapy of the age.

Enema use dates back to ancient Egypt and is mentioned in many ancient texts throughout several cultures including the Sumerians, Chinese, Hindus, Greeks and Romans. Initially enemas were a tool used by the medical community under the supervision of physicians. The practices of taking enemas (then called clysters) were very popular among the privileged class and it was not uncommon for some to have as many as three to four infusions a day. History records that Louis XIII received as many a 200 enemas a year. As time passed, enemas popularity faded, improvements were made and by the early 19th century, colon hydrotherapy was once again a province of the medical community.

Colon hydrotherapy, since the turn of the century, has experienced periods of popularity alternating with periods of inaction. The factors that contributed to this ambivalence primarily were due to the practice of colon hydrotherapy by the untrained and unskilled, which was very detrimental to its professional growth. When the therapy gained the attention of such physicians as James A. Wiltsie, M.D. and Joseph E.G. Waddington, M.D., great value was again placed on the therapeutic benefits of this modality. Historically, we recognize two unequivocal conclusions: first, there is something of value to this therapy or it would have been conclusively withdrawn; and second, that through lack of professional control and study, colon hydrotherapy never received the attention and recognition it justly deserves.

Environmental Health Technologies
Solar Is Finally Affordable

If you want to cure dis-ease you must stop doing all those things known to cause it and start doing all those things to help heal yourself. Anything that will contribute to cleaning the air we breathe, will help prevent a litany of dis-eases.

One reason we have so many lung dis-eases in the United States is because of our air quality. One thing that makes our air so toxic comes from burning fossil fuels for electricity. The answer to this dilemma has always been with the sun. Solar energy is one key to saving the planet and ourselves. Going "solar" is *finally* affordable.

During the time I lived in Maine, I was privileged to meet many talented and interesting individuals. One was Naoto Inoue an inventor, environmental activist and visionary. He's the kind of guy that can do anything he puts his mind to. If he doesn't know how to do something, he studies, researches, experiments and then gets it done. Back in the late 80s, he even built an all-electric solar car from the ground up, just to see if he could.

Going to his house was a learning experience in itself. The entire house was solar; panels in the back yard and on top of the roof, a windmill five stories high, a composting garden, goats for weed abatement, you name it and Naoto had it.

One thing that impressed me the most was Naoto's concern for the earth and its people. He always said he would one day make solar energy affordable. True to his word, that day has finally come.

His companies are called *Solar Market of Arundel*, *Talmage Solar Engineering, Inc* and *Blue Link Solar*. The following information I took off of his website by the same name. As we know, "If you are not part of the solution, you are part of the problem." If we really want to make a difference in this world, we must *stop* polluting it. With *Blue Link Solar,* we can begin.

www.BlueLinkSolar.net

Electricity use in the United States comes from many

different sources feeding the transmission grid. The current mix is roughly 50% coal, 21% petroleum and natural gas, 7% hydroelectric and solar power accounts for 0.001% of the electricity generated in this country. Because of our dependence on fossil fuels to produce electricity and to operate our machinery, mankind is creating a certain economic crisis, not to mention a life-threatening situation for the entire planet and all of its inhabitants.

The American Lung Association estimates that more than 64,000 Americans die prematurely each due to air population. The burning of coal and oil are major contributors to airborne heavy-metal pollutants such as lead, arsenic and mercury. The *World Health Organization* (W.H.O.) estimates that 6% of the total 50 million annual deaths around the world are attributed to air pollution from energy use.

According to the W.H.O.; the burning of the above fuels for electricity, have polluted the atmosphere to the extent of adversely affecting the climate. As an example the atmospheric concentration of carbon dioxide has increased by 31% since pre-industrial times, causing more heat to be trapped in the lower atmosphere. Emissions of carbon dioxide are still increasing.

It is estimated that the earth originally had about 2,000 billion barrels of oil and mankind has used about 1,000 billion of those barrels to date. The world consumes about 30 billion barrels per year which means that we have approximately 33 years worth of oil left at our current rate of consumption, probably even less with growth of countries like China and India demanding more use of fossil fuels. There is no question that there is a great need for alternative energy sources in this country but there seems to be little if any movement on the political scene to effect a change in our current use of fossil fuels or search for alternative energy.

Now many environmentally conscious companies are taking the lead in the area of alternative energy. There is one company (with three names) that is really taking the lead in the solar energy industry: Talmage Solar Engineering, Inc., Solar Market and Blue Link Solar, headquartered in Arundel, Maine.

Since 1975 *Solar Market* has been designing and installing renewable energy systems for a wide range of applications. Solar Market offers pre-engineered systems to provide clean energy for a wide range of applications and is committed to providing practical and reliable renewable energy. Solar Market is trying to do more than just make money, they trying to create positive returns for society and the environment as well. Their company value statement is built upon the balance of nature, humanity, and technology.

Solar Market recognizes the intrinsic value of nature. They embrace humanity, our uniqueness and our interconnection to each other and they work towards a healthier, more compassionate existence. Solar Market has developed a unique concept that involves a sophisticated technology called *Blue Link Solar Network*, a concept that could just be the answer to eliminating our nation's dependency on fossil fuel.

The National Renewable Energy Laboratory recommends our electricity generation mix include 10% solar power by 2030. Providing 10% of our power from solar energy will shut down over 300 coal-fired plants. For the individual, as with the country, providing 100% of electricity demand from solar power is expensive and challenging - anywhere from fifty to one hundred thousand dollars. So much so that it discourages any action. In contrast, 10% solar power is affordable, easy, and meaningful. Providing 10% of your own electricity from solar power means using 10,000 times the amount of clean, solar electricity you used before. *Blue Link Solar Network* is a grassroots, community effort seeking widespread education about and adoption of solar power. With the Blue Link 480, many of us can achieve the 10% goal today, paving the way for bigger accomplishments tomorrow.

What is *Blue Link Solar Network*? Blue Link 480 component contains a PV panel that converts sunlight directly into electricity. An inverter that converts the solar electricity (DC) into standard grid current (AC), Blue Link 480 feeds clean electricity into the grid at the building load center. It takes less than 30 minutes to install: position facing south, fold out the array, wire into a load center, and flip the switch. Specifications: Rated Power: 480 watts DC and Power Output: 120 VAC split phase pure sine wave power works with all household appliances.

At homes and buildings across the country, Blue Link systems connect to the grid, adding clean electricity whenever the sun shines. Together, these systems form Blue Link Solar Network, a Virtual Power Plant, with generation equipment distributed around the country. Clean electricity produced by Blue Link Solar Network decreases output from polluting, unsustainable fossil fuel power plants. As the network grows and produces clean electricity, the network page tracks electricity production, environmental benefits, and the community that makes it possible.

Capturing the full monetary value of solar power is difficult, which explains in a large part why more businesses and individuals aren't using it. The most attractive benefits of Blue Link Solar Network are pollution reduction, using a renewable resource, supplying power during peak demand, and reducing strain on the utility grid. In addition, by increasing participation in and awareness of solar electricity, Blue Link Solar Network creates a virtual circle that will reduce costs and other barriers so that more solar energy can benefit the country. Most of these positive externalities are not easily traded for money, although gradually this is changing.

Some of the economic benefits associated with solar energy include: reducing acid rain, particulate pollution and/or global warming. In addition, saving lives, medical costs, habitat, property, and ecosystems are equally as important. Although the benefits are not easily quantified, it is clear that we need to invest in clean, renewable energy, if for no other reason than the cost of not doing so will be devastating.

Without considering any of these benefits, a Blue Link 480 located in the northeast U.S. will save about $80 per year in electricity. In the sunniest parts of the country or where utility rates are high, it might save $120 per year or more. Savings increase as electricity rates increase. Over its 35 year expected life it is possible the 480 system will pay for itself several times over. A few utility companies vary rates according to time of use, making solar electricity even more valuable as demand, rates and solar production all peak at the same time. In some areas of the country rebates or tax incentives for solar power decrease the initial cost. Currently in California, there is a $1,800 rebate for the Blue Link solar system retailing at $4,600. This means you can have a solar system for your home or office for around $2,800. Perhaps someday government rebates will happen on a national level. For more information go to www.dsireusa.org to see what benefits are available for you.

Blue Link 480 from Solar Market and Blue Link Solar is an exciting and great opportunity for this nation to cut its dependence from fossil fuel use and to do something positive to clean our environment and to positively impact the general health of the world. I am thankful my friend Naoto is playing his part in saving a place for his children and yours. (See Index E-*Resources*) or call 1-877-785-0088. If you mention reading my book, they'll give you a *discount* as a courtesy.

Cost of Prevention: It's All About Priorities

In the 1800s our ancestors lived off the land. It took very little to get by. Since electricity hadn't been invented, we had no electrical appliances and therefore no electric bills. We had no automobiles and therefore no car payments, up-keep, oil, gasoline, insurance, registration, licenses or other related expenses.

Most people acquired their land by homesteading. There were no property taxes, sales taxes or income taxes. There was no such thing as a Federal Reserve Note since there was no Federal Reserve. In fact, our money was backed by silver and was actually a United States Silver Certificate or U.S. dollar.

Water was free because we were allowed to drill our own water wells. If we lived in the city it was supplied at no or little charge. Most people lived in the country and grew their own food.

Those in the city had to pay for it. For the most part, we did not need money or very little of it. We lived by what we could grow or raise ourselves.

Times have changed and are continually changing, however, some things *never* change. From the beginning of our existence, humans have always wanted a better life. Separate from the basic necessities of food, water, clothes and shelter, we seek health, peace, love, joy, happiness and success. What we seek becomes a priority.

I remember an older patient of mine coming to my clinic when I had just raised my office visit from $17 to $25. She was complaining to my office staff how expensive it was to come and see me. This women did not have a lot of money or so I thought. As a matter of fact, she was on my holiday list for that year to receive a gift. Every year I would take my accounts receivables and find those individuals that I thought were struggling financially. I would copy their statement showing what they owed me and then showing a zero balance with the words: "May God continue to bless you as you are a blessing."

I pulled this woman into my office to talked to her about my new fees and her perception of my value. I was planning on reducing her fee right on the spot. However, for the first time, I noticed how meticulous she was.

Her hair was that silverish-blue you see so many older women have done at a hair salon. Her fingernails were a beautiful light pink and her clothes we freshly pressed or cleaned. Her husband was in the car and became agitated while waiting, so he "honked" the horn to get her to come out. I decided to go out and see what kind of car they were driving. It was an older Cadillac, but in mint condition. There wasn't a spot on it. I even commented on how clean the car was. Her husband said he had it washed every week and waxed every month.

I asked him if I could talk to his wife for just a few more minutes. He agreed, so his wife and I returned to my office.

We had a quick lesson on re-establishing priorities. She

paid her bill and never complained again.

In a nutshell, most people take *better* care of their cars, homes, pets and possessions than they do their own health. In other words, they put themselves on a *low* priority. This woman could easily afford a $25 visit once per month. Her problem wasn't money or even perceiving my service as having value, her problem was she had other priorities above her health.

Now a days, we budget all the basics needed for survival plus those things we *feel* we *can't* live without. Cell phones, home computers, high speed access to the Internet, a second car or motorcycle, cable or satellite TV and on and on. People even pay $500 to $600 or more monthly for "health" insurance only to find out when they need it, they have an outrageous deductible they're not prepared to pay for.

As you now know, to obtain optimum health it takes *education* and *effective action*. Part of that action is to stop doing all the things known to be unhealthy and start doing all the things known to be healthy. Part of what you need to do is eat all organic food, drink pristine or charged distilled water, detoxify the body on a regular basis, exercise, rest, relax, forgive and if you live in "civilized" society, ensure your nutritional needs with organic, whole-food nutraceuticals containing vitamins, minerals, enzymes, amino and essential fatty acids, antioxidants and stabilized oxygen.

For we, the *People of the World*, these suggestions cost money. Some of you will not be able to afford them on your current income. You will either have to earn more money, borrow it or do without. For others it may not be so difficult.

Are you worth spending a couple of hundred dollars or more on preventing cancer, heart dis-ease, diabetes or any other degenerative condition? Perhaps you think it's cheaper to wait until you get sick and then treat it? It's all about priorities. I'm sure if my mother were alive today, she would be re-prioritizing.

Notes

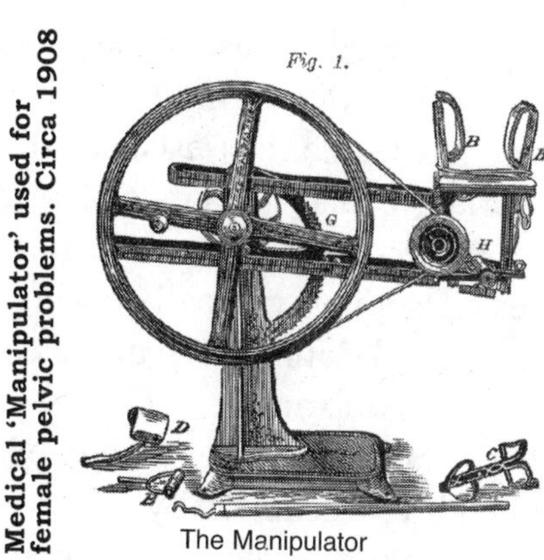

Medical 'Manipulator' used for female pelvic problems. Circa 1908

The Manipulator

CHAPTER 5 - *EXPERIMENTAL* ORTHODOX MEDICAL TREATMENT: DRUGS AND POLITICS

"Doctors are men who prescribe medicines of which they know little, to cure diseases of which they know less, in human beings of whom they know nothing." **- Voltaire**

The only thing more confusing than the *cause* and *cure* of disease is the unified string theory and quantum physics. Actually, even that is easier to comprehend. The "intellectual" health gurus create their own language designed to bewilder those not in their "club," least the masses just might understand the simplicity of complexity. In other words, there is a whole lot of mist in mysticism and there is a tremendous amount of *misinformation* concerning health and healing.

Most of this confusion is deliberate. It is created to keep people in the dark about their own health and choices so they can't exist without the litany of "health" practitioners and their potions, there to prey upon one's ignorance and finances. Shedding light on this *misinformation* is one reason why I wrote this book.

My mother was cleverly duped into believing everything her doctors told her. Even I could not convince her differently. She believed her doctors wore white coats because they were pure, honest, trustworthy and dependable. Besides that, they accepted health insurance, which made it easy to be "treated" by the system

Dis-ease is defined as lack of ease or harmony, it is NOT the same as "disease," a medical term for illness treated by medicine.
NEVER attempt to stop or reduce your medication without the supervision of your medical doctor.

they created dubiously called "healthcare."

In addition, my mother was brought up to believe doctors were like Catholic priests, one of God's messengers. Of course, we now know this is absolutely false. Although I don't think doctors are universally being found guilty of molesting children, the only message they typically bring is that which represents the pharmaceutical industry and the AMA, not God.

Insurance

Have you ever wondered why there is an insurance policy called life, when it really only becomes effective after you die? It's death insurance, not life insurance. Sounds better to call it life, doesn't it? What about health insurance, isn't it really sickness insurance? Doesn't it kick-in when you are sick or at least it's supposed too? Let's face it, there really isn't any insurance company encouraging or teaching us to stay healthy, they just pay for specific treatment when we are ill. They make money by charging for their coverage and finding ways not to honor that coverage when you need it. The world is full of oxymorons: those things that really don't make any sense, similar to warring or killing for peace. So it is with the orthodox "health" industry.

Osteoporosis: One Example

After months or years of malnutrition, dehydration, toxemia, stress and lack of proper exercise, the pH of the body will often shift to acid. What we eat and drink and how we think determines whether we accumulate hydrogen or oxygen. Organic fruits and vegetables, charged distilled water and positive, healthy thoughts keep us alkaline, most everything else makes us acid.

When considering pH, the range is 1 to 14. The number seven represents neutral. Under seven is acid and over seven is alkaline. Normally, the pH of the body runs about 7.2 or slightly alkaline. The blood ranges from 7.35 to 7.45. Outside of this blood range we quickly die. It is therefore vital to keep the body on the alkaline side.

If your diet contains sufficient amounts of minerals, specifically calcium, the minerals will buffer dietary acids and shift the pH back to alkaline. However, with a mineral deficiency, especially bio-unavailable calcium, the body will simply take calcium from the bones and teeth. Instead of seeing this condition as a *sign* or *signal* of a nutritional, hydration, lack of exercise, toxin, stress challenge, orthodox medicine merely names it osteoporosis. It is now classified as a legitimate "disease," which is then insurance reimbursable and treatable, with a host of new drugs and therapies. Incidentally, no one on the planet may claim to treat osteoporosis but your symptom-treating allopathic doctor, your MD. It's called trade-union protectionism and the AMA has mastered it.

That's right. If you are not a drug-prescribing medical doctor, other doctors will be arrested and thrown in jail for possessing or using anything other than a drug for the prevention, treatment or cure of any "disease," including osteoporosis.

The Line in the Sand

What we have is a major division between natural healing and orthodox medicine. On one hand, we have a discipline that states one's lifestyle and a mineral deficiency have caused a condition whereby bone is de-mineralizing suggesting a lifestyle change and an inexpensive mineral supplement. On the other hand, we have a discipline that takes the *signs* and *signals* of imbalances and deficiencies and converts them into a list of symptoms thereby attaching them to a "disease" they call osteoporosis, which is really only a description of a process. Osteoporosis literally means porous bone. Of course with orthodox medicine there is no cure only treatment using expensive drugs, tests and therapies. With the governments stamp of approval, orthodox medicine has set up a monopoly in all facets of American life, including the military, which we pay for out of our tax dollars.

What a scam. The pharmaceutical companies use the AMA and their union members to promote and distribute drugs and then have their lobbyists infiltrate the United States government convincing it to only use their system of so-called "healthcare." If that's not bad enough, just in case you try to compete by using anything but their system, the FDA (Food and Drug Administration), made up of former drug company employees, becomes the legal arm for the drug cartel to arrest, prosecute convict and incarcerate you. Wouldn't you love to start a business with that kind of protectionism?

The Common Cold

What about the so-called common "cold"? What is a cold anyway? Is it a viral or bacteria infection? If so, why and how do we recover? If bacteria cause a cold, when are we *not* exposed to them? The answer is simple: We are ALWAYS exposed to pathogens such as viruses, bacteria, parasites, fungus and germs of all types. They are in our food, water and air. They only proliferate in the body when the internal terrain or internal environment is toxic enough to attract and harbor them.

Since germs, virus, bacteria and fungus are scavengers, they are attracted to toxins and undigested, putrefied food. Toxic people are actually a food source for them. Just like a vulture attracted to carrion, pathogenic scavengers are attracted to anything unhealthy and/or decaying.

Once they have consumed their fill, they themselves become slow, sluggish and vulnerable to our immune system. However, if that immune system is *not* healthy enough to begin with, the invaders can kill the host which eventually kills them as well. If you are *not* filled with toxins and undigested putrefied food or have no other H O N S T E C contributing factors, your immune system should be healthy and strong. If you are then exposed to a heavy dose of pathogens by someone sneezing in your face, you still will not get sick because 1) you don't have the pathogen's toxic, putrefied food source and 2) if your immune system is healthy to begin with it will destroy the pathogens on contact.

Only when someone is toxic with a compromised immune system, will they be at risk for an infection caused by one or more of life's scavengers. Truly, **"Only sick people get sick."**

So what *theory* do you subscribe to? Statistics show more and more people are moving away from slash, burn and drug therapy opting to try natural healing because it's safe and effective.

Germs

Ask yourself. Do germs actually cause sickness? If every time we see a dead animal on the side of the road decomposing and filled with parasitic maggots, should we blame the parasites for killing the animal or did they come after the fact of the animals death? I suggest they came after the animal died.

My mother used to say in her sweet Italian manner, "Jimmy, don't go outside with your hair a wet, you'rr gonna catch a cold." Even as a young boy, I questioned everything. I'd ask my mom, "What happens to all the people swimming in the ocean during the summer, mama? They're outside. Will they all catch a cold?" She would reply, as she slapped me up side the back of my head, "I don't know about them, I just know about you."

As I have already discussed, germs, viruses and other opportunistic pathogens come *only* after one is toxic enough to attract them and the immune system is compromised enough to harbor them. In other words, **"Only sick people get sick."** We don't catch colds. We get rid of toxins, which give us the *symptoms* we call a cold - which are really *signs* and *signals* of The H.O.N.S.T.E.C. SYNDROME. And so it is for *every* condition.

Doctors and More Doctors

Since we all have heard about medical doctors taking the Hippocratic oath, I thought I would reproduce the classical form word for word.

Hippocrates, known as the *Father of Medicine,* lived from 460 to 377 B.C. As of this date, it is approximately 2,465 years ago. Apollo was the Greek god of music, poetry, prophecy and *medicine*. Aesculapius was a word found in the Chaldean language which meant man (ashe), instruct (skul), snake (aphe). It literally meant *man-instructing snake.* The medical emblem called the Caduceus is the winged staff (used as a symbol of authority) of an ancient herald (one who proclaims news) with two serpents or snakes (meaning unclear) coiled about it, carried by Mercury (messenger's of the gods).

In *The Golden Wand of Medicine: A History of the Caduceus Symbol in Medicine*, by Walter Friedlander - an unknown medical publisher in the 19th century used the symbol prominently on their texts and thereby began the association of the caduceus with medicine, an association made firm by the prevalence of the image in the American Medical Corps work during World War I; circa 1914.

In his oath, Hippocrates swore he would give no "deadly medicine," which means he would not knowingly give anything of a harmful or destructive nature. This is why current medical doctors say they have taken the Hippocractic oath to "First, do no harm." Tell me, how are they doing? Hippocrates also said, he would "not give a woman a pessary to produce abortion." It seems medical doctors are flagrantly violating their oath on a daily basis. Hippocrates' methods of treatment were used until the year 1500 A.D. During this time no "regular" physician would attempt chemical poisoning of the body (see oath at end of this chapter).

The *classical* Hippocratic oath was replaced in 1964 with one written by Louis Lasagna, Academic Dean of the School of Medicine at Tufts University. His version is the version medical students and doctors now recite. Oddly enough, there is little to none of the original intent remaining in the Lasagna version as opposed to the one written by Hippocrates almost 2,500 years ago. Of course, the part where it once said, **"I will give no *deadly* medicine to anyone if asked, nor suggest any such counsel; and in like manner I will not give to a woman a pessary to produce abortion"** has subtly been removed. Perhaps that's why our "doctors" are not adhering to the original oath?

As a law professor once told me, "What we don't say can often be more revealing then what we do say."

As you now know, in their search for answers, *experimental* orthodox medicine has blamed evil spirits, bugs, germs, viruses, prions and now genetics for all our "diseases." If they can't blame it on one or more of those villains, they claim it's all in your head. But fear not, they have a doctor that can take care of that too.

Dis-ease is defined as lack of ease or harmony, it is NOT the same as "disease," a medical term for illness treated by medicine.
NEVER attempt to stop or reduce your medication without the supervision of your medical doctor.

By dividing the body into separate, unrelated parts, we now have "specialists" that can treat everything. Heart problem? Go to a cardiologist. Lung infection? Check out a pulmonologist. Hemorrhoids? Don't worry, you can see a proctologist. Then there are epidemiologists, gastroenterologists, allergists, dermatologists, internists, podiatrists, oncologists, rheumatologists, gynecologists, endocrinologists, neurologists, obstetricians, pediatricians, oral surgeons and on and on.

Other than emergency treatment for accidents, injuries and a few other crisis situations, there is really only one problem with orthodox medicine. *It doesn't work.* If it did, we wouldn't have more people visiting natural healers today than our medical counterparts, and according to government statistics the numbers are growing.

Since its inception, the medical profession has strived to compartmentalize the human body into multiple areas, parts and divisions. From specialties to sub-specialties they have forgotten, assuming they knew in the first place, how every part of the body, mind and spirit are related in balance and harmony. How could they be so far off from common sense and logic? Who or what lead them in a direction so disconnected from the natural order?

It's Called the AMA

Most medical doctors belong to a union. It's called the American Medical Association or AMA. As unions are required, they are there to protect their members, to make sure everyone that wants to is working and that their fees for service are profitable. The AMA was first formed in 1847 at the Academy of Natural Sciences in Philadelphia by Dr. Nathan Smith Davis.

Did I say natural? What an oxymoron that is. Nothing is farther from nature than the "healthcare" treatment the American Medical Association promotes. And no organization has been as relentless as they vehemently attack natural healing.

It's All About Money

The AMA and their *experimental* orthodox medical approach really hasn't changed much from its unionized origin.

Dis-ease is defined as lack of ease or harmony, it is NOT the same as "disease," a medical term for illness treated by medicine.
NEVER attempt to stop or reduce your medication without the supervision of your medical doctor.

In the days of Davis, medics (medical doctors) used blood letting, leeches, surgery and toxic drugs such as mercury, arsenic and lead to treat diseases. Remember how the medics of the day killed President George Washington with blood letting and mercury? Today, they use toxic drugs, invasive surgery, cancer-causing burning radiation and immune destroying chemotherapy to treat "diseases."

Regardless of their current complementary medicine advertising campaign that supposedly embraces all disciplines of medicine, the AMA and their drug-promoting sales force have been fighting natural healing for over two hundred years. Fight they must for there are billions and billions of dollars at risk and don't you think they know it.

Whether attacking homeopathy, chiropractic, osteopathy, naturopathy, acupuncture or Ayervedic, the AMA has viciously and continuously attempted to degrade, ridicule and condemn all other medical disciplines that do not owe its allegiance to them. Even the osteopaths have buckled under pressure and sold out becoming *pseudo* M.D.s, prescribing drugs and performing surgery. The "new" naturopaths are on the same road. They even started their own "club" where they declare only graduates of their *schools* may be licensed, approved or legal. A case in point is Bastyr University in Seattle, Washington.

Reportedly, Dr. John Bastyr became a chiropractic doctor in Seattle, Washington after graduating from the Seattle College of Chiropractic in 1931. In 1936, he acquired a Sanipractic Degree (Natural Healing) from the Northwestern College of Chiropractic in Seattle, Washington. In 1956, Dr. Bastyr founded the College of Naturopathic Medicine in Seattle, Washington. In 1957, Dr. Bastyr was allowed to convert his Sanipractic Degree to a naturopathic degree after completing courses given at Grace University. In 1978, along with Les Griffith, N.D., Bill Mitchell, N.D., Joseph Pizzorno, N.D., and Sheila Qinn, he started Bastyr University in Portland, Oregon, a four-year program offering students a degree in naturopathy.

Unfortunately, Bastyr University, along with The Southwest College of Naturopathic Medicine and Health Sciences and The University of Bridgeport College of Natural Medicine have formed an alliance whereby only their graduates may "legally" practice naturopathy. They infer that all other naturopathic schools such as Christopher and Clayton are inferior and that their graduates are potentially dangerous to the public.

If that is the case, who taught the first graduates of Bastyr? Wasn't it naturopaths like Griffith, Mitchell, Pizzorno and even Bastyr? If their education was good enough to teach others, isn't it good enough to be licensed, approved or legal?

What we have is the beginning of a 'good ole boys" club. My colleagues have forgotten their roots. There wouldn't be a Bastyr or Pizzorno without Sebastian Kneipp (1821-1897), Benedict Lust (1872-1945), Henry Lindlahr (1853-1925), Bernarr Macfadden (1868-1955), John H. Tilden (1851-1940) and the most profound natural healer of our time, John Christopher (1909-1983).

This is protectionism plain and simple. The medics started it against everyone, especially the homeopaths, the osteopaths claim it against the chiropractors and the naturopaths claim it against their own kind! Eventhough it is under the auspices of health, it is really all about *fear*. Since there is only so much money people are willing to spend on healthcare, these "clubs" fear they won't get the biggest piece of pie.

I suppose, if Jesus were alive today, he would be persecuted and prosecuted all over again, but this time it would be for practicing medicine or chiropractic (he used his hands) or naturopathic (he suggested herbs) *without* a license. After all, no one, including Jesus, can claim to heal anyone unless they belong to a "club." The exception to this is under our Freedom of Religion clause in the United States Constitution. However, they would still get him for organizing a *non-chartered* religion, plus, it's against the law to ride a donkey in the city, especially without a driver's license. If you belong to a religious order, you may claim certain healings, but not without a "legal" charter granted by the government. It's all about control and manipulation. It's *really* all about money.

One of the best books I have ever read on how, what and why the AMA and OMIC (Organized Medical Industrial Complex) have created a monopoly in medicine, was written by Daniel Haley entitled, *Politics in Healing.* Introduced by one of very few medical doctors I respect, Dr. Julian Whitaker, Mr. Haley's book takes a deep look into the history of the AMA and its influence in politics and medicine.

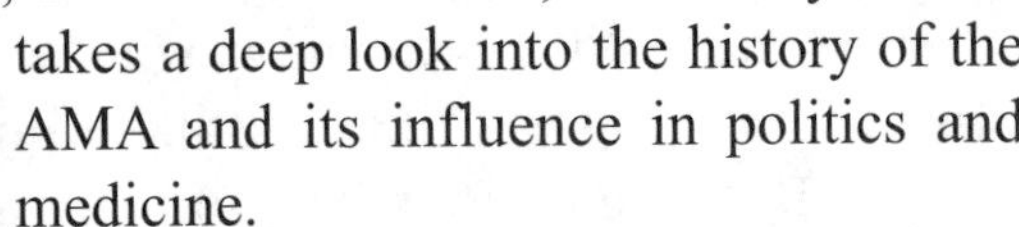

From suppressing natural healing cures such as those discovered by Drs. Hoxsey (Formulae), Koch (Glyoxylide), Rife (Frequency), Ivy (Krebiozen), Jacob (DMSO), and others, to the strategies of the AMA to dominate medicine, this book covers it all.

The Hoxsey Formulae

The Hoxsey formula was discovered by Dr. Harry Hoxey's greatgrandfather. The year was 1840, when John Hoxsey put one of his horses out to pasture to die. Apparently, the horse had incurable cancer and rather than put him down, Mr. Hoxsey let him go.

However, the horse began to heal and John Hoxsey noticed each morning the horse grazing in a particular area. When the tumor dried and fell off, Hoxsey gathered every plant and herb the horse had been eating and then experimented on his neighbors sick animals with the same success.

The formulae was passed down from son to son, using it on farm animals and humans throughout the area, without too much fanfare. No one was ever charged a fee by the Hoxseys nor were they ever turned away. Donations were accepted and by word of mouth news was spreading. No one seemed to care until Dr. Hoxsey started to see *too many* people.

Dis-ease is defined as lack of ease or harmony, it is NOT the same as "disease," a medical term for illness treated by medicine. *NEVER* attempt to stop or reduce your medication without the supervision of your medical doctor.

The herbal formulae his great grandfather created is a simple concoction of specific herbs all known to kill cancer cells.

Dr. Hoxsey, a traditional naturopath, was so successful curing people with cancer the AMA approached him with a deal. They said they wouldn't prosecute him for practicing medicine without a license if he would give them his formulae and never treat another patient again.

When he found out the AMA intended to set up high end expensive clinics using his formulae, he declined their offer. That was the beginning of a thirty-year vendetta against Dr. Hoxsey from court to jail, fines and back to court, until they closed his clinics in 1957. Moving to other states, proved to be futile as the AMA followed Dr. Hoxsey in their smear-and-destroy campaign.

In 1962, Dr. Hoxsey moved his clinic to Mexico where freedom of expression and unorthodox medicine were still allowed. Dr. Hoxsey continued to treat and cure cancer patients until his death in 1974. Known as Centro Bio-Medico, it was one of the first natural healing clinics to go into Tijuana along with the Centro Medical Delmar opened by Dr. Ernesto Contrereas. Dr. Hoxsey's clinic is still there, still curing cancer. I bet you have never heard about it. Why do you think that is?

You may be saying, "This happened a long time ago. It does not happen now." I wish that were true. Unfortunately, it is still happening and in greater numbers. You don't hear about it, because main stream media is part of the "club."

Have you ever thought who decides what gets aired on television? Someone makes a decision to run the stories they do. When dog attacks are declared interesting, all the networks will cover them. If they can't show the truth, they make it up. Even our government has perfected and legalized the use of misinformation. If you doubt me, I suggest you see the movie *Wag the Dog* with Dustin Hoffman.

Several years ago, I got a call from a friend who owned a company making a highly concentrated organic Aloe Vera liquid called T-Plus. Dr. Allen Hoffman, was a biochemist and natural healing researcher. After years of trial and error, he discovered how to reduce sixty gallons of aloe vera juice to just two ounces while keeping the bio-active nutrients intact. The net result of this "tincture" was a cancer cure.

Although Dr. Hoffman only used his T-Plus for cancer in Mexico, it was sold in the United States as a food supplement. When the FDA made contact, they asked him to dilute it. They said at his current concentration it was *too* effective. By diluting it, his product would be as ineffective as all the rest of the liquid extracts.

Like Dr. Hoxsey, Dr. Hoffman refused the government's offer. He is now spending five years in a federal penitentiary. He lost his business, home and all of his money. Even the farmer that grew his aloe was sent to prison.

I spent over 25 years, sending patients to Mexico as well as working with them there. Just twenty years ago, you could receive three weeks of full care and board for under $2,000. After the GATT and NAFTA treaties were signed during the Clinton administration, the United States FDA claimed jurisdiction 200 miles beyond the Mexican border. All clinics and hospitals were order to raise their prices so the United States could be more competitive. However, price or no price, Americans are still not allowed to receive the same kind of medical care in the United States that one receives in Mexico.

From Hoxsey, Gerson, Contrereas, Rife, Hoffman and all other innovators of medicine and natural healing, the only reason why these people went to Mexico is because of the AMA, FDA and our government's suppression of natural healing.

Of all the current facilities operating in Mexico today, I highly recommend *The Oasis of Hope Hospital* in Tijuana, Mexico. Although Dr. Ernesto has passed away, his son, Dr. Francisco, is carrying on the tradition of excellent natural healthcare. Being a German-trained medical doctor and surgeon, Dr. Francisco also incorporates orthodox medicine, but it is not experimental. It is always with respect to the natural balance of the body. For more information, see Index E-*Resources* in the back of the book.

Money

by
Eric C Wyndham

They say it doesn't grow on trees, yet it comes from them.
Money, a medium of exchange, a unit of production,
evidence of ideas in currency.

Although the principle in acquiring it
is somewhat difficult to grasp, once in the flow,
it is easily attainable in greater and greater abundance.

Money is *not* the root of all evil as so often said.
It is the *love* of money that circumvents
the prosperity principle,
thus bringing spiritual torment without recourse.

It is what governments, companies, organizations
and individuals are willing to kill and die for.
It brings people to Lucifer on bended knee,
selling their soul for the opportunity
to acquire more "stuff."

The consciousness of enlightenment
is expressed in us
through our creative imagination.
When we clear our mind of mundane affairs,
we empower ourselves,
finding answers to all our concerns.

Money? It's just something we use
to do the things we choose to do.
Without it, we are merely forced to be more creative.

The Classical Hippocratic Oath

"I swear by Apollo physician and Aesculapius, and Hygieia, and Panaceia, and all the gods and goddesses, making them my witnesses, that I will fulfill according to my ability and judgment, this oath and this covenant:

To hold him who taught me this art as equal to me as my parents, and to live my life in partnership with him, to share my substance with him, and to look upon his offspring in the same footing as my own brothers, and to teach them this art, if they shall wish to learn it, without fee or covenant; and that by precept, lecture, and every other mode of instruction, I will impart a knowledge of the art to my own sons, and those of my teachers, and to disciples bound by the covenant and oath according to the law of medicine, but to none others.

I will apply dietic measures for the benefit of the sick according to my ability and judgment; I will keep them from harm and injustice.

I will give no *deadly* medicine to anyone if asked, nor suggest any such counsel; and in like manner I will not give to a woman a pessary to produce abortion. With purity and with holiness, I will guard my life and practice my art.

I will not cut persons laboring under the stone, but will leave this to be done by men who are practitioners of this work.

Into whatever houses I enter, I will go for the benefit of the sick, and will abstain from every voluntary act of mischief and corruption; and further, from the seduction of females or males, of freemen and slaves.

Whatever I see or hear in the course of treatment, which ought not be spoken of abroad, I will not divulge, as all such said should be kept secret. While I continue to keep this oath unviolated, may it be granted to me to enjoy life and art, respected by all men, in all times; but should I trespass and violate this oath swearing falsely, may the reverse be my lot.

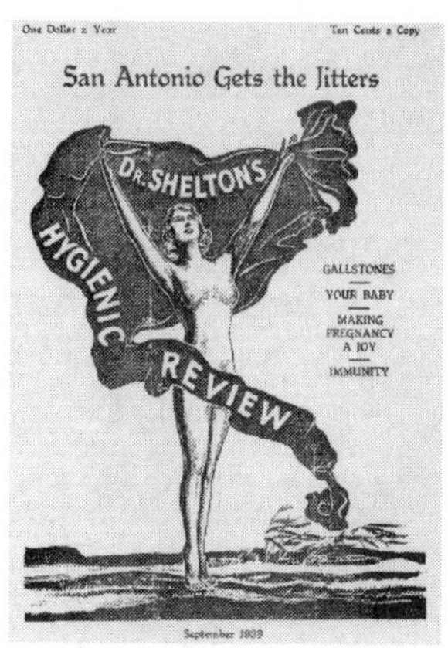

CHAPTER 6 - THE CHAPPELL PROTOCOL FOR HEALTH & LONGEVITY: A STEP-BY-STEP *INTENSIVE* CLINICAL PROGRAM

"We all would love to play piano. Unfortunately, only few of us are willing to practice." **- Liberace**

The following protocol is *extremely* thorough and very complete. In fact, it is *intense* to say the least. Having said that, it is also a culmination of the best programs of every healing center I know of. After reading this chapter, you will know why *experimental* orthodox medicine doesn't work, yet is still first choice when one is seeking to find temporary relief.

Taking powerful drugs that are designed to cover up symptoms is a lot easier to do than going on an all-inclusive healing program like the one contained herein. Some drugs can give instant relief, as aspirin does for most headaches. Unfortunately, if your headache is *caused* from a toxic liver, aspirin won't help, but a coffee enema along with a good detox and nutritional program, should.

Before we jump into the core of my protocol, I again need to give you a *mandatory* governmental warning. You won't find such a warning in an *experimental* orthodox medical doctor's book, but we in natural healing are forced to print the following if the book provides real information about healing yourself:

Dis-ease is defined as lack of ease or harmony, it is NOT the same as "disease," a medical term for illness treated by medicine. *NEVER* attempt to stop or reduce your medication without the supervision of your medical doctor.

United States Government
WARNING

The statements found within the pages of this book and especially this chapter, have not been evaluated by the United States Food and Drug Administration (FDA) or The American Medical Association (AMA).

(The FDA is allegedly a non-bias governmental agency created to protect American citizens from toxic and/or unsafe food and drugs. This is the agency that has approved the thousands of drugs found in the over 3,000-page Physician Desk Reference (PDR), much of which is devoted to the adverse, life-threatening, TOXIC side effects of drugs. Confused? You are not alone.)

(Remember: The AMA is a private corporation serving as a union to protect its members made up of medical doctors. A medical doctor is one that practices medicine as dictated by the AMA limited to using the FDA approved toxic drugs, including chemo-therapy, mutilating surgeries and carcinogenic radiation. The AMA uses the FDA and other governmental agencies to enforce their medical monopoly on the unsuspecting and uniformed public. Both the FDA and AMA are part of the Organized Medical Industrial Complex (OMIC) which is controlled by the major pharmaceutical and petro-chemical companies.)

This book is published under the First Amendment of the United States Constitution, which grants us the right to discuss openly and freely all matters of public concern and to express viewpoints no matter how controversial or unaccepted they may be. However, medical groups and pharmaceutical companies have finally infiltrated and violated our sacred constitution. Therefore, we are FORCED to give you the following WARNINGS:

If you are ill or have been diagnosed with any disease, consult a medical doctor before attempting to use any natural healing program or nutraceutical/botanical formulae explained in this book. (As ludicrous as that sounds and knowing medical doctors know nothing about natural healing, your government has been lobbied by the above organizations to force us, for your own good, I am sure, to warn you):

I, Dr. James Chappell, am *not* a licensed medical doctor (nor do I want to be) therefore my opinions, assumptions, suggestions, beliefs and advice are based solely on my 34 years of research, education, investigation and clinical experience in the natural healing field. Although I have specialized in educating people with severe, chronic and so-called "terminal" illnesses, my opinions, experience and beliefs are *not* accepted by medical (drug) doctors, medical associations (AMA) and the accepted medical "scientific" community.

Many foods, herbs or other natural substances that I may reveal herein, can occasionally cause or have dangerous allergic reactions in some people. As an example, there have been individuals that have died from allergic reactions to peanuts and strawberries. According to your government, any one of the nutraceutical/botanical formulae or natural healing programs in this book could be potentially dangerous, even lethal, especially if you are seriously ill or pregnant. Therefore, any formulae or natural healing program you learn about in this book theoretically may cause harm, instead of the benefit you seek.

Nothing in this book is intended to diagnose, treat, cure or prevent any "disease," even if it does. (The FDA and AMA want you to know that only a medical doctor can do that. Although it is agreed that members of OMIC can diagnose and treat anything they want, we are still waiting for their cure or prevention of anything, even the so-called "common cold.")

(Although some of what you are about to read may be repetitive, it is worth repeating. It has been said, it takes seven exposures to a thought or idea before it really imprints in our memory. With that in mind, you may want to read this book or at least this chapter several times just to make sure you thoroughly understand how important this information is. After that, start doing whatever feels comfortable to you, but get started.)

A Word from One Who's Been There

While others write about miracle doctors *curing* so-called "incurable" diseases, Dr. "Jimmy" Chappell is the kind of doctor they are writing about. I call Dr. Chappell "Jimmy" because when I first met him over 40 years ago, that's who he was.

Jimmy was a bright-eyed, scrappy kid with a good singing voice. I was the manager of a local teenage band looking for someone to replace our bass player who quit the group. As luck would have it, I happened to be one of the judges in a battle-of-the-bands contest where 15-year old Jimmy was competing. After the contest, I approached him and asked if he would like to audition for my group. He did and soon became a member.

For over three years, I knew what kind of life Jimmy had at home. I even used to go dancing with his parents, drinking and smoking until all hours of the night. I got to know Jimmy's folks, very well.

After years of abusing my body, I finally came down with throat and lung cancer. Even though my family and I knew Jimmy had become a natural healing doctor, I was brought up to have faith in the orthodox medical approach, so I tried them first.

Of course, after removing the cancer in my throat, preventing me from ever speaking again and going through chemotherapy and radiation, the doctors gave me up for dead. It was at that time, my daughter Linda called Jimmy.

Without a second thought, Dr. "Jimmy" immediately came to see me at the VA Hospital in San Diego, California. In spite of my death sentence, he told me if I would commit to his *intensive* protocol, I had a chance of not only surviving, but to actually beat this thing called cancer.

Let me tell you, his program *is* intense, but I am here today because it absolutely works. Thanks to Dr. Jimmy's help and with my wife and daughter's love and devotion, it has been eight years and I am still cancer free. He promised me I would and I am.

I always knew Jimmy was special.

Carl Semon

Dis-ease is defined as lack of ease or harmony, it is NOT the same as "disease," a medical term for illness treated by medicine.
NEVER attempt to stop or reduce your medication without the supervision of your medical doctor.

I. THE *CAUSE* OF DIS-EASE

A. Affecting the Physical Level:

As we discussed in detail in Chapter 2, the common denominator in all dis-eases is a condition called The H.O.N.S.T.E.C. Syndrome®. It includes the following:

H - Hydration or the lack thereof;
O - Oxygen/Tissue deprivation;
N - Nutritional deficiencies and/or excesses;
S - Spinal/Structural/Neurological aberrations;
T - Toxic waste accumulation;
E - Emotional/Energetic blocks or release; and
C - Creation Consciousness

As it is now known, all life is Energy (spirit) in a physical form. Although there are physical reasons for illness as described above, the underlining real *cause* can always be traced back to displaced vibratory energy. Displaced harmonious energy leads to vibratory chaos. Vibratory chaos leads to dis-harmony and this ultimately leads to dis-ease. Those spiritually aligned seem to handle any and all of the components of The H.O.N.S.T.E.C. Syndrome® more easily. When we lose our "connection," spiritually speaking, we become susceptible to this world and its environment.

II. PSYCHOLOGICAL PREREQUISITES TO GETTING WELL

A. Attitude and Perception :

You may have heard or even believe; "You have cancer or AIDS etc., and there is *no* cure. You have three months to live." Once you realize that this image you call "you" is actually a projection of Energetic, Spiritual, Vibratory Consciousness of which you control, then life takes on a whole new meaning and so does regaining your health.

To become your new attitude, try writing a new *script* of who you are and what you want to do in this life. See yourself healthy, happy and at peace. If you can think it, you can create it.

B. Eliminating Stubbornness:

Without question, one's reluctance to expand their paradigm (consciousness), will inherently keep them from realizing their full healing potential. Have you ever said, "This is too good to be true, after all, if this really worked, why haven't I heard this before or why hasn't *my* doctor told me about this." Or what about, "*My* doctor said natural healing is *quackery*."

Now that is an interesting statement. Do you really know what a *quack is* anyway?

After being called a *quack* by our illustrious medical establishment more times than I'd prefer to remember, I decided to find out the history behind this word and meaning.

Theophrastus von Hohenheim was known as the *Father of Pharmacology*. He was born in 1490 and died in 1541 A.D. Although the Chinese reportedly used mercury (a metallic mineral) for the treatment of ulcers over 2,000 years before, Hohenheim was the first person at that time to give the toxic metal to his patients.

From 460 B.C. the year of Hippocrates' birth, to 1500 A.D., we have *no* record of anyone giving large doses of poisonous minerals for the cure of dis-ease until Hohenheim thought of using them.

The giving of mercury, also called quicksilver or *Quack Salber* resulted in the naming of physicians who treated patients with this toxic substance, *quacks*. This was the start of toxic metals, minerals and potions for the treatment of dis-ease. Our current *experimental* orthodox medical system has merely expanded on this archaic practice of applying toxic substances to humans with their litany of drugs. The only doctor that could ever be called a *quack*, is the medical doctor prescribing poisonous pills.

Although herbal medicine was the first system of healing historically recorded several thousands years B.C., with the plague-like convergence of *quacks* and their toxic minerals (drugs), herbs fell out of favor.

What we have now is a world fooled by quacks (medics) peddling their toxic drugs to an unsuspecting populace. Of course, more and more of us are becoming enlightened on all levels, including that which relates to health and healing.

When I am asked what the number one reason why someone does *not* get well, in my opinion, it is always because of their stubbornness. If we would simply, "Throw our heart over the bar, our body would follow." If you really want to be well, you must be willing to do whatever it takes, including forgiving the unforgivable and doing the following intensive program.

III. PROTOCOL TO HEAL YOURSELF OF *ALL* DIS-EASES.

(For *all* suggested products, go to the *Resources* page in the back of the book).

A. Physical Level:

1. Open the Elimination Channels - One reason why so many natural healing protocols do not work is because they are initiated *out of order*. You cannot destroy a tumor or a pathogen and expect to get well, if you have not opened the pathways to allow the body to remove the destroyed material. And so it is for parasites, viruses, bacteria and pathogens. Only after the elimination channels are open can you depolarize the blood and lymph and then detoxify the entire body. Once this has been accomplished, you can rebuild and repair the immune system that will then go after pathogens, carcinogens and other infectious agents. The first channel that must be open is the colon:

a. Colon - The first and most important part of any true natural healing protocol is to purge or clean the colon. The best way to do this is with either a high enema or colon therapy. Using organic coffee water in a high enema not only flushes out the colon, but will help to purge the liver and gallbladder. (See how to do a proper coffee enema on page 271 in this chapter). Additionally, take one or more capsules of *Intestinal Stimulating Compound #1* at night. Increase the dose nightly until you have a tremendous bowel movement in the morning. Reduce dose until you find the minimum amount that allows the same action. Additionally, take two *CellBiotics* capsules orally every night.

b. Kidneys - One way to open the kidneys is to take an herbal tincture called *Goldenrod & Horsetail Compound.* This formulae increases the flow of urine and disinfects the kidneys and bladder. One dropperful three times per day in a cup of *red clover tea* (a blood purifier) will start the process.

c. Liver - *Milkthistle & Dandelion Root* tincture will help to open, repair, rebuild and protect the liver. As with the above, take one dropperful three times per day in the same red clover tea.

d. Lungs - *Lobelia & Fenugreek* tincture will dilate the bronchial tubes, work as an expectorant and dry excessive mucous from the lungs. Dosage is the same as above in the same cup of red clover tea.

e. Skin - The skin is actually the largest detoxifying gland in the body. Before your morning shower: hydrotherapy, do a dry skin brushing, then get in the shower and alternate hot and cold.

To do a dry skin brushing you simply use a natural bristle brush with a long handle. Start at your feet and brush your skin always towards the heart. From your legs, brush your arms, back, chest and buttocks. The purpose of a dry skin brushing is to stimulate your blood and lymphatic circulation.

Take as hot of a shower as you can for about 10 seconds, then cold for about 10 seconds or more, then turn the hot water back up for about 10 seconds. Do the hot and cold routine for six or seven times each. Always end with cold.

You can take a hydrotherapy shower one to three times per day. After the shower, apply an apple cider vinegar and distilled water solution to the entire body. I recommend *Bragg's Apple Cider* at four ounces to one gallon of distilled water. Apply to a sponge and then to your body.

2. Depolarize and Liquefy the Blood and Lymph - When we are sick, our blood and lymph (the sewer system of the body) becomes very thick. This condition is called agglutination or polarization. If you look at a sample of blood with a darkfield microscope, you will see the red blood cells looking like a "string of pearls." This is actually called rouleau. In order to actuate a true healing or recovery, one must depolarize and liquefy the blood and lymph. Here are a few ways known to really get the job done:

a. Stillingia Root and Red Clover Compound (Hoxsey Formulae) - Even if you open the elimination channels, unless you depolarize and liquefy the blood and lymphatic circulation, you will not be able to remove toxic waste from the body. Take this tincture as with the above herbal tinctures, same dose, in cup of red clover tea.

b. Beck's Lymphatic (Magnetic Pulser) and Blood (Pulser) Depolarizer - The magnetic pulser helps to increase lymphatic flow. The blood pulser does the same for the blood. By electrifying it, it also kills bacteria, viruses, parasites and other pathogens. The blood pulser can also make colloidal silver.

c. Skilling's Harmonic Pulser - A 728 Hz healing frequency modulates a 28.322 MHz Radio-Frequency generating a large amount of harmonics. These frequencies have a positive effect on one's well-being. It has been known to reduce tumors.

d. Dinshah's Light Emitting Diode (LED) - The LED assists the body to achieve a free flow of proteins within the cell, providing for the body to re-establish its 'fluid flow' and release hemo-toxins. The LED, a non-invasive technology, uses specific light waves to provide compatible frequencies used by the cell in correcting its out-of-balance condition. Disassociation from the binding agent, which contributed to the swelling and blockage, is accomplished with the cell's toxic flow pattern re-established.

3. Detoxify, Purify and Oxygenate the Body

From the beginning of my career, I have told people to simple stop doing those things that make them sick and start doing those things that will help them get well. One of the easiest ways of detoxifying the body is to replace eating junk food with all-organic (toxin and chemical free) fruits, vegetables, nuts, seeds, sprouts and legumes. In addition, drinking charged distilled water and plenty of it, will not only detoxify the body, it will help purify

Dis-ease is defined as lack of ease or harmony, it is NOT the
same as "disease," a medical term for illness treated by medicine.
NEVER attempt to stop or reduce your medication without the supervision of your medical doctor.

and oxygenate. Just doing these two simple things will improve your health greatly.

a. Flor Essence by Flora - Originally formulated by the Ojibwa Indians in Canada, this herbal compound has a tremendous effect on purifying and detoxify the body. Dr. Charles A. Brusch, the personal physician of President John F. Kennedy, has stated unequivocally that *Flor Essence* is a *cure* for cancer. He should know: he cured himself of liver cancer using it. Take 1 to 3 oz. per day.

b. Charged Distilled Water - Remember, adults need to drink half of their body weight in ounces per day. Distilled water is pure H2O. Mix 1/2 teaspoon of Zeta Crystals® to one gallon of distilled water to charge it.

c. Red Clover Tea & Green Tea - Both are strong, blood-purifying herbs. They are also used to put most of the other herbal tinctures in. Drink 3 cups per day alternating each herb every other day.

d. Intestinal Drawing Compound - This is a major detoxifier. Take four capsules in a glass of charged distilled water every night. It contains activated charcoal, slippery elm and other drawing elements. If you have toxic metals in your body, like mercury or aluminum, this is an excellent first step.

e. Bio-Oxidative Therapies - The FDA and the AMA want you to know that regardless of how many people throughout the world are using bio-oxidative therapies, including medical grade ozone machines and 35% hydrogen peroxide, it is only safe in Mexico and other specific countries and possibly Nevada. Outside of those areas, it's illegal in the United States.

Ozone and 35% food or medical grade hydrogen peroxide stimulate the production of white blood cells, which are necessary to fight infection. They are virucidal. They increase oxygen and hemoglobin disassociation, thus increasing the delivery of oxygen from the blood to the cells. They are anti-neoplastic, which means that they inhibit the growth of new tissues like tumors. They oxidize and degrade petrochemicals and increase red blood cell membrane distensibility, thus enhancing their flexibility and effectiveness. They increase the production of interferon and tumor necrosis factor, which the body uses to fight infections and cancers. Ozone increases the efficiency of the antioxidant enzyme system, which scavenges excess free radicals in the body. Ozone accelerates the citric acid cycle, which is the main cycle for the liberation of energy from sugars. This then stimulates basic metabolism. It also breaks down proteins, carbohydrates and fats to be used as energy.

Finally, oxygen therapies increase tissue oxygenation, thus bringing about patient improvement. 35% hydrogen peroxide: Dose: 5 to 10 drops in 8 oz of water three times per day. Ozone: In Mexico, the doctors apply ozone using either I.V. or vaginal and rectal insufflation.

f. Wormwood Compound - According to the world-famous researcher and natural healer, Dr. Hulda Clark, most dis-eases and *all* cancers are associated with parasites. Not just "worms" that you can see, but microscopic parasites you cannot see without the help of a microscope. Dr. Clark recommends Wormwood Compound per instructions on the label for at least two months.

4. Nourish and Rebuild the Body and Immune System

There are SEVEN food consumption nutritional levels:

1. Poor - defined as those eating mostly carbohydrates; beans, rice, pasta, bread, cereals etc. Junk food; donuts, cookies, pies, cakes, chips, candy, ice cream and others daily. There is no concern if GM, irradiated or pesticide sprayed food "stuffs" or alcohol is consumed.

2. Typical - defined as those eating mostly carbohydrates along with a large amount of animal: pork, beef and some poultry. Very little fruits and vegetables are consumed. Junk food and liquid candy - sodas and coffee-drinks are also part of this level. Again, toxic-sprayed food is not a concern, nor copious amounts of alcohol.

3. Optimum - defined as those eating mostly

organic fruits, vegetables, nuts, seeds, sprouts, legumes, grains, limited dairy, free-range chicken and turkey only. No junk food is ever eaten. Alcohol is always in moderation.

4. Ideal - defined as those not only eating an optimum diet, but whereby strict food combining and eating according to the seasons is practiced. I do NOT believe only vegetarians or vegans can attain ideal health. According to Dr. William Kelly and others, there are several distinctive classifications of metabolism, from vegetarian, carnivore to mixed, your genetic make-up plays a major role in what types of foods are best for you.

5. Therapeutic - defined as those eating mostly fruits, vegetables, nuts, seeds, sprouts and legumes. When someone is ill, they need to conserve energy and rapidly change their pH from acid to alkaline. Animal protein takes a lot of time and energy to digest. It also acidifies the body. Grains also acidify the body. Therefore, animal and grains are not recommended in a therapeutic diet.

6. Intensive - defined as those eating organic vegetables only. They may only drink organic vegetable juice and eat organic soups and salads. Nothing else is allowed.

7. Extreme - defined as those drinking organic vegetable juice only. This nutritional level is primarily for those individuals either very ill or having gone through orthodox medical treatment such as chemotherapy and radiation.

(Note: The more ill one is, the more restrictive their diet should be. After you have established your diet level from the therapeutic, intensive and extreme levels, the following basic nutritional recommendations apply).

Juice and Supplements

a. Only after the elimination channels are open, the blood and lymph have been depolarized and the body is detoxifying, will you be able to rejuvenate the immune system and rebuild/repair the body. When someone is ill, they need all the energy they can acquire to get well, to include the energy that is expended while eating. For that reason and others, most natural healing protocols have an individual drink (really chew) organic vegetable juice all day long. The best organic vegetable juice is carrot, beet and spinach with the juice of two cloves of garlic. Added to your morning organic vegetable juice will be one tablespoon or more of QCI's Super Kamut (part of QCI's LifePack System®) and 1/8 teaspoon to as much as you can take of cayenne powder. You may also add one tablespoon of Brewer's yeast and/or wheat germ, if you wish and Omega 369 Flaxseed oil.

b. Along with your morning drink, take one capsule of ProDigestives and one capsule of Coral Blend, then again two more times during the day.

c. To build your T-cell count take d-Lenolate, 3 capsules per day or Aloe Immune at the same dose. There are also several other effective immune enhancers available. See under Index E-*Resources*.

d. For Vitamin A and DHA/EPA take one to two capsules of Neptune Krill Oil daily.

e. For Vitamin C take one scoop of Ultra C three times per day in a glass of ozonated, charged distilled water with 10 drops of Stable O.

f. The best form of B-17 is apricot kernels. If you need this nutrient, eat 1 kernel per ten pounds of your ideal weight per day; that is, 150 lbs. = 15 kernels daily. You can also alternate apricot kernels one day and up to six bitter almonds the next. If your health is compromised, just eat the apricot kernels, daily.

g. There may be additional herbal tinctures or remedies, nutraceutical products and/or electronics needed. See product list in attached catalog for additional items.

h. One of the most important additions to a complete health plan are Probiotics and HSO's or homeostatic Soil Organisms. Take one capsule three times per day of PB8 and one scoop, one time per day of Primal Defense.

IV. Important Tests

This is covered in detail with several of the best diagnostic tests available in Chapter 8 - Health Questionnaire & Effective Evaluations.

V. Level-One Adjunctive Additions:

A. Chiropractic and acupuncture are extremely important healing modalities. Have one or both a couple of times per week until well or balanced.

B. General and lymphatic massage is very helpful at least three times per week. Even relatives can learn how to give a good massage, thereby reducing the expense.

C. Castor and olive oil packs are fantastic decongestive aids. Apply to the affected area each night using flannel or cotton soaked in a piece of old flannel or new in a cake pan. Place over area and cover with plastic wrap. Leave on all night.

D. The Rebounder (a small trampoline) helps to stimulate the blood and lymphatic circulation. Use it about 10 to 20 minutes daily.

The Cold-Sheet Treatment: Inducing a Fever

Mankind suffered greatly when the Black Plague struck Europe during the dark ages as well as the many times these types of flu or influenza have returned to the world. Today, AIDS is known as the plague and feared at the same level. But fear not, for what you are about to learn, just may keep you healthy.

In natural medicine, a fever is given to a person to assist in healing the body that has become toxic, *causing* a dis-ease. Fever is like a fire, which can warm your body and save your life or burn your house down and kill you. If the fever is properly controlled and skillfully handled it will clean the poisons, toxins and surplus mucus from the body and bring on a healing crisis. If not controlled properly the fever can kill the patient.

With the information you are about to learn, many lives can be saved should an induced fever be necessary. Water therapy has been used for centuries to heal the sick. Reverend. S. Kneipp, the great natural doctor of the old country, had published books on "water cures." Many doctors and authors have written volumes on this subject, and why not? The body is made up of over 75% liquid. However, when the fluids in the body become toxic - loaded with "bad" cholesterol, mucus, parasites, viruses, bacteria, etc., we must detoxify. By properly replacing toxic fluids with healthy ones, we have an opportunity to achieve optimum health.

As a story goes, many years ago a peasant was walking home with miles to go. He was sick with a fever, upper-respiratory infection ("cold") and sciatica or what was then called lumbago. While crossing a stream using a log for a bridge, he slipped and fell into the icy cold water and was drenched to the "bone." It was a bitterly cold day and the man had to walk home in the cold in sloppy wet clothes. By the time he arrived home, his clothes were nearly dried out. His fever had risen, to a point of a healing climax and was down to nearly normal at the end of his journey. The sciatica and fever were gone.

I guess since he never got to the *cause* of his problem, the next time he got sciatica with a fever he knew the cure: he would return to the stream, fall in and walk home again.

What I am about to tell you will have the same net effect of "falling into a stream" relative to having and losing a fever, but it will be something you can do at home. It is called The Cold-Sheet Treatment.

This program will take a little time and effort for the one doing the nursing. If you are interested in seeing a sick friend, patient or loved one healed, you will never regret the time spent learning this procedure, because The Cold Sheet Treatment has literally saved many lives. Even some of those who were given up as hopeless, left to die, were brought back to good health with this program. Follow it to the letter and don't be afraid. You are not the first to induce a fever.

Step One: Coffee Enema

Coffee enemas have been used for hundreds of years to detoxify the liver, purge the gallbladder and clean the colon, including bowel pockets. Here's a safe way of doing one:

1. Prepare the bathroom with towels on the floor, a pillow, candles, incense and a CD/Tape machine with your favorite relaxing music.

2. Make two cups of organic coffee using distilled water.

You can buy organic coffee and distilled water at any good health food store. Any coffee maker will do. Read instructions.

3. Pour two cups (mugs) of coffee into an enema bag. You can buy a bag at most pharmacies. After pouring the coffee water in the bag, fill the rest of the bag with warm distilled water. Make sure the hose valve is clamped so the coffee water does not leak out.

4. Placing the bag on a coat hanger, hang the enema bag on the inside of the bathroom doorknob.

5. Turn on your music, light a candle and the incense (unless you want to go without).

6. Lie down on your left side and apply a little olive oil on the rectal tip at the end of the enema bag hose and a little olive oil on your anus.

7. Insert tip into the anus and release the valve on the bag hose. As the coffee water is entering the colon, massage the left side of your abdomen. Once you have allowed enough fluid to enter, based on pressure felt, close the valve, remove tip and hold the coffee water for at least three to five minutes, then void contents in toilet. Deep breathing during this time helps to relax you and lessen cramping.

8. Lie down on the floor again, this time on your back. Repeat the same process, however, this time massage the center of your abdomen. Again, breathe deeply; hold coffee water for a few minutes and then void.

9. Finally, get on the floor on your right side down. Repeat the same process as above, however, this time massage the right side of your abdomen. Again, hold for a few minutes and void. If you have a tremendous amount of fecal matter coming out, repeat the whole process using just distilled water.

(NOTE: If coffee water is too stimulating, you can use the juice of two lemons mixed in the same amount of distilled water, instead).

Now that you have learned how to do a proper coffee enema, give the patient an enema. A *cold* enema will cause the anus and rectal area to contract and retain the fluid until it reaches body temperature. This allows the liquid to stay in the body longer which softens more dried waste matter, causing it to become loose. However, you can use a warm water enema if you wish.

Step Two: Garlic Injection or Implant.

In herbology an injection is *never* a needle; it is a syringe-type application. For this part you need a baby rectal syringe or bulb. Into a pint of one-half Bragg's Organic Apple Cider Vinegar and one-half distilled water, blend in two finely grated or pressed garlic cloves. Have the garlic liquid still thin enough that it will pass through the orifice of the syringe. If you use a blender just drop in cloves of peeled garlic, one at a time, until the proper amount is used where it still flows from the syringe without clogging.

With the patient lying on the bathroom floor on a towel, using the baby rectal syringe, implant/inject the garlic solution into their rectum (a pint for adult or less for children), encouraging the patient to *retain as long as possible* before voiding. However, most people can *not* hold garlic for longer than a minute or so. Keep the patient well covered while waiting. You will find it is easier for the patient to hold in the liquid if lying on a slant board or with buttocks elevated with pillows. After the garlic mixture has been voided, go to next step.

Step Three: Seal the Tissue.

Before the patient is placed in a bathtub, apply petroleum gel to the sensitive parts of the body: vagina, rectum, penis (orifice) and nipples. Then place the patient in the tub full of hot water, as hot as as possible (without blistering or scalding the flesh, of course). Once they have entered and become equilibrated with the temperature of the water, add three very finely ground diaphoretic herbs, namely an ounce or more of *cayenne*, an ounce or more of *ginger* and an ounce or more of dry *mustard*. It may be best to place all three herbs in a clean white sock then swish the sock around in the hot water.

These three herbs will assist greatly in speeding up the perspiring of the patient, which is very important. This program creates an artificial fever or increases the fever they already have, to a higher degree. This is being done to bring an incubation condition into place and to cause the WBCs (white blood cells) to multiple and move as rapidly as is possible, and the pathogens to neutralize toxins. Remember, germs are scavengers that live on toxins, mucus, poisons and filth. They are nature's perfect garbage men. We should work with them, not against them. With the moist incubation, they multiply faster and faster. To live they must eat, and the only thing they can consume is the filth of the body. When all the garbage is cleaned up they die, because they have nothing more to live on.

A pathogen or germ cannot consume or live on a good live-cell structure. If they could, then they would literally consume us. But after cleaning out the body of our sickness - debris and accumulated waste, the germ finishes its job and leaves us with a healing climax.

If we take shots, inoculation and/or oral medication to kill "germs," pathogens, virus or bacteria, we have defeated the purpose of nature. It is like having a sanitation strike in a large city. We have seen this several times in our travels, and in one large city it was estimated that three thousand tons of garbage was stacked up on the streets each day. When we kill our garbage men (germs) in the human body, we still have the original filth they were trying to consume, plus continual additions and the corpses of all the germs we have killed.

This causes the heart to labor, trying to pump the sludge through the system, pulling calcium from wherever it can to help in this extra labor. Then when we are faced with a calcium deficiency, which can develop rheumatic fever (causing a rheumatic heart and a weakened body). It can even (one day) go into polio, stroke, multiple sclerosis, muscular dystrophy, etc. The rheumatic fever condition leaves a calcium weakness that can lie dormant for years and then with a new loss of calcium at some future date, can develop into a worse condition.

The purpose of a Cold-Sheet Treatment is to build a fever as fast as possible with moisture. A dry fever is a killer, causing infantile paralysis, brain fever, etc., but *moist* fever can go much higher and if used properly can only do good as the "Maker" of this human body intended.

Step Four: Herbal Teas.

To assist increasing the fever, give the patient diaphoretic teas. This can be any good sweating tea such as yarrow (Achillea millefolium), blessed thistle, camomile (Anthemis nobilis), pleurisy root (Asclepias tuberose), boneset (Eupatorium perfoliatum), thyme (Thymus vulgaris), Hyssop (Hyssopus officinalis), garden sage (Salvia officinalis), catnip (Nepeta cataria), spearmint (Mentha viridis) or other good diaphoretic (sweating) herbs.

When the patient begins to sweat in the tub, give only hot yarrow or one of the other teas, unsweetened, but stay with one type of tea to drink if possible, like yarrow or boneset or whichever you have. Have them drink as much as is possible or at least four cups.

During the sweating, the patient may get lightheaded and feel like fainting. If so, place a cold towel or washcloth on the forehead. Leave the patient in the hot tub as long as is possible, then have them step out or lift them out of the tub.

Step Five: The Cold Sheet.

Wrap a large white sheet, dripping wet from being soaked in a bucket of ice-cold water, around the standing patient. The patient wrapped and then put into a bed that has been prepared by having a rubber or plastic sheet protecting the mattress, with a cotton sheet over it. Then a dry cotton sheet covers the patient (still wrapped, of course in the cold wet sheet), and natural fiber blankets are put over the top sheet for warmth and to help continue the sweating routine.

The reason for using natural fibers to cover the patient is that synthetic cloth will not breathe. It will not allow oxygen, the breath of life, to get into the body. Approximately 60 percent of all breathing done by the human body is from the neck down. This is done through the skin, and if the skin is covered with material that cannot permit breathing, the individual will eventually suffocate.

Step Six: Garlic Foot Paste.

Having already prepared the garlic paste by blending crushed or finely grated, peeled cloves of fresh garlic into Vaseline (petrolatum) about half and half. The low-vibration Vaseline will not be absorbed into the skin, as will anhydrous lanolin or vitamin ointment. The Vaseline holds the garlic in suspension - where the high-vibration ointments would be absorbed and leave the garlic exposed to the bare skin to thus blister it.

Before applying the garlic paste, the feet, from the ankles down, must be thoroughly massaged with olive oil. Allow as much of this oil to be absorbed into the skin as possible, covering the sole, sides and entire foot area.

After the oiling is accomplished, the next step is to use about one-half inch thick or more of the garlic paste and spread it on gauze or a cotton or wool cloth and apply over the entire sole of both feet. Do not allow the paste to get up on the sides on top of the foot only on the sole. The sole is the area where the major part of reflexology (zonal therapy) is applied, and here is where the nerves end from the entire body, including all the organs. By being applied to the soles of the feet, the garlic will be able to disperse its oxygen-carrying power throughout the body for healing.

Use two-inch gauze or torn white cotton strips as a bandage to hold the garlic paste on the sole of the foot. When this is in place, gently pull a large cotton or wool white sock over the foot and bandage to aid in holding in place.

Put the bandaged feet back under the cold wet sheet and pin the bottom of the sheet together so the patient will be in a wet sack. Use a large double sheet (instead of small) because it will allow the patient to roll or turn around as we often do at night without being too closely confined.

The patient should now sleep all night, in most all cases, and you will not have to worry about the problem of wanting to get up to urinate (because of drinking all that tea). If they have to, they can while in the sheet. In addition, the subconscious mind will automatically build up more artificial fever to warm the body. Here we continue the incubation process and use up the teas and moisture accumulated in the body to warm the outside of the wet body. This process causes perspiration and draws heavily on the body for moist heat. While this is being done it breaks loose old toxins, drugs and medicines, mucus and poisons of the past which have accumulated, and will, with the sweating, carry these unwanted materials to the outside of the body.

With the heat generated the wet sheet will become dry. With the poisons and old drugs being removed from the body, the patient will rest better and their sleep will be a much more satisfying one than can be imagined.

Step Seven: Morning Sponge Bath.

In the morning after the patient awakens from their deep sleep, take them out of the bed and sponge them down thoroughly with 50 percent Bragg's Organic Apple Cider Vinegar and 50 percent warm distilled water. This is to remove any sticky poison mucus that has worked its way out of the body. Some of it will still be in the pores and on the skin. Sponging off the body this way will allow the body to breathe again through the skin.

The patient will now feel fantastic as though all the weight of the world has been lifted off their shoulders (with poisons and toxins removed). Put fresh clothing on them and make up the bed with fresh bedding and have them go back to bed and relax to gain back their strength.

The large white "cold" sheet should be stained with dye from old drugs and toxins from as far back as childhood. The dye from these drugs will be of various shades and colors from pastel to dark. It is far better to have these inorganic drugs and poisons on the sheet, rather than inside the body.

Note: This process has been used successfully to aid in removing the cravings for nicotine, alcohol, as well as other drug problems. The person to be helped must want to have this aid and must cooperate with the program.

Step Eight: Juice.

By this time the patient may have a desire for something to drink or to eat. This is a very important because we can gain or lose ground at this time. Cravings from the past may crop out; the patient will want a steak, full meal, processed beverages, ice cream, gooey pastries, junk "food," etc. Do not let them eat this junk. Give the patient fresh fruit or vegetable juices or bottled or fresh grape juice, apple juice, etc., with no additives.

Each mouthful of juice should be swished (chewed) thoroughly to mix it with the saliva for good assimilation. By chewing, there will be no adverse action on the pancreas, thereby being helpful instead of reactionary as in cases of diabetes or hypoglycemia.

Do not mix the juices, but let them drink (chew) as much of any one kind they want or feel comfortable with. If a change of juice is desired, wait at least one half hour before using a different one. After a few hours, if the patient is really hungry, let them have a little local ripe fresh fruit, but it must be chewed to a liquid before swallowing, During the day it is good for the patient to have as much charged distilled water as desired and good herb teas. Add a little honey to the teas, if desired.

Personal Case:

Many years ago I received an emergency call from a male patient of mine asking me to come to his house immediately. He said his wife had a high fever and was hallucinating. I asked him a few questions concerning drug use, allergies, etc., to rule out other contributing factors, but since he did not want her to go to the hospital, I went to see her.

Upon arriving, I noticed an extremely agitated women in her mid 30's. She was in bed with her nightclothes soaked through and through from a sulfur-smelling perspiration and fever. She told me she had not had a bowel movement for ten days and had a fever for the last three.

I had seen patients like this on many occasions before, I asked her husband and son to leave the house. I knew what was about to take place and I didn't need her family to come to her rescue.

I made her a cup of organic red clover and red raspberry tea. While she was sipping the tea, I drew a hot bath with two cups of Epsom Salts mixed in and started a fresh brew of organic coffee. I told her I was going to give her a coffee enema until her colon was completely clean. As expected, she went ballistic. She yelled, screamed, spit and cursed. It reminded me of the scene in the Exorcist.

I had to throw her over my shoulder while she kicked and scratched all the way to the bathroom. I could have really used some help, but I was alone.

I am sure I violated some rule, ordinance or law relative to the doctor-patient code, but I didn't have time to think about it. This woman could have easily had a stroke, seizure or heart attack. I had to do something quick and I knew just what to do.

I sat her down on some towels I had placed on the floor in the bathroom. I again told her what I was going to do. She started crying for her husband. Crying I can handle, spitting, scratching and screaming is another thing. I held her in my arms while she begged me not to do anything. I told her we were alone and that I was not leaving until her colon was clean. I explained that she had auto-intoxication from not having a bowel movement for over ten days. Her fever and hallucinations were coming from toxins.

The first enema released nothing but dark water. The second enema released four or five small rock-like particles. It took six high enemas before the "plug," a large putrefied bolus came out. The first five enemas had virtually no smell. Once the bolus was released, the stench was so strong it made her vomit, while I went outside for some fresh air.

To drop her fever, I used ice water mixed in the brewed coffee. After her colon was clean and the fever gone, I placed her in the warm bath with a cold cloth on her head. I gently and thoroughly washed her with Dr. Bronner's Castile Soap. After shampooing her hair and brushing her teeth, she was dried off and placed on her couch wrapped in blankets.

While she rested, I changed the sheets and put her back into her bed. I used a product I created for athletes and others with muscle-joint problems called Penatrol®. I gently massaged the Penatrol® into her legs and back. I used a eucalyptus ointment on her chest and by the time her husband and son got home, she was sitting up with color back in her face, no fever, no hallucinations and no pain.

The whole family thought it was a miracle. There have even been books written about doctors like me - calling procedures like that, miracles. The truth is, what I did, old-time knowledgeable nurses did everyday. It's called natural healing.

Several days later, the entire family came to my clinic to learn how and why she became so ill. I explained the H.O.N.S.T.E.C. Syndrome and how to achieve optimum health. Although I received greeting cards for years, I never saw this lady again. She did not need me.

Conclusion

Here is where short-sighted doctors of all kinds make a mistake: They are afraid of patient independence. They fear losing their income if the patient knows how to prevent illness. I learned along time ago, doctors should strive to work themselves out of a job. Their goal should be to get people well, not create an endless stream of income from the same chronically ill people.

Good doctors will never be out of work. As people get well they will tell their friends and so on. It is better to have an office full of new patients then to see the same sick people forever. If that is what your doctors are doing, how helpful are they?

The following pages are concerned with the dose recommendations of my *LifePack System®* thoroughly discussed in Chapter 4 - *Curing Dis-ease with Food, Herbs, Supplements, Exercise, Electronic Frequency Devices, Therapy & More.*

Dose Recommendations for
Dr. Chappell's LifePack System®

First and foremost, the seven items of Dr. Chappell's LifePack System® have been designed to enhance, through supplementation, a good nutritional foundation based on eating organic, healthy food, breathing non-contaminated air/oxygen and drinking charged distilled water with Zeta Crystals®. Assuming one is at least trying to do that, it is imperative we supplement our mineral and nutrient depleted food, organic or not, with superior whole food nutritional supplementation. It is for that reason Dr. Chappell's LifePack System® was developed.

This system supplies every known vitamin, mineral, amino and essential fatty acid, enzyme, antioxidant and even stabilized oxygen. It is one of the most comprehensive and complete nutritional programs ever formulated. You will *never* find anything comparable to its *quality* and *value* in any healthfood store or anywhere else. If it can nourish those individuals with chronic, severe and so-called "terminal" illnesses, it can nourish you.

Here are the dose recommendations for the average size adult; 125 to 150 lbs. For children, always adjust to one's weight:

1. Super Kamut -Protein/Vitamin Powder

Each morning mix one to two tablespoons of Super Kamut in almond or rice milk, fruit or vegetable juice. You could use a blender and put fresh fruit, berries or a banana in it when using the milks or fruit juice, thereby making it a smoothie, however, don't use any fruit if you have Cancure® and you are on my *Intensive* or *Extreme* diet.

2. Coral Blend

Take one capsule three times per day with or without meals.

3. ProDigestives

Take one capsule three times per day with or without meals.

4. Omega 369

Mix one tablespoon of Omega 369 in the above morning smoothie. Note: If you are on a Cancure® program, in addition to adding the oil to your morning smoothie, The Budwig protocol calls for two tablespoons of organic low-fat cottage cheese mixed with one tablespoon of Omega 369 flaxseed oil and one tablespoon of freshly ground HC Flaxseeds in a bowl and consumed daily.

5. Ultra C

Mix one scoop (1.3 grams) of Ultra C in an 8 oz. glass of charged distilled water (Zeta Crystals®) and take three times per day away from meals.

6. Stable 'O'

Squirt 10 to 20 drops of Stable 'O' in the above 8 oz. glass of Ultra C and *charged distilled water with Zeta Crystals each time you drink it; three times per day minimum.

7. Acai Plus

Take one capsule three times per day with or without meals.

8. CellBiotics

Take two capsules at night, just before bedtime.

This is not a one-a-day, synthetic, isolated, vitamin pill program. This is serious whole-food nutritional supplementation. My system is the 'crème de la crème' of all current nutraceuticals on the market today. Nothing is more comprehensive. Nothing contains the all-synergistic ingredients I have formulated. If you seek optimum health and longevity, Dr. Chappell's LifePack System is for you.

Note: To maintain quality control and guaranteed availability, my products are *only* available by membership. I have enough product for a limited amount of customers. I would rather have fewer *satisfied* customers then thousands of unsatisfied ones.

I guarantee you will not find any better whole-food nutritional products anywhere in the world. I know my patients depend on effective products, some of them with their lives. Rest assured, my products are all that I say they are and more. You have my promise, they really work!

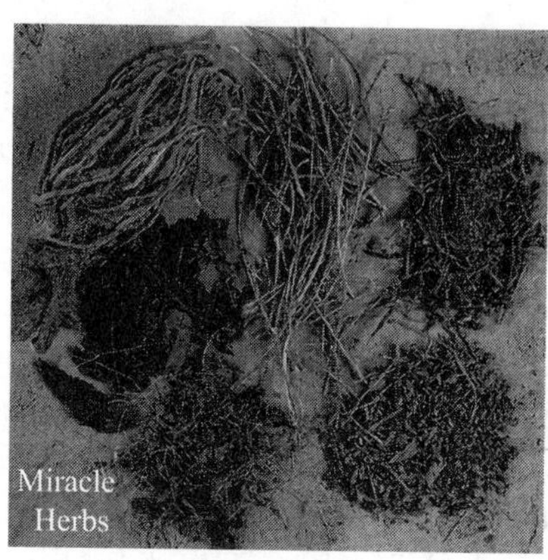
Miracle Herbs

CHAPTER 7 - SEVEN MIRACLE ELEMENTS SCIENTIFICALLY PROVEN TO *CURE* DIABETES

"No physician can ever say that any disease is incurable. To say so blasphemes God, blasphemes Nature, and depreciates the great architect of Creation. The disease does not exist, regardless of how terrible it may be, for which God has not provided the corresponding cure."

- Paracelsus

As you have read, there are many effective remedies being withheld and suppressed from the people that need them the most. In a nutshell, the politics of medicine and OMIC decide what is available to us and what we are allowed to learn. The following six herbs and one mineral have not only been used for up to thousands of years, but they have been currently *scientifically* proven to normalize, regulate and lower glucose, thereby *reversing* diabetes. In my opinion and by definition, this compound along with what you have learned in this book, will actually *cure* diabetes.

Of course this language sends chills throughout all those vested interested groups living off your dependency on their products or services. After all, NO ONE may state they *cure* any "disease" other than the medical profession using their "approved" treatments, specifically their drugs.

Well, excuse me, but I forgot to step in line. My mother died waiting for their *cure*, so I had to discover it myself.

Over 30 years ago, I learned about the health benefits of *fenugreek* and *chromium*, especially how they affect sugar in the body. Many years later, I learned about *American ginseng* and *Nopal cactus* doing the same. About 10 years ago, I discovered *Gymnema sylvestre*. And finally just within the last year or so, I was introduced to activated *cinnamon* and *bitter melon*. After I combined these six herbs and one mineral, I discovered the most profound synergistic, adaptogenic health benefits of any herbal compound I had ever used or experienced. Unfortunately, our trusted government has barred me from commercially making this product for you. The only thing I can legally do is write about it. You will have to seek out those companies that sell the individual components and make this formulae yourself, unless of course you can find a compounding herbal pharmacy that can blend the ingredients for you. You just need to keep searching.

For now, let's start with the most recent addition to this all powerful *miracle* formulae:

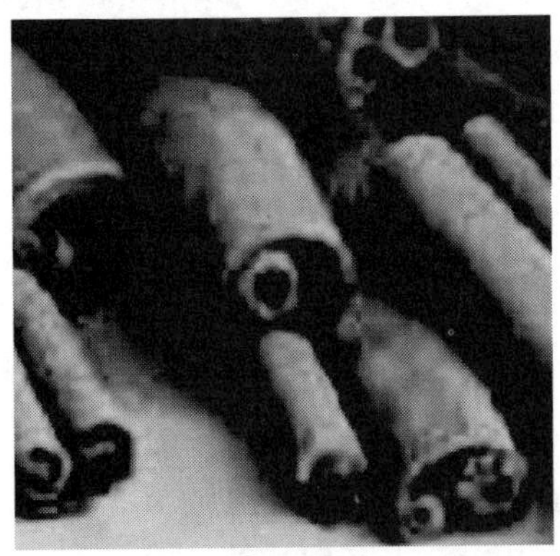

1. Cinnamon - is found in many parts of the world from India, China, Madagascar, Brazil to the Caribbean. The use of cinnamon dates back as long ago as 4,000 years. It has a broad range of historical uses in different cultures, including the treatment of diarrhea, rheumatism, as an antibacteria, digestive aid relieving gas and bloating as well as certain menstrual disorders. But the most significant use recently discovered by Dr. John Anderson of the United States Department of Agriculture (USDA), is for *regulating* glucose.

As you know, sugars and starches in food are broken down into glucose, which then circulates in the blood. The hormone insulin helps the cellular receptor sites attract glucose to be used as energy or made and stored as fat.

Dr. Anderson discovered a water-soluble polyphenol compound called MHCP in cinnamon that actually mimicked insulin and activated the cells receptor site. Testing it in several clinical trials, he not only discovered cinnamon could lower glucose, but it appeared to lower blood levels of fats and "bad" cholesterol. It also neutralized free radicals.

If glucose builds up in the blood, it causes *signs* and *signals* of fatigue, weight gain and blurred vision. Eventually, fat and muscle cells lose their ability to react to insulin all together, thereby leading one to develop Type II diabetes. Apparently, cinnamon rekindles the ability of fat and other cells to react to insulin.

One very interesting observation made by Dr. Anderson and his team of scientists took place *after* the clinical trial had ended. It appears that the health benefits of cinnamon lasted for at least 20 days *after* people stopped taking it.

Dr. Frank Sacks, an allopathic physician and professor of nutrition at the *Harvard School of Public Health* said, "I don't know of any drug or product whose effects persist for 20 days, cinnamon must be an exception."

Alam Khan, Ph.D. with the *Agricultural University in Peshawar*, Pakistan, stated, "Cinnamon can improve glucose metabolism and the overall condition of individuals with diabetes; thereby improving cholesterol metabolism, removing artery damaging free radicals from the blood and improving function of small blood vessels."

Even the president of the *American Diabetic Association*, Dr. Eugene Barret said, "If the results hold up in additional studies (concerning cinnamon), the impact could be significant."

Again, Dr. Anderson excitedly said, "Cinnamons medicinal properties demonstrate the most significant nutritional discovery I have seen in 25 years." He continued saying, "There were significant decreases in fasting serum glucose by 18 to 29%, lowered triglycerides by 23 to 30%, lowered total cholesterol by 12 to 26% and LDL cholesterol by 7 to 27%." All after just taking cinnamon for 40 days.

We now not only have thousands of years of anecdotal testimonials, but we have major universities, hospitals and even our own federal government agency, the USDA, scientifically *proving* that cinnamon mimics insulin and helps drive glucose into the cells. As good as this sounds, it gets even better. Next we have bitter melon.

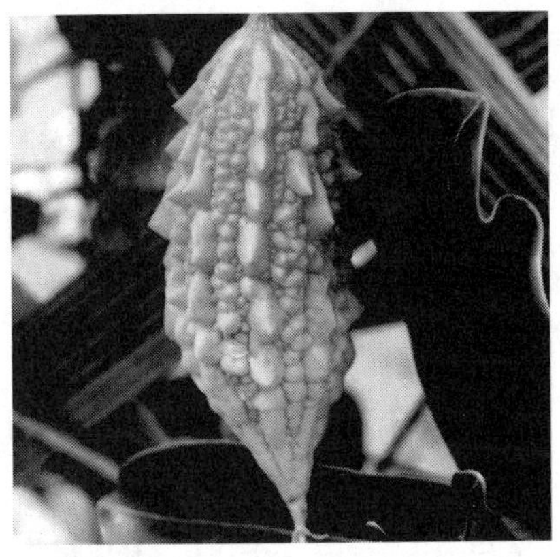

2. Bitter melon - grows in tropical areas, including parts of the Amazon, eastern Africa, Asia and the Caribbean. It is also cultivated throughout South America as a food and medicine. Its use dates back over 5,000 years in China. In the Amazon it is being used for expelling worms, intestinal gas, stimulating and promoting menstruation, as an antiviral for measles and hepatitis, but it is especially used for diabetes or "sweet urine."

In Brazilian and Mexican herbal medicine, bitter melon is used for tumors, wounds, malaria, vaginal discharge, inflammation, menstrual problems, colic, fevers and worms, but again, it is specifically used for diabetes.

Bitter melon contains an array of biologically active plant chemicals including triterpenes, proteins and steroids. In numerous studies, at least three different groups of constituents found in all parts of bitter melon, have clinically demonstrated hypoglycemic properties. To date, close to 100 in vivo (human) studies have demonstrated the blood sugar-lowering effect of this bitter fruit. The fruit has also shown the ability to enhance a cells uptake of glucose, to promote insulin release and to potentiate the effect of insulin. The fruit and leaf are best used, not the seeds.

Researchers believe bitter melon lowers blood sugar by increasing the activity of hexokinase and glucokinase - enzymes in your body that convert sugar into glycogen stored in the liver.

In the *Journal of Nutrition*, April 2003 issue, Drs. Q. Chen and Li Et from the *University of Hong Kong*, The People's Republic of China, were quoted as saying, "Bitter melon appears to have multiple influences on glucose and lipid (fat) metabolism that strongly counteract the effects of a high-fat diet."

Even the prestigious *Memorial Sloan-Kettering Cancer Center* recognizes bitter melon stating, "Bitter melon has been used to treat diabetes, cancer, viral infections and immune disorders. Data suggests it has a significant hypoglycemic effect."

However, the most notable statistical reference came from the *Journal of Phytotherapy*, December 2003, when Drs. W Jia, W Gao and L Tang state, "Pharmacological and clinical evaluations indicate that bitter melon had a.significant blood glucose lowering effect and that the long term use may be advantageous over chemical drugs in alleviating some of the chronic diseases and complications caused by diabetes. The use of natural agents in conjunction with conventional drug treatments, such as insulin, permits the use of lower doses of the drug and/or decreased frequency of administration which decreases the side effects most commonly observed."

This is an extremely significant finding. They are saying bitter melon not only had an impressive blood glucose lowering effect, but even if this herb doesn't totally lower one's glucose to normal limits, it allows the diabetic user to lower their insulin medication where they have little side effects from that medication.

It is *not* advisable to use bitter melon during pregnancy or breast feeding since it is a weak uterine stimulant. As with other herbs, taking bitter melon for 27 days, then discontinuing for 3 days or so and then repeating, is the best use approach. Continuous use only causes homeostasis thereby lessening the medicinal effect.

When I combined cinnamon with bitter melon, the effects were even more impressive, but we're not even one third of the way into the *Seven Miracle Elements*. Next is gymnema sylvestre or gurmar from India.

3. Gymnema sylvestre - is a woody climbing plant that grows in the tropical forests of central and southern India. The leaves are used in herbal medicine preparations. The plant, when chewed, actually blocks the sugar receptor sites, which explains the Hindi name gurmar or "sugar destroyer." Gymnema has been used in India for the treatment of diabetes for over 2,000 years. The leaves were also used for stomach ailments, constipation, water retention and liver disease.

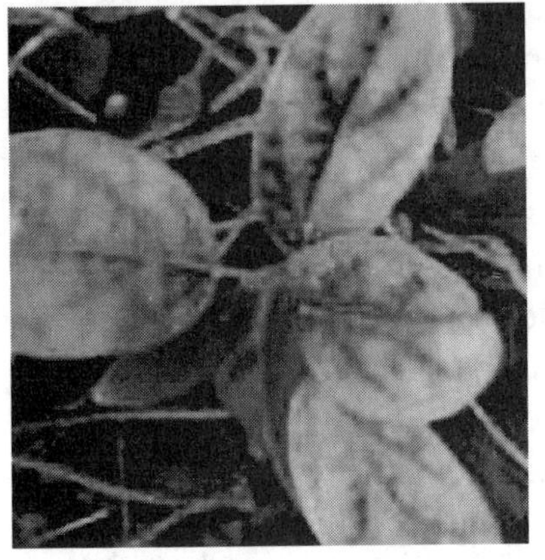

According to current research, gymnema improves uptake of glucose into cells and prevents adrenaline from stimulating the liver to produce glucose, thereby reducing blood sugar levels.

Even the notable *Harvard Medical School* in conjunction with the *Natural Standard*, an organization that produces scientifically based reviews of complementary and alternative medicine topics, states, "There is evidence to suggest that gymnema can lower blood sugar levels in people with Type I and Type II diabetes." This is significant to say the least. Harvard is saying gymnema sylvestre can even affect the glucose levels of those with Type I diabetes!

Remember, approximately 2 million people have Type I diabetes in America today. This condition involves the pancreas not producing enough insulin. Most so-called authorities claim Type I is a genetic disorder with no hope of correcting except for using insulin. I guess they have never heard of gymnema?

Then, we have the *Yale University* publication called *Yale New Haven Health*. Therein they state, "Gymnema sylvestre will often improve blood sugar control in diabetics. Although no interactions have been reported, gymnema may decrease the required dose of insulin."

From the *Journal of Endocrinology* November 1999 at the *School of BioMedical Sciences*, King's College, London, England, Drs. SJ Persaud and PM Jones state, "Results confirm the stimulatory effects of gymnema sylvestre on insulin release indicate that this herb acts by increasing cell permeability."

Finally, from the *Journal Ethnopharmacol*, October 1990, Dr ER Shanmugasundaram, et al, from the *University of Madras*, India, states, "Gymnema sylvestre therapy appears to enhance endogenous insulin, possibly by regeneration and/or revitalization of the residual beta cells in insulin-dependent diabetes mellitus."

Again, we are taking about Type I diabetes, the kind of diabetes that normally requires one to inject insulin for life. Now we have *Harvard Medical School* and the *University of Madras* in India telling us gymnema sylvestre lowers glucose in Type I diabetics through possibly regenerating beta cells! This is truly exciting.

You might think I had enough evidence to stop right here. But I wasn't finished with my research. From cinnamon, bitter melon to gymnema, I wanted more insurance. I wanted something that would *always* lower glucose. So I kept experimenting and decided to add Nopal cactus.

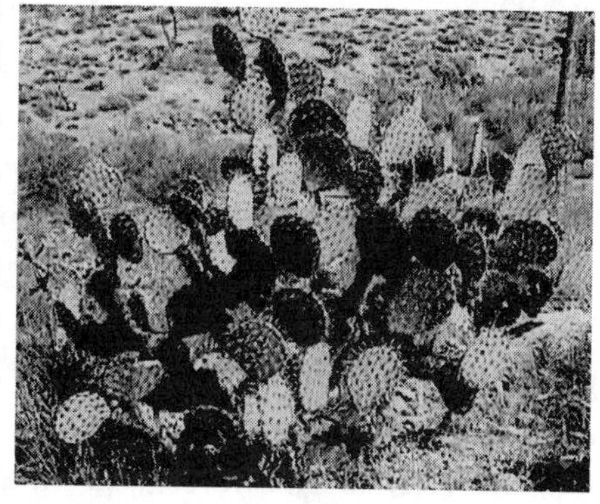

4. Nopal Cactus - has been used in Mexico to treat diabetes, stomach problems, fatigue, shortness of breath, easy bruising, prostate enlargement and liver disease for over 1,000 years. It has been thoroughly documented for over 500 years. Legend has it, the Aztecs consumed the "prickly pear" to control or actually cure "sweet urine" (diabetes) disease in adults. Nopal cactus continues to be a traditional treatment of diabetes in Mexico and other Latin American countries.

Nopal lowers blood sugar levels by blocking absorption of sugar in the intestinal tract. It lowers overall cholesterol levels, improves the ratio of HDL to LDL cholesterol and lowers triglycerides by preventing the conversion of blood sugar into fat and by eliminating excess bile acids, which would ultimately be converted to cholesterol. It also lowers blood pressure and curbs the appetite and facilitates the breakdown and excretion of fat.

In the 1991 issue of Archives of Medicine as reported by the Department of Internal Medicine, Mexico, Drs. AC Frati, N Diaz Xiloti, et al., state, "Diabetic patients had a significant decrease of serum glucose reaching from 41 to 46%" when taking nopal cactus.

From cinnamon, bitter melon, gymnema sylvestre to nopal, my formulae was becoming more and more effective. I had patients on insulin reducing their medication by 5, 10, 20 and 50 percent. However, I wanted even a better formulae, one that main stream medicine could accept as scientifically proven beyond a doubt to lower glucose. I looked into American ginseng.

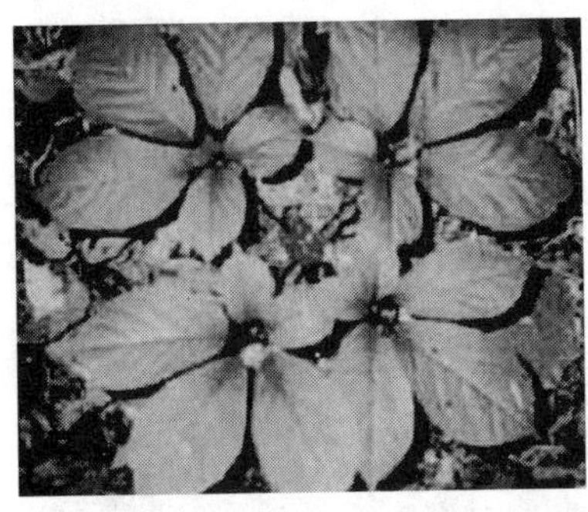

5. American ginseng -Asians consider ginseng the king of all herbs. American ginseng is similar enough to Asian ginseng to chemically have the same effects.

In 1718, American ginseng brought $5 a pound in Canton, China. Today, it costs around $20 per pound for non-organic and $100 to $600 per pound for organic. In 1773, 55 tons of American ginseng were sold to the Chinese. In 1824, 380 tons were exported. Today, thousands of tons are bought and used all over the world. Why is this herb so popular? Why is it called the king of all herbs?

Whether American, Asian or the Russian/Siberian ginseng, all three ginsengs are regarded as adaptogens, each one is used for similar reasons. Ginseng is useful in the treatment of diabetes, fatigue, for alleviating stress and during convalescence. It increases stamina and well-being, therefore athletes take ginseng to increase both endurance and strength. It helps to focus your thoughts, enhance memory, learning and behavior in patients with Alzheimer's and other dementias. It is anti-viral and antibacterial. Best of all there are no known adverse side effects.

For an anti-diabetic remedy, American ginseng is very effective. In the *Archives of Internal Medicine* (2000), it was reported by the *University of Toronto*, Canada, that American ginseng produces a "significant reduction" in blood sugar in people with diabetes.

Even at the *Pritzker School of Medicine, University of Chicago,* Dr. Jing-Tian Xie, reported in the *Pharmacology Res.* 2004, "American ginseng possesses significant anti-hyperglycemia and thermogenic activity and may prove to be beneficial in improving the management of Type 2 diabetes." He also said, "American ginseng berry possesses significant antihyperglycemic and antiobese effects."

From a 2,000-year-old history of the Chinese using Asian ginseng, to our 300-year-old history using American ginseng, there is plenty of evidence that ginseng absolutely lowers glucose. Now comes the magical herb fenugreek.

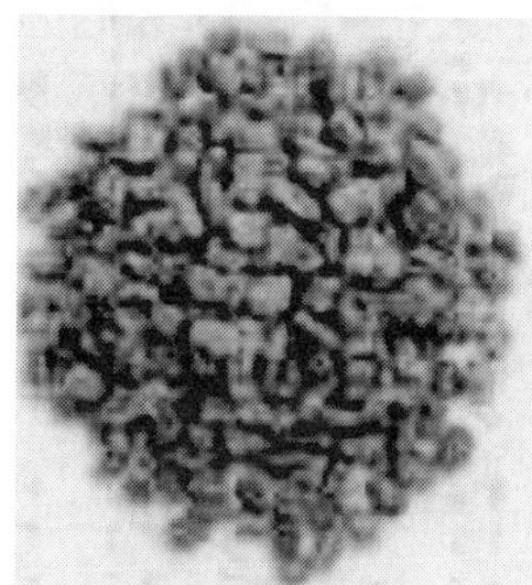

6. Fenugreek is used as a spice and medicinal herb throughout the world. Traditional Chinese herbalists use it for a multitude of conditions including kidney problems, male reproductive infections, constipation, atherosclerosis, high triglycerides and high cholesterol. However, the number one reason fenugreek is used universally, is for diabetes and sugar-intolerance problems.

After exhaustive scientific research, the European Scientific Cooperative on Phytotherapy lists fenugreek as an adjuvant therapy in diabetes and for hypercholesterolemia. It also has an effect on lipid peroxidation thereby lowering free-radical damage.

Even the German Commission E, the equivalent to our FDA, recognizes the benefits of fenugreek and has listed it as one of their approved herbs for medicinal purposes, including breaking down (dissolving) mucous and other secretions, increasing blood flow and inhibiting growth of infectious organisms.

In the *European Journal of Clinical Nutrition* 1990, Drs. R.D. Sharma, T.C. Raghuram and N.S. Rao from the *National Institute of Nutrition, Council of Medical Research*, Hyderabad, India report, "Fenugreek significantly reduced blood sugar and improved the glucose tolerance test with a 54 percent reduction in 24-hour urinary excretion.

Again, from India at the Jaipur Diabetes and Research Centre and reported in the *India Journal Association of Physicians,* Drs. A. Gupta, R. Gupta and B. Lal report "Use of fenugreek seeds improves glycemic control and decreases insulin resistance in mild Type 2 diabetes.

Finally, our own Sloan Kettering Cancer Center states, "Fenugreek exhibits hypocholesterolemic, hypolipidemic and hypoglycemic activity in healthy and diabetic humans and animals." They continue saying it is the defatted seed that seems to be of benefit. This is a very important point since many manufacturers use the regular, less-effective seed. I recommend *only* the defatted seed. The final element known to lower glucose is the trace mineral chromium.

7. Chromium - In the 1950s it was found that chromium was necessary for the maintenance of normal glucose tolerance. Although it used to be found in many foods - whole grains, cereals, spices, mushrooms, raw sugar and meat Brewer's yeast is the best source available. Chromium increases insulin binding and cellular insulin receptivity.

Knowing that the plasma chromium levels are at least 40% lower in 100% of diabetics, The *American Diabetes Association* admitted in 1996 that "chromium supplementation has no known benefit in patients who are *not* chromium deficient." This is a convoluted way of saying chromium benefits all diabetics.

As reported in numerous clinical trials, subjects taking chromium demonstrated significant improvement of fasting glucose and postprandial (after eating) glucose.

Yale New Haven Health, a medical research and hospital facility states, "Chromium is an essential trace mineral that helps the body maintain normal blood sugar levels. Chromium picolinate increases fat loss and promotes a gain in lean muscle tissue." The suggested dose is 400 mcg of chromium picolinate daily. Although helpful for weight loss, depression, athletic performance, Syndrome X, insulin resistance, high triglycerides, hypoglycemia and high cholesterol, it is primarily beneficial for diabetes. Once found in abundance in the earth's soil, commercial farming and food processing have all but destroyed it. Our only chance for replacement is with supplementation.

There you have it. Six herbs that have been used for up to thousands of years, on several continents, by millions of people for a list of conditions, including diabetes, with virtually no side effects. Now, modern science has come along and analyzed every component including the molecular structure of these time-tested herbs only to prove they absolutely lower glucose. And not to forget a little trace mineral called chromium.

When combining these miracle elements with eating a good diet, doing effective exercise, drinking pristine charged distilled water, getting plenty of rest, sunshine and relaxation, meditating daily and most of all, forgiving the unforgivable, you have everything you need to *cure* yourself of diabetes and most of the other so-called "diseases."

You will never know, unless you try. You have nothing to lose and everything to gain. I hope by now, you have learned enough to overcome your fears and step into the world of natural healing. Once you are comfortable making a few changes in your lifestyle, more advanced approaches to health and longevity will be easier to accomplish.

SUMMARY OF HERBAL COMPOUND AND TRACE MINERAL TO *CURE* DIABETES

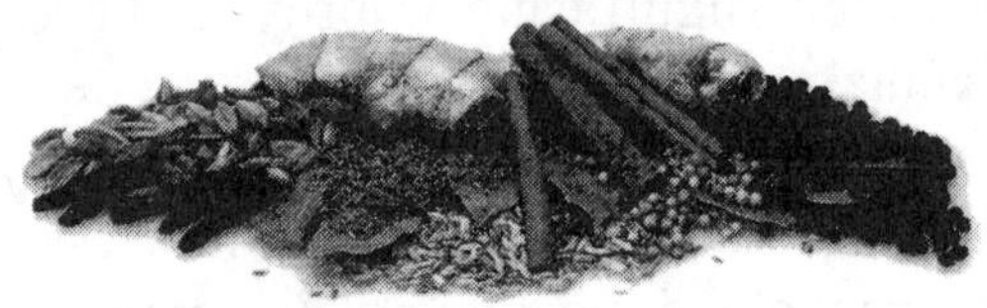

I have found the ingredients that have been scientifically and historically proven to reverse (*cure*) diabetes are:

1. Cinnamon
2. Bitter melon
3. Gymnema sylvestre (Gurmar)
4. Nopal cactus
5. American ginseng
6. Fenugreek
7. Chromium picolinate

A quick search on the Internet will give you dozens of sources for each ingredient or you may try your local health food store. I have also included in Index E-*Resources*, a list of herbal companies that sell individual herbs and make compounds, Herbal Promise being one. Make sure you buy <u>*only*</u> organic, non-fumigated, irridated or genetically engineered herbs. Any combination of the above, *respecting therapeutic values*, should be effective. Chromium picolinate is well tolerated at 50 mcg/per cap.

Since writing this book, the FTC and FDA have *barred* me from manufacturing or having financial interest in *any* product that lowers glucose. Relative to diabetes, I am a health researcher and author. I write informational and educational material under the *Freedom of Speech* clause in the United States Constitution.

Although I do have non-specific nutraceuticals (vitamins, minerals, enzymes, amino and fatty acids) and botanicals, no product treats diabetes and no claims are made. Therefore, I may participate in growing, producing, manufacturing, promoting and selling *those* products. If you are interested in knowing more, see Index E-*Resources* in the back of the book under QCI Products®.

God's Cure for Cancer, Tumor and Goiter

Many years ago, I acquired a small pamphlet allegedly written sometime between 1890 and 1910 entitled, *"God's Cure for Cancer, Tumor and Goiter"* by Mrs. Julia A. Shelhammer.

Sponsored by a church, the contents of this little pamphlet is strongly faith based, however, it demonstrates the simplicity of complexity I referred to in my book. Mrs. Shelhammer gives excellent, timeless advice, much of which mirrors what I was taught as a natural healer. As far as I know, I have the only copy remaining of this precious gift.

I have included the entire pamphlet in the following pages to demonstrate how natural healing was applied in the 1800s. Although I do not necessarily subscribe to Mrs. Shelhammer's faith, I do concur with her approach to helping the infirmed.

Remember, these remedies came from natural healers prior to Mrs. Shelhammer. They worked during her life time and still work today, with some exception relative to the aforementioned loss of some of the herbs' powers.

In the old days, herbs were found and harvested in the wild. They were *extremely* powerful. The soil was thriving with minerals and microbes. When you read the texts from one hundred or two hundred years ago, they talk about the *ease* by which these herbs worked. This is *not* the case today.

Even organic herbs may not be as strong as those used by our ancestors. Commercial, non-organic herbs are even less effective and most don't work at all.

I have been in the natural healing field longer than most. I have seen the degradation of my beloved profession and it saddens me. It is not for myself I weep, it is for my precious daughter and your children's children.

Once we lose the ability to heal ourselves, life as we know it, will cease to exist. The planet and all its inhabitants will perish. And for what, I ask? Greed, contempt, power and control seem to rule the world, while most of us just want peace. I pray we find what we seek in my lifetime.

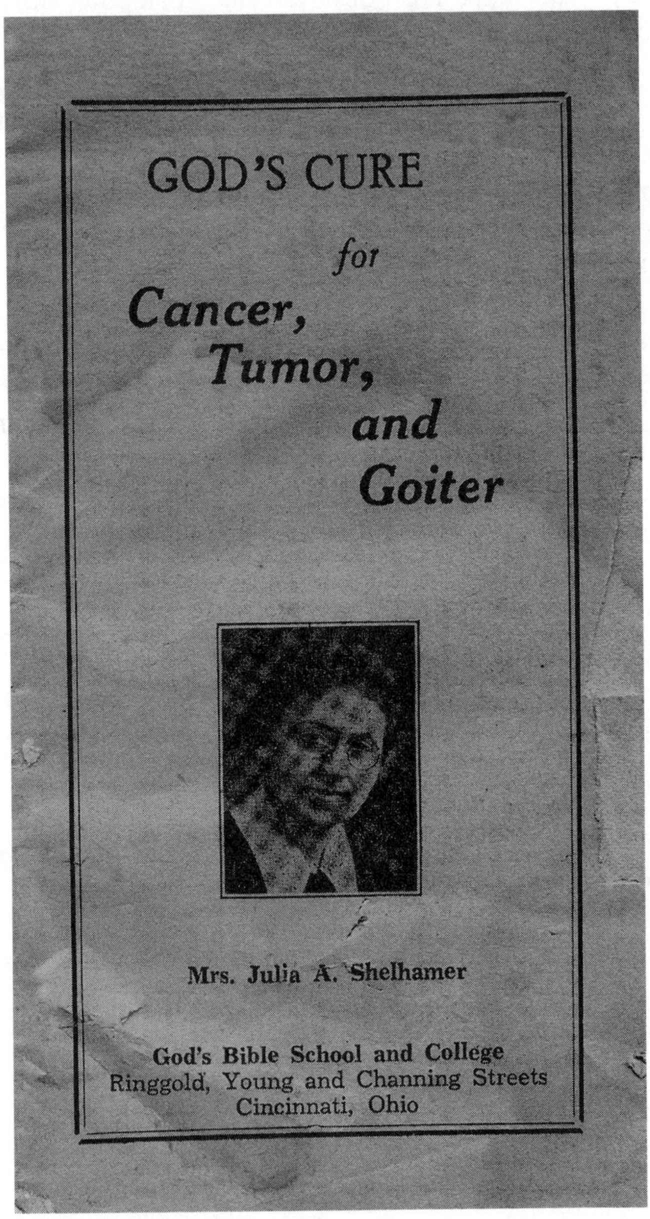

GOD'S CURE

for

Cancer, Tumor, and Goiter

Mrs. Julia A. Shelhamer

God's Bible School and College
Ringgold, Young and Channing Streets
Cincinnati, Ohio

Dis-ease is defined as lack of ease or harmony, it is NOT the same as "disease," a medical term for illness treated by medicine. <u>*NEVER*</u> attempt to stop or reduce your medication without the supervision of your medical doctor.

INTRODUCTION

I am not a doctor or a nurse. My training has been along other lines, and I do not wish to be consulted as either. In these pages I am simply giving a few simple remedies for cancer, tumor, and goitre which I have gathered from our travels in this and other lands.

When God asked me to open a new mission station in Africa, I told Him that I did not know how to get the money. His answer was, "You have been twice around the world and have learned many things that would be very helpful to people. You know how guilty you feel when you hear of a person's dying with cancer while in your hand you have a number of fine home cures you have found here and there. Why not write up a list of these and present to the public?"

"But, Lord," said I, "there would not be enough money in that, though such a publication would be worth many millions of dollars to some."

"Help them and then let them help you support that mission station. Make no charge for the booklet; but after people have read it, let them mail you an offering for missions," said the Master.

So I am simply obeying God in sending out this small book, trusting that it may carry a message of peace and health for soul, mind, and body to those who read.

Chapter I.

CANCER IN THE FAMILY

Cancer was in my mother's family. She had a lovely sister who died with it after having three operations. Of course, the disease was still in the system and a surgeon's knife could not remove it in its entirety, for cancer is not local. It is in the blood stream.

When removed, my aunt's cancer always returned and with greater force, as though to take vengeance on anyone for disturbing it.

I had an older sister—a lovely sister, who took tender care of me when I was a baby and was a pal to me in my teen age.

She was a fine help-meet to her ministerial husband, taking charge of the young people of his circuit. She always seemed to know just how to advise them and many were led to Christ by her untiring efforts.

Well, later, a hardness appeared in her forehead and a little below one eye. It was rather yellow in color and had a defined boundary line. The best medical aid was secured but all to no avail.

Oh, that I had known then what I know now! She was not old enough to die, but a stone marks the grave on which are the words **"A Saint."**

Her husband, Rev. D. W. Rose, did his best, regardless of the cost. He took her regularly to Pittsburgh, Pa., where were the great cancer specialists. The tissue of Lucia's face was not broken at that time. The great doctor brought out a tiny piece of radium the size of a dime, which was valued I believe at $10,000, and applied it to her face

(3)

right under the eye. Then he lent it to her without security to take to her home in a distant city. The radium drew her face all out of shape, pulling the eye wide open so it could never close, and left an unhealing sore. The hardness never melted from her forehead and she was so unsightly that she never looked into a mirror again to the day of her death. It is strange, how little some great men know! If doctors lived nearer the heart of God and prayed for hours over their work and their difficult cases, cures would be revealed to them never before known in the medical world, for our Lord is a God of revelation and He loves us.

When in Africa, doctoring thousands of ulcer patients, our little daughter Esther (nineteen years of age) saw the need of a more effective and speedy remedy for those hideous tropical ulcers that eat to the bone, sometimes taking off the toes. She knew little about medicine but was thrown right into the position of superintendent of the large new dispensary and just had to do something in the name of Jesus Christ, for the mission was new and there was no one else to do the work.

She knew that her Heavenly Father knew what would cure those dreadful ulcers, so asked advice of Him and it came. Quickly she compounded something, tried it and, lo and behold, she had the cure. It was marvelous how soon her patients recovered, and so popular did she become that people came from far and near to be treated. Our Heavenly Father knows, why not ask Him?

In Job we read, "He that is perfect in knowledge is with you." Let us take Him into our business and professional work and make Him partner and give Him a control-

Dis-ease is defined as lack of ease or harmony, it is NOT the same as "disease," a medical term for illness treated by medicine. *NEVER* attempt to stop or reduce your medication without the supervision of your medical doctor.

ling interest. Then, ah, then, things will bloom out like morning-glories and you will wonder at your amazing success.

My oldest sister, Mary, once developed a lump in her breast. Her husband took her to a number of physicians in Atlanta, Georgia, the "New York of the South." Every one pronounced it cancer, and wanted to operate **"at once."**

Not satisfied with the verdict, I put on my hat and took her to several more doctors of the city. Among these was a cancer specialist. They all with one consent voiced the same opinion as the others. Mother was not satisfied. She did not want an operation and believed that there was some way to avoid it.

Finally, Mary went with her husband to Kansas and there met an old friend of Mr. Beeson who had once been a physician, but now was in the ministry. He diagnosed Mrs. Beeson's case and pronounced it cancer, advising an operation.

Now, something had to be done, and **done at once**, for every day meant that the plague was going deeper, and the examination of so many physicians had done it no good, but rather inflamed it.

Mary was distressed and did not know what to do. She finally decided on a certain sanitarium and began to make preparations to go, but dear Mother continued to talk against it. Poor Mary was in a quandary. Every day meant danger, for the tumor could now be removed and there was some chance of life, but if she waited it might be too late.

Mary was always very respectful to her parents, so against her judgment abandoned

Dis-ease is defined as lack of ease or harmony, it is NOT the same as "disease," a medical term for illness treated by medicine. *NEVER* attempt to stop or reduce your medication without the supervision of your medical doctor.

the idea of going to a doctor, just to please Mother.

That threw the whole responsibility of her case into Mother's hands but with a firm determination and with faith in her God, she went to work and planned the following program:

1. Take a daily tub-bath. As we were in the country this had to be taken in a large washtub.

2. Keep the breast, on and around the tumor, saturated with olive oil.

3. Take long walks in the country.

4. The diet must be very simple and consist largely of cranberries, not boiled down into jam but cooked only a few minutes. They must be sweetened sparingly as sugar hinders a cure. Honey and brown sugar are best.

Mother had read that cranberries would cure cancer, so laid in a good supply. Mr. Beeson found large quantities of them at a reduced price, so we canned them by the gallon. Mary ate cranberries at nearly every meal and often made almost a whole meal of them.

Any scientific mind can easily see the value of such food. It is a **solvent,** dissolving hard lumps in the body, scattering congestion. During that time, we had, I believe, no steaks or chops or roasts, or rich gravies or pastry. We baked no cakes or doughnuts, but lived mostly on fruit, vegetables, cereals, milk and brown bread.

5. Mother's fifth prescription was prayer. Perhaps I should have put this first. Oh, how Mother prayed! Often I heard her sweet voice off in the attic, pleading with God to bless the simple, natural means she was using to the good of her first-born child, who was now a minister's wife and

needed her health. Her prayers were not little weak ones. They were strong in their sincerity—strong in their earnestness—strong in their logic and strong in their faith.

Mother was a spiritual merchant in a heavenly exchange, driving rich trades for the treasure of health. That was prayer. What a rebuke to our cold devotions! This is walking with God. And busy as God was at that time, He never heard the last of those prayers until something was done.

One day, Mary discovered that the ugly lump had lost its defiant hardness and had softened. I cannot remember just how long this was after Mother began treating her patient. It may have been four or five months, but—I do know that we all were happy.

I took her then to the cancer specialist just to see what he would say. He looked wisely at the weakening tumor and exclaimed, "Why, what have you been doing to that?" After we had tried to tell him, he said, "I would advise you to keep up that treatment."

That was some years ago. Mrs. Beeson is alive and well, having suffered no recurrence of the trouble. Rev. Beeson has gone to Heaven but his dear wife, assisted by our sister Helen, is doing pastoral work!

She labors for her poor people hard enough and skillfully enough to demand two thousand dollars a year salary, but, instead, she usually gets less than a dollar a week. She would go without molasses on her corn bread to be able to buy a stamp to write to you, but if you want to be sure of an answer it might be well to enclose an offering. Her address is Mrs. Mary A. Beeson, Hendricks, W. Va.

(7)

Dis-ease is defined as lack of ease or harmony, it is NOT the same as "disease," a medical term for illness treated by medicine. *NEVER* attempt to stop or reduce your medication without the supervision of your medical doctor.

Chapter II.

SIMPLE HOME REMEDIES

God's medicine includes an outdoor life. He never intended man to be shut in behind four square walls. The Indians lived a roving life and had wonderful health. Cancer is scarcely known among the primitive natives of Africa. They have but one or two meals a day and are usually hungry. It is only after they become civilized that they get the white man's diseases. Automobiles do our walking for us and we lose the art. High-heeled shoes make it difficult to travel far on foot.

And now may I tell you of some of the wonderful cures of which we have learned in our travels—cures for the incurable except by operation?

No. 1—While in Australia holding a revival for Reverend Jolley in his large Baptist Church, we met a fine-appearing lady whose husband was one of the deacons there. She had been very ill for nine years, having had a complication of inward troubles. Her doctor pronounced her case hopeless. In the list of diseases was what seemed to be cancer.

But she had faith in God and left her case with Him. Soon He sent to her a friend who prescribed the following which cured her in a few months' time. Her diet was simple. The juice of twelve citrus fruits each day. Lemon, grapefruit, and orange make a wonderful drink. Added to this were two quarts of vegetable soup without salt or meat; the soup to be made of about eight different kinds of vegetables always including onion. The only addition to this diet was plenty of water to drink between meals. All her complications left her until she was young and strong again though somewhat advanced in years.

No. 2—Grapes are a cure for cancer as well as for goitre and tumor. The wonderful story of the healing of a lady doctor, Johanna Brandt, by this means is given in her marvelous book, "The Grape Cure," which you may have by sending one dollar and fifty cents to us or to Harmony Centre, 604 W. 112th Street, New York City. After suffering from cancer of the stomach for nine years, Dr. Brandt cured herself in six weeks' time by living alone on grapes. Later she discovered their value in treating other diseases.

Dr. Arthur Vos, 537 Howell St., Cincinnati, O., has a sanitarium where he cures his patients without operating, by means of **"The Grape Cure."**

No. 3—When one's body has become abnormal so that lumps or kernels have formed, the first thing to do is to cleanse the system by baths, enemas, and a diet of hot water, taking nothing else for several days. Hot water is a food, i. e., it serves as a food in the following way. When one is fasting, it satisfies, keeping up a degree of strength while softening the tissues of the body, relieving congestion, inflammation and high blood pressure.

In the body is stored sufficient fat or other material to nourish one for some time. Those congested portions which we call tumor, goitre, or cancer are surplus supplies of protein and carbohydrates which the body does not need. Because of a lack of exercise, the blood did not distribute them evenly through the body, so they lodged at the weakest place as ice or driftwood flows down the

Dis-ease is defined as lack of ease or harmony, it is NOT the same as "disease," a medical term for illness treated by medicine. *NEVER* attempt to stop or reduce your medication without the supervision of your medical doctor.

river until it comes to an irregularity in the bank and there lodges, causing trouble. To keep the blood stream clear and clean, one must not overeat. It is surprising how little one really needs.

Hot water enables the congested tissue to dissolve and to be properly absorbed by the body. As long as one eats, that tumor or goitre keeps enlarging, for there is no outlet—no chance for it to be absorbed. If the surgeon's knife cuts it away, it causes inflammation and excitement all through the system. The blood hurries here and there, not knowing what to do with its surplus food and eventually, weary with its burden of too much protein and carbrohydrates, dumps them off anywhere it can and a new kernel is formed. Such lumps are merely unnatural storehouses for food that the body did not need, and unless emptied quickly before they become malignant, are difficult to remove.

Why Bears Live All Winter without Eating

"One-half of the answer to this is: As bears sleep most of the time in a warm place in winter they do not need so much food as when they are active. The other half is that they eat themselves. In the summer months they eat greedily, a great deal more than they need at the time. This extra food is stored up in their bodies in thick layers of fat. This fat keeps the sleeping bear warm. Food is fuel. As he is very warm in his blanket of fat, a bear needs less food. And gradually he eats the blanket. The fat is absorbed into the blood to feed all the other tissues of the body. In the spring the bear comes out thin and poor.

Many other animals hibernate in the

Dis-ease is defined as lack of ease or harmony, it is NOT the same as "disease," a medical term for illness treated by medicine.
NEVER attempt to stop or reduce your medication without the supervision of your medical doctor.

winter. Snakes store up fat to live on. You see, there is little food for them in the winter, so nature taught them how to stock up their internal pantry shelves for hard times. When you are sick and cannot eat as much as usual, you, too, live partly on the fat stored in the body. That is why you become thin. And that is why, when you begin to get well, you are as "hungry as a bear."

There are doctors who perform wonderful cures with water alone. They use what they call the water cure, cleansing the system by means of baths (cold and hot), enemas, and drinking water.

People swarm to the Hot Springs of Arkansas and other such places where sanatariums and hotels are situated to accommodate sick ones who have come to bathe and to drink their way to health. They stand around those hot gushing springs by the hour, sipping the water from their individual cups. I suppose at these resorts one drinks about a gallon of water a day. No wonder they derive benefit! Try it yourself at home and see how much better you feel.

If your surgeon presses you to hurry and have an operation now before the trouble gets beyond control, don't get excited. Remember, NO DISEASE CAN PROGRESS WHILE ONE IS FASTING. Continue to fast and to drink hot water, a glass full every hour for two or three days. Then take citrus fruit juice without sweetening, all you want. Keep the system flooded with these nourishing, cleansing fluids and in a few days you will notice that your symptoms are less.

Milk may later be added to this diet, also tomato juice and all other kinds of fruits. But give your system a thorough cleansing

(11)

first by using gallons of hot (or cold) water while fasting.

No. 4—The fourth cure was one I just stumbled onto under the following circumstances. My husband and I were holding an evangelistic campaign in Lakeland, Florida, when one day a dear little lady came greatly distressed over the fact that she and her three little children had all been badly exposed to smallpox. They had spent considerable time day after day in a neighbor's sick room before any one knew what was wrong with the patient.

I told her to try an old remedy which is said never to fail; not only to cure, but also to prevent smallpox when one has been exposed. It had been impressed on me so strongly that it was a never failing remedy that I gave it to her with considerable confidence, though I had never seen it tried.

The remedy was as follows: Pour boiling water over cream of tartar in the proportion of one quart to about four teaspoonsfuls. Let it stand until cool. Drink this freely and often, using no other water day or night until all danger is passed—about ten days.

She tried it, supplying plenty for the family. In a few weeks she came to tell me that none of them had taken the smallpox and, more than that, a growth in her cheek of three years' standing had disappeared as a result.

This is scientific: Cream of tartar is one of the best blood purifiers known and is used by physicians.

No. 5—We are indebted to the "Physical Culture" for the following remedy for cancer, which is merely a strict diet of fruits and milk. This is said to be so effective that

(12)

when used but seven days the offensive odor of a cancer disappears.

Chapter III.

INWARD GOITRE

To have to give up to die so young was hard, but the doctors had said there was nothing more they could do, so Mrs. Blank lay in bed thinking. That inward goitre had troubled her for years and now it had grown to such proportions that she was almost choked. The surgeon had wanted to remove it but her heart was weak and he declined.

Must she wait until that goitre grew so large she would actually choke to death? It was a horrible thought and the young wife lay there feeling desperate at times, then again more submissive to her fate.

Was there no way to cure without the knife? Surely there should be! Strange that no one knew! Her doctor constantly affirmed that hers was a hopeless case without an operation. What ignorance! What cruelty!

Well, to pass the time away Mrs. Blank sat up in bed reading magazines. She came across one which gave a simple, harmless cure for goitre. It was:

(1) A daily bath.
(2) Physical culture exercises.
(3) A strict diet of milk and fruit juices only.

Oh, what joy to think of finding a road to health other than by way of the operating table. She would try it. It could not make her any worse. There are always skeptical friends around when one decides

Dis-ease is defined as lack of ease or harmony, it is NOT the same as "disease," a medical term for illness treated by medicine. *NEVER* attempt to stop or reduce your medication without the supervision of your medical doctor.

to do anything unusual, but she reasoned that she must die anyway and an experiment like that would not hurt her.

She began. The nurse helped her bathe. The physical exercises were limited to perhaps the fingers and the wrists at first, for any extra exertion caused the heart to palpitate. The diet she liked. It appealed to her as cooling and refreshing. It did not leave that full choking feeling after eating. Her whole system began to feel clean and clear. There was less pressure of the goitre and less around the heart. She realized that she had at last struck a gold mine of health. In a few days she began to feel so much better that she was able to sit up part of the time. The heart beat more regularly and life began to gather interest once more.

The milk and fruit juices were taken regularly at short intervals. She was conscientious and would taste nothing else.

Later Mrs. Blank was up around doing a little work. It was not long until she had so far improved that she was doing her own cooking and when four months had elapsed she was well. The goitre was all gone and she was feeling like her old self except of course a little weak. Her husband came in one day for dinner and found her frying chops. He stopped and kissed her, saying she looked just like she did when he married her. The roses had returned to her cheeks and her complexion was beautiful. He urged her to dine with him but she declined, saying that she had vowed that she would continue on that diet for six months and though apparently well, she would stick to her promise. She did so and could always thank God for nature's cure for her goitre. Thus

(14)

Dis-ease is defined as lack of ease or harmony, it is NOT the same as "disease," a medical term for illness treated by medicine. *NEVER* attempt to stop or reduce your medication without the supervision of your medical doctor.

health was brought about by taking God's medicines. The simple kind that He always supplies. The kind that requires no cooking, no frying in indigestible fat—so different from pastries, rich gravies, cake or puddings. Just the pure unsweetened juices from the garden of Eden.

Chapter IV.

WHAT ABOUT DIVINE HEALING?

Sometimes God takes the short-cut to health and heals miraculously after doctors have failed. Why not? He is omnipotent and asks, "Is there anything too hard for me?" (Jer. 32:27.) It is a most sensible thing to believe that the Creator of the universe is able to cure disease.

Perhaps every physician has met with cases of Divine healing which have compelled him to say in his heart that God can do what nature cannot. Mrs. M. G. Standley, Editor of "God's Revivalist," was recently near death with the strepticoccus germ in the blood. She had several blood transfusions, and according to medical science there was absolutely no hope. Her case attracted the attention of many of Cincinnati's physicians. The family was in mourning and deep distress. Finally, a notice was put into the periodical of which she is editor, and has about 40,000 subscribers, asking for special prayer. God answered and Mrs. Standley recovered. Shortly after that, one of her physicians came to see her. He was so surprised to see the improvement in her health that he could hardly believe his eyes, and remarked, "Mrs. Standley, you ought to be

Dis-ease is defined as lack of ease or harmony, it is NOT the same as "disease," a medical term for illness treated by medicine. *NEVER* attempt to stop or reduce your medication without the supervision of your medical doctor.

dead," meaning that there was no reason why she was living, except for Divine interposition. Some months later, while riding on a train, I picked up a newspaper and read a beautiful story of Mrs. Standley's healing, written by a newspaper correspondent. Thus, the news has gone far and wide, and today Mrs. Standley is back at her post of duty editing "God's Revivalist."

Recently news came over the radio from a certain commercial announcer, testifying that God had miraculously healed him of pneumonia, adding that his little daughter had been very low with the same disease but that, in answer to prayer, God had marvelously healed her.

Yes, God answers prayer. He has no respect of persons and can help you, dear reader, if you exercise simple faith in Him.

I was once holding services in a certain town in the East, and, wanting to get everybody possible to pray regardless of his religious belief, I put into the newspaper the following display ad, which attracted some attention.

WHAT ARE YOU DOING FOR THE SALVATION OF YOUR UNSAVED LOVED ONES?

When death has claimed them will you have any regrets? Is ten minutes a day too much to spend in prayer for them? If not, will you join us at ten o'clock each day in earnest prayer at your home for a revival of old time salvation in ....?

MRS. E. E. SHELHAMER.

The ladies of the Lutheran Church commented on it in one of their services and

(16)

Dis-ease is defined as lack of ease or harmony, it is NOT the same as "disease," a medical term for illness treated by medicine. *NEVER* attempt to stop or reduce your medication without the supervision of your medical doctor.

joined in praying for a general revival all over the town. In fact, such a spirit of prayer and of old-fashioned faith in God settled down over the community that many were encouraged to pray.

On his way to work one morning was a gentleman who was suffering from rupture. As he passed his church (which happened to be Catholic) the inspirational faith that impregnated the atmosphere of the town seized him and he entered the church, knelt alone at the altar, and was instantly healed of his troublesome rupture. Yes—God is no respecter of persons or of churches. He loves us all alike. Let us have faith in Him.

Conditions of Divine Healing

The only condition of Divine healing is faith. "If thou canst believe, all things are possible to him that believeth." (Mark 9:23.) But healing faith is not always easy to obtain. It is the gift of God and comes alone from Him. It has its conditions, for instance:

1. Perfect resignation to the will of God, who will not give faith for healing to a rebel against Himself. One must put away rebellion and submit to his Creator if he wishes his prayers answered.

2. All sin must be renounced and abandoned. The Bible says, "God heareth not sinners." (John 9:31); that is, He will not hear unrepentant sinners, but He does hear the prayer of all who humbly ask. Any sinner may get an answer to his payer if his heart is submissive to God's will and if he is willing to obey the Lord. "Let the wicked forsake his way, and the unrighteous man his thoughts: and let him return unto the Lord, and He will have mercy upon him;

Dis-ease is defined as lack of ease or harmony, it is NOT the same as "disease," a medical term for illness treated by medicine. *NEVER* attempt to stop or reduce your medication without the supervision of your medical doctor.

and to our God, for he will abundantly pardon."

3. Tithing our income. Many people read Malachi 3:10 but fail to read the next verse. As surely as you meet the conditions in verse ten, you have the right to claim the promise in verse eleven. Get your Bible and read it now.

Chapter V.

WORRY

It is impossible to be well if one worries. All the medicine in the world cannot cure the body if the mind is distressed.

Worry is of two kinds, first, distress over one's self, second, over others.

1. Worry over one's self. The deepest worry is caused by a guilty conscience. This is the cause of a great deal of poor health and premature old age. It saps one's beauty and vitality. No amount of exterior care can counteract the evil effects of a guilty conscience. There is only one thing to do and that is to get rid of it. It is like a thorn in the flesh—the wound will not heal until the thorn is removed. How can this be done? Confess your sins to God. Renounce them all and let Him free you from their bondage. Accept His forgiveness, for it has been bought for you on Calvary. He says, "Him that cometh unto me I will in no wise cast out."

2. **Worry over others.** Are you in distress over your loved ones? Cast that care upon the Lord.

Are you mistreated or neglected or forgotten? Tell it to Jesus. He understands and

Dis-ease is defined as lack of ease or harmony, it is NOT the same as "disease," a medical term for illness treated by medicine. *NEVER* attempt to stop or reduce your medication without the supervision of your medical doctor.

says, "As one whom his mother comforteth, so will I comfort you."

Recently a very dear friend was telling me how she got rid of her worries and here is her story; she says, "Prayer is the key which unlocks Heaven's door. When one prevails in prayer the door is opened, sometime, somewhere. I remember going through great sorrow. Husband was not regularly employed and I was having to go out to work. Besides this, some very heart-rending disappointments came into my life. One was that my companion would visit gambling places and forget to come home till the wee hours in the morning, then his eyes were red and blurred from drink and dissipation. I had always said I would never live with a man that would gamble or drink, but here I was married to one who was even worse. He was untrue to me! Husband had made me believe, when he was courting me that he was a Christian and had been brought up a Christian, for he carried his testament to make me believe this fact.

"I knew at that time I was away from the Lord but we both promised when we got married to get right. He did attend church with me for a while and made a profession when I did, but sad to say he gave up by the time we reached home. This was a dreadful shock to one that had her hopes built so high. I struggled along for more than six years, weeping and praying, running to my friends and unloading my troubles but after I had told them my sorrows I still went home with a heavy burden. Soon the strain was more than my body and mind could bear; my health failed. I then suffered as never before, for my husband's neglect was cruel and his scolding when I was a helpless invalid was still worse.

(19)

"One night while he was out I remembered that the Scripture said, 'Whatsoever things ye desire, when ye pray, believe that ye receive them, and ye shall have them.' Then I know the Word said, 'Cast all your cares upon him, for he careth for you.' With my Bible in my hand and quoting such promises to the Lord as would come to my mind, I entered into earnest prayer. I became desperate, and prayed until the midnight hours and then kept on praying. I asked the Lord to let me cast that burden on him and leave it on Him never to take it up again. I became willing for the Lord to handle the situation. I found that my weeping and unloading upon others did not help the case; it only gave the devil a chance to club me. Had I known to carry my burdens to the Lord, my prayers might have been answered sooner. However God heard my cry and unlocked Heaven's doors between the hours of 2:30 and 3:00 in the morning. I felt the burden leave; the Lord took it and left me with joy. I was as free as a bird and as happy as a lark. Very soon husband returned seemingly very much excited and instead of scolding me for not having gone to bed, he was kind and promised on his own volition to stop going out at nights. Very soon he got a steady job and stopped living the way he had. He has had work all the time when thousands have been idle. My home has been refurnished and everything paid for and the Lord has used me to witness for Him to my neighbors. Best of all, God has restored me to perfect health.

"Discouraged ones, take your burdens to the Lord and leave them with Him and be willing to accept whatever He sends and He will lighten your path for He still answers prayer."

(20)

Chapter VI.

IN HEAVEN

(The following will explain why I am interested in foreign missions.)

Who was that tall, handsome gentleman who met me at Heaven's gate just as I entered? He had the appearance of being extremely intelligent and had the most superb manners. He bowed and smiled modestly while graciously thanking me for something I had once done for him on earth. I did not know the man, did not remember of ever having seen him, but as I looked at him it suddenly dawned on me who he was and what it was that evoked his expression of gratitude.

It was while my husband and I were in Urundi, Central Africa, visiting our little daughter Esther, that we went early one morning to the missionary dispensary. It was cold and damp. In the crowd of waiting natives I saw a poor emaciated baby. His eyelids drooped from weakness and pain, and his little limbs looked like lead pencils, while his stomach had the appearance of a watermelon. He had been deserted by his mother and was the very picture of neglect as he cried piteously because of the cold—for he hadn't a thing on his naked body. His head seemed too large, and was scaly with dirt. His nose was too long and his high forehead badly wrinkled, as though he carried too many burdens. In all he was about as ugly a looking child as one ever sees, and when I spoke of doing something for him, someone said, "Oh, don't bother. He will soon be dead, for the worms are eating him up inside."

"Well, I can't meet him at the Judgment

(21)

if I don't do something for him."

So saying, I asked for a pan of warm water, and immersed the little one in a comfortable bath. He screamed when I put him in as it was likely the first he had ever had. After giving him a good soak from head to foot, I took him out, wrapped about him a soft cloth, sat down by the fire and commenced to doctor his feet—a job for an experienced surgeon; but a native woman came to our help as I tried to remove the pus and layers of hardened filth. Of course, this hurt a little, though we were very careful. Then we began on his fingers—trimming those hard, long nails and removing pus from around them. Clean water was brought and I gave the little one a second bath. This all happened out on the ground outside the dispensary, while a motley crowd of men, women, and children looked on. Inside, a long line of poor suffering people stood, waiting to be served by Esther, who was conversing pleasantly with them in their native language.

Crowding in behind her table with the little patient in my arms, I asked her to stop long enough to put some medicine on his poor, bleeding feet and fingers. She did so and I soon had them bandaged. While being treated, the little one called loudly for bananas. This made the natives laugh, but they carried the news to Sister Ila Gunsolus who came from the mission home and brought the child what he wanted.

From Australia, I had brought in my suitcase twenty-four baby dresses which had been given us for Africa by a dear lady who has since gone to Heaven. One of these soft garments was now put on my baby. Though very weak, he tried to stand so as to be able

(22)

to see how he looked in the first garment he had ever owned. After I had finished with the little one, a native woman carried him back to his dingy hut in the banana forest and I went to our room in the mud home occupied by Miss Gunsolus and Esther, happy to have been able to do a tiny bit for "one of these little ones."

While alone with God, Jesus Himself drew near and whispered, "Inasmuch as ye have done it unto one of the least of these. . . ye have done it unto me." Then I saw myself in a vision just entering Heaven and met by the strange man mentioned above who was thanking me for what I had done for him. A second glance proved that he was the babe I had just dressed, as he would look a few years hence. Either he had grown to manhood and entered that blissful abode, a redeemed soul, or he had died young but developed in Heaven. I do not know which, but his appearance now was so striking that I felt insignificant in his presence. He was no longer black, but of the same complexion as others, and, oh, so handsome and heavenly. His appearance was absolutely indescribable.

I was amazed to see how every little deed of kindness or of unkindness is registered for or against us in Heaven. Then I thought how ashamed I would feel to meet that cultured gentleman there had I taken the advice of one and neglected him because he would soon be dead! I fully realized in the presence of Eternal Majesty that this redeemed native would remember as he saw me at the gate, had I passed him by and failed to help him, just because I was doing other work that perhaps seemed more important. Since then my spirit shudders when

(23)

Dis-ease is defined as lack of ease or harmony, it is NOT the
same as "disease," a medical term for illness treated by medicine.
NEVER attempt to stop or reduce your medication without the supervision of your medical doctor.

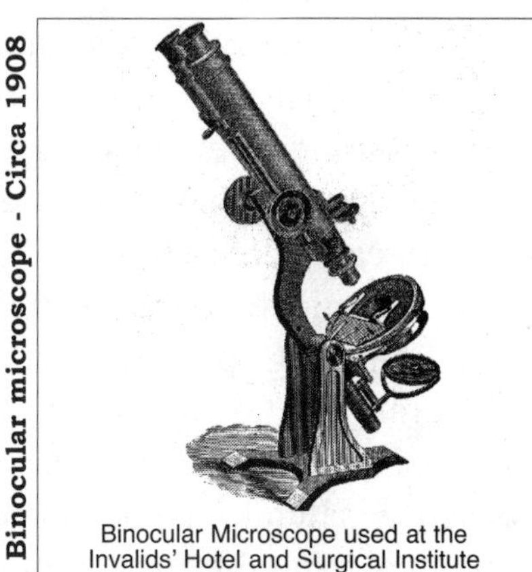

Binocular Microscope used at the Invalids' Hotel and Surgical Institute

CHAPTER 8 - HEALTH QUESTIONNAIRE AND EFFECTIVE EVALUATIONS: THE FIRST STEP TO KNOWING YOUR HEALTH STATUS

"A new scientific truth is not usually presented in a way to convince its opponents. Rather, they die off, and a rising generation is familiarized with the truth from the start."

- Max Planck

The follow questionnaire and other analytical tests are similar to what I used in my clinic and career for over 34 years. By truthfully answering the following questions, you will be able to evaluate 29 different body areas and 11 different systems. Simply add up the points in each section and apply them to each part. The No and Yes answers will either be a zero, a three or a specific number as indicated in brackets ( ). They key to understanding what the questionnaire means is at the end and is rated by a low, moderate to high score relative to your risk factors.

As an example, if under cardiovascular-circulation, you rate a 13, you are in the high rating for circulation problems. However, this questionnaire is not definitive in itself. It merely gives you a glimpse at what you might be experiencing relative to your health. If you are concerned about any signal (symptom) your body might be demonstrating, you should seek a competent natural healing doctor for additional tests, exam and consultation.

This questionnaire, along with a CBC blood test, toxic-metal hair analysis and the *Optimal Wellness Test* or urine/saliva profile, should give you a good picture of your health status. Once your health status has been ascertained, an effective natural healing protocol can be created.

Practicing good health principles and eating all organic food, drinking pristine water, exercising daily, praying or meditating and taking my LifePack System®, may help many areas of concern you may have. For any health challenge remaining, consult a natural healing doctor using time-tested classic and/or aboriginal natural healing protocols and condition specifics.

Instructions: Circle the number which best describes the intensity of your symptoms (signals). If you do not know the answer to a question, leave it blank.

0= Symptom not present 1= Mild 2= Moderate 3= Severe

Part I

Section A:

1. Burping.......................	0	1	2	3
2. Fullness for extended time after meals......	0	1	2	3
3. Bloating	0	1	2	3
4. Poor appetite..............	0	1	2	3
5. Stomach upsets easily	0	1	2	3
6. History of constipation......	0	1	2	3
7. Known food allergies......	0	1	2	3

Score_____

Section B:

1. Abdominal cramps.........	0	1	2	3
2. Indigestion 1-3 hrs after eating...	0	1	2	3
3. Fatigue after eating...........	0	1	2	3
4. Lower bowel gas..............	0	1	2	3
5. Alternating constipation and diarrhea...	0	1	2	3
6. Diarrhea.......................	0	1	2	3

7. Roughage and fiber causes

constipation…	0	1	2	3
8. Mucous in stools…………	0	1	2	3
9. Stool poorly formed………	0	1	2	3
10. Shiny stool …………………	0	1	2	3
11. Three or more large bowel movements/day	0	1	2	3
12. Foul smelling stool…………	0	1	2	3
13. Dry, flaky skin and/or dry brittle hair…….	0	1	2	3
14. Pain in left side under rib cage…	0	1	2	3
15. Acne………………………	0	1	2	3
16. Food allergies………………	0	1	2	3
17. Difficulty gaining weight…	0	1	2	3

Score____

Section C:

1. Stomach pains………………	0	1	2	3
2. Stomach pains just before and/or after meals	0	1	2	3
3. Dependency on antacids……	0	1	2	3
4. Chronic abdominal pain……	0	1	2	3
5. Butterfly sensations in stomach	0	1	2	3
6. Difficulty belching…………	0	1	2	3
7. Stomach pain when emotionally upset…….	0	1	2	3
8. Sudden, acute indigestion…	No			Yes
9. Relief of symptoms by carbonated sodas….	No			Yes
10. Relief of stomach pain by drinking cream…	No			Yes
11. History of ulcer or gastritis……	No			Yes
12. Current ulcer……………………	No			Yes (10)
13. Black stool when not taking iron supplement…	No			Yes (10)

Score____

Dis-ease is defined as lack of ease or harmony, it is NOT the same as "disease," a medical term for illness treated by medicine. *NEVER* attempt to stop or reduce your medication without the supervision of your medical doctor.

Section D:

1. Seasonal diarrhea..............	0	1	2	3
2. Frequent and recurrent infections (colds)...	0	1	2	3
3. Bladder and kidney infections...	0	1	2	3
4. Vaginal yeast infection......	0	1	2	3
5. Abdominal cramps...........	0	1	2	3
6. Toe and fingernail fungus...	0	1	2	3
7. Alternating diarrhea constipation	0	1	2	3
8. Constipation....................	0	1	2	3
9. History of antibiotic use......	No			Yes
10. Meat eater....................	No			Yes
11. Rapidly failing vision.........	No			Yes

Score____

Part II

Section A:

1. Intolerance to greasy foods...	0	1	2	3
2. Headaches after eating......	0	1	2	3
3. Light-colored stool...........	0	1	2	3
4. Foul-smelling stool...........	0	1	2	3
5. Less than one bowel movement daily......	0	1	2	3
6. Constipation........................	0	1	2	3
7. Hard stool..........................	0	1	2	3
8. Sour taste in mouth.............	0	1	2	3
9. Grey-colored skin................	0	1	2	3
10. Yellow in whites of eyes........	0	1	2	3
11. Bad breath..........................	0	1	2	3
12. Body odor...........................	0	1	2	3
13. Fatigue and sleepiness after eating.....................	0	1	2	3
14. Pain in right side under rib cage.............	0	1	2	3
15. Painful to pass stool.........	0	1	2	3

16. Retain water.................	0	1	2	3
17. Big toe painful..............	0	1	2	3
18. Pain radiates along outside of leg...........	0	1	2	3
19. Dry skin/hair.................	0	1	2	3
20. Red blood in stool...........	No			Yes (6)
21. Have had jaundice or hepatitis..............	No			Yes
22. High blood cholesterol and low HDL........	No	Unkwn		Yes(10)
23. Is your cholesterol level above 200?...........	No	Unkwn		Yes
24. Is your triglyceride level above 115?..........	No	Unkwn		Yes

Score____

Section B:

1. Swollen eyes (bulging)......	0	1	2	3
2. Strong-smelling urine......	0	1	2	3
3. Thick skin and finger nails	0	1	2	3
4. Dry skin.......................	0	1	2	3
5. Sensitive to the cold.........	0	1	2	3
6. Cold hands and feet.........	0	1	2	3
7. Excessive menstrual bleeding................	0	1	2	3
8. Chronic fatigue..............	0	1	2	3
9. Trouble waking up in the morning...........	0	1	2	3
10. Depressed or apathetic......	0	1	2	3
11. Low sex drive.................	0	1	2	3
12. Puffy wrinkly skin...........	0	1	2	3
13. Sugar causes irritability & mood swings......	0	1	2	3
14. Premenstrual tension.........	0	1	2	3
15. Constipation.................	0	1	2	3
16. Thinning/loss of outside of eyebrow...	No			Yes

Dis-ease is defined as lack of ease or harmony, it is NOT the same as "disease," a medical term for illness treated by medicine. *NEVER* attempt to stop or reduce your medication without the supervision of your medical doctor.

17. Gain weight easily............... No Yes
18. Anemia un-effected by taking iron...No Yes
19. Axillary (armpit) temperature below 97.6... No Yes
20. Slow reflexes..................... No Yes
21. Infertility........................ No Yes

Score____

Part III

Section A:

1. Sensitive to exhaust fumes, smoke, smog or petrochemicals.....................	0	1	2	3
2. Periodic constipation............	0	1	2	3
3. Cannot tolerate much exercise	0	1	2	3
4. Depression or rapid mood swings............	0	1	2	3
5. Dark circles under the eyes......	0	1	2	3
6. Dizziness upon standing.........	0	1	2	3
7. Lack of mental alertness.........	0	1	2	3
8. Catch colds easily when weather changes....	0	1	2	3
9. Headaches.....................	0	1	2	3
10. Difficulty breathing.........	0	1	2	3
11. Water retention....................	0	1	2	3
12. Eyes sensitive to bright light...	0	1	2	3
13. Feel weak and shaky...........	0	1	2	3

Score____

Section B:

1. Inflamed or bleeding gums......	0	1	2	3
2. Running nose....................	0	1	2	3
3. Get boils or styes..............	0	1	2	3
4. Nose bleeds....................	0	1	2	3
5. Loss of smell.................	0	1	2	3
6. Throat infections..............	0	1	2	3
7. Cold sores, fever blisters......	0	1	2	3
8. Loss of taste....................	0	1	2	3

9. Poor wound healing...........	0	1	2	3
10. Hair falls out....................	0	1	2	3
11. Swollen lymph glands.........	0	1	2	3
12. Ear infection....................	0	1	2	3
13. Hair grows slowly..............	0	1	2	3
14. Slow to recover from cold or flu	0	1	2	3
15. Catch colds or flu easily.........	0	1	2	3
16. Bumpy skin on back of arms...	0	1	2	3

Score____

Section C:

1. Itching of nose or eyes.........	0	1	2	3
2. Itching of roof of mouth or throat...........	0	1	2	3
3. Migraine headaches...........	No			Yes (10)
4. Entire body aches, painful to touch..........	0	1	2	3
5. Swollen joints....................	0	1	2	3
6. Food sensitivity or allergy......	0	1	2	3
7. Certain foods make you sick, depressed or jittery..........................	0	1	2	3
8. Chronic pain....................	0	1	2	3
9. Painful stomach and/or intestine.............	0	1	2	3
10. Alternating constipation and diarrhea........	0	1	2	3
11. Mucous in throat..............	0	1	2	3
12. Post-nasal drip.................	0	1	2	3
13. Discharge from eyes...........	0	1	2	3
14. Watery eyes....................	0	1	2	3
15. Puffiness or dark circles under eyes..........	0	1	2	3
16. Ear discharge or ears stuffed up	0	1	2	3
17. Nasal congestion..............	0	1	2	3
18. Running nose....................	0	1	2	3
19. Breathe through mouth.........	0	1	2	3

Dis-ease is defined as lack of ease or harmony, it is NOT the same as "disease," a medical term for illness treated by medicine. *NEVER* attempt to stop or reduce your medication without the supervision of your medical doctor.

20. Swollen tongue..................	0	1	2	3
21. Difficulty swallowing.........	0	1	2	3
22. Bedwetting.........................	No			Yes(5)
23. Hyperactivity..................	0	1	2	3
24. Chronic lung congestion......	0	1	2	3
25. Use aspirin, Tylenol or Motrin regularly.....	No			Yes
26. Wheezing....................	0	1	2	3
27. Skin rashes.................	0	1	2	3
28. Sneezing....................	0	1	2	3

Score____

Part IV

Section A:

1. Difficulty breathing at night...	0	1	2	3
2. Chest pain while walking...	0	1	2	3
3. Heaviness in legs..............	0	1	2	3
4. Calf muscles cramp while walking..........	0	1	2	3
5. Heart pounds easily...........	0	1	2	3
6. Feel jittery.....................	0	1	2	3
7. Heart misses beats or has extra beats.........	0	1	2	3
8. Swelling of feet and ankles...	0	1	2	3
9. Rapid beating heart............	0	1	2	3
10. Heartburn after eating.........	0	1	2	3
11. Pain in left arm.................	0	1	2	3
12. Exhaust with minor exertion...	0	1	2	3
13. Do you do aerobic exercise?......	No			Yes
14. Have you ever exercised regularly?.........	No			Yes
15. Drink 5 or more cups of coffee daily...	No			Yes
16. Severe cough....................	No			Yes
17. Has a doctor ever told you that you have heart trouble?....................................	No			Yes (6)

Score____

Section B:

1. Cold hands and feet...........	0	1	2	3
2. Slurred speech..................	0	1	2	3
3. Calf muscles cramp while walking...........	0	1	2	3
4. Headaches.......................	0	1	2	3
5. Numbness in extremities......	0	1	2	3
6. Poor concentration..............	0	1	2	3
7. Ringing in ears.................	0	1	2	3
8. Ear canal hair.................	No			Yes
9. Tingling and/or burning in hands or feet....	No			Yes
10. Spider veins on nose and/or face	No			Yes

Score____

Section C:

1. Pain when getting up in morning in back of neck and head.................	0	1	2	3
2. Dizziness.......................	0	1	2	3
3. Vertigo..........................	0	1	2	3
4. Blushing with no apparent cause	0	1	2	3
5. Is your blood pressure high?........	No			Yes(10)

Score____

Part V

Section A:

1. Dizziness when standing suddenly............	0	1	2	3
2. Loss of vision when standing suddenly.......	0	1	2	3
3. Crave sweets....................	0	1	2	3
4. Headaches relieved by eating sweets or alcohol.......................	0	1	2	3
5. Feel shaky or jittery...........	0	1	2	3
6. Irritable if a meal is missed...	0	1	2	3

7. Wake up in middle of night

craving sweets..	0	1	2	3
8. Feel tired or weak if a meal is missed.........	0	1	2	3
9. Heart palpations after eating sweets..........	0	1	2	3
10. Need to drink coffee to get started............	0	1	2	3
11. Impatient, moody or nervous...	0	1	2	3
12. Feel tired 1 to 3 hours after eating...........	0	1	2	3
13. Poor memory....................	0	1	2	3
14. Feel faint.......................	0	1	2	3
15. Poor concentration...........	0	1	2	3
16. Forgetful.........................	0	1	2	3
17. Calmer after eating........	No			Yes

Score____

Section B:

1. Night sweats....................	0	1	2	3
2. Increased thirst................	0	1	2	3
3. Lowered resistance to infection	0	1	2	3
4. Fatigue..........................	0	1	2	3
5. Boils and leg sores..............	0	1	2	3
6. Lesions, cuts take a long time to heal.........	0	1	2	3
7. Overweight....................	0	1	2	3
8. Feel pick up from exercise......	0	1	2	3
9. Failing eyesight.................	0	1	2	3
10. Crave sweets, but eating sweets does not relieve symptoms..............	0	1	2	3
11. Family history of diabetes...	0	1	2	3
12. Sugar in urine.................	No			Yes

Score____

Part VI

1. Chest pain.......................	0	1	2	3
2. Chronic cough.................	0	1	2	3

3. Difficulty breathing...........	0	1	2	3
4. Coughing up blood...........	0	1	2	3
5. Coughing up phlegm.........	0	1	2	3
6. Pain around ribs...............	0	1	2	3
7. Shortness of breath...........	0	1	2	3
8. Rattling mucous when you breathe...........	0	1	2	3
9. Sensitive to smog...........	0	1	2	3
10. Infections settle in lungs......	0	1	2	3
11. Live or work around people who smoke.....	0	1	2	3
12. Bronchitis.......................	No			Yes (10)
13. Exposed to chemicals and radiation	No			Yes (6)
14. Smoker..........................	No			Yes (6)

Score____

Part VII

1. Frequent urination...........	0	1	2	3
2. Frequent bladder infections......	0	1	2	3
3. Rarely need to urinate.........	0	1	2	3
4. Urination when you cough or sneeze.........	0	1	2	3
5. Painful/burning when passing urine..........	0	1	2	3
6. Difficulty passing urine......	0	1	2	3
7. Dripping after urination......	0	1	2	3
8. Can't hold urine..............	0	1	2	3
9. Rose-colored (bloody) urine	0	1	2	3
10. Cloudy urine.................	0	1	2	3
11. Strong smelling urine.........	0	1	2	3
12. Back or leg pain associated with dripping after urination.................	0	1	2	3
13. History of kidney or bladder infections.......	No			Yes
14. Have used antibiotics to control urinary tract infections.................	No			Yes

15. Back pain in kidney area......	0	1	2	3
16. General water retention.........	0	1	2	3

Score____

Part VIII - MALES ONLY

Section A:

1. Difficulty urinating...........	0	1	2	3
2. A sense of bladder fullness...	0	1	2	3
3. Increased straining with smaller and smaller amount of urine passed	0	1	2	3
4. Rose colored (bloody) urine	0	1	2	3
5. Pain or burning while urinating	0	1	2	3
6. Wake up to urinate at night......	0	1	2	3
7. Dripping after urination......	0	1	2	3
8. Pain or fatigue in the legs/back...	0	1	2	3
9. Lack of sex drive...........	0	1	2	3
10. Ejaculation causes pain......	0	1	2	3

Score____

Section B:

1. Difficulty attaining and/or maintaining an erection....................	0	1	2	3
2. Low sexual drive..............	0	1	2	3
3. Premature ejaculation........	0	1	2	3
4. Pain/coldness in genital area......	0	1	2	3
5. Infertile.........................	No			Yes (5)
6. Varicose veins on scrotum......	No			Yes
7. Low sperm count..............	No			Yes(5)

Score____

Section C:

1. Discharge from penis.........	0	1	2	3
2. Past or present rash on penis...	0	1	2	3
3. Swollen genitals..............	0	1	2	3
4. Swelling in groin..............	0	1	2	3
5. Venereal disease; gonorrhea, syphilis, herpes or other.................	No			Yes(9)

Score____

Part IX - FEMALES ONLY

Section A: Circle if you experience any of these symptoms within approximately 2 weeks (ovulation) prior to menstruation.

Section A:

1. Monthly weight gain.........	0	1	2	3
2. Depression........................	0	1	2	3
3. Moodiness/irritability.........	0	1	2	3
4. Bloating and swelling............	0	1	2	3
5. Nausea and/or vomiting......	0	1	2	3
6. Suicidal feeling..............	No			Yes (10)
7. Anxiety...........................	0	1	2	3
8. Leg cramps and tenderness...	0	1	2	3
9. Asthma attacks..................	No			Yes(10)
10. Headaches........................	0	1	2	3
11. Easily distracted..............	0	1	2	3
12. Anger..........................	0	1	2	3
13. Tender breasts....................	0	1	2	3
14. Low backache.................	0	1	2	3
15. Other symptoms____________	0	1	2	3

Score____

Section B:

1. Vaginal itching.................	0	1	2	3
2. Vaginal discharge..............	0	1	2	3
3. Low or no desire for sex......	0	1	2	3
4. Dislike for intercourse.........	0	1	2	3
5. Missed periods.................	0	1	2	3
6. Over 15 years of age and have not begun menstruation....................	0	1	2	3
7. Unable to get pregnant......	No			Yes
8. Miscarriages....................	No			Yes
9. Abortion....................	No			Yes

Score____

Section C:

Circle if you have experienced any of these symptoms during menstruation. (Section C Only)

1. Low abdominal pain.........	0	1	2	3
2. Dull ache radiating to low back or legs.......	0	1	2	3
3. Increased urinary frequency......	0	1	2	3
4. Pelvic soreness..................	0	1	2	3
5. Diarrhea..........................	0	1	2	3
6. Headaches........................	0	1	2	3
7. Abdominal bloating...........	0	1	2	3
8. Menstrual pain....................	0	1	2	3
9. Nausea and/or vomiting.........	0	1	2	3
10. Have to lie down on first 1-2 days of period	0	1	2	3
11. Craving for sweets..............	0	1	2	3
12. Insomnia....................	0	1	2	3
13. Light scanty blood flow.........	0	1	2	3
14. Pain and cramps without blood flow.........	0	1	2	3
15. Heavy menstrual bleeding......	0	1	2	3
16. Anxiety about menstrual cycle	0	1	2	3
17. Pain during period is progressively getting worse with time..............	0	1	2	3

Score____

Section D:

1. Vaginal bumps and sores......	0	1	2	3
2. Pubic area sore.....................	0	1	2	3
3. Ovarian cysts.................	No			Yes(10)
4. Uterine cysts....................	No			Yes(10)
5. Pain in ovaries....................	0	1	2	3
6. Breast lumps.................	No			Yes (10)
7. Breasts sore to touch...........	0	1	2	3
8. Breasts painful.................	0	1	2	3
9. Water retention.................	0	1	2	3
10. Swollen feeling.................	0	1	2	3
11. Premenstrual breast pain or discomfort......	0	1	2	3

Dis-ease is defined as lack of ease or harmony, it is NOT the same as "disease," a medical term for illness treated by medicine. *NEVER* attempt to stop or reduce your medication without the supervision of your medical doctor.

12. Mother used D.E.S. (hormones) while pregnant...........	No			Yes
13. Recent pap smear positive...	No			Yes (15)
14. Family history of breast cancer	No			Yes

Score____

Section E:

1. Hot flashes.....................	0	1	2	3
2. Night Sweats.....................	0	1	2	3
3. Hysterectomy.................	No			Yes
4. Depression/mood swings......	0	1	2	3
5. Insomnia.......................	0	1	2	3
6. Craving for sweets..............	0	1	2	3
7. Heavy bleeding two weeks per month........	0	1	2	3
8. Sweating throughout the day...	0	1	2	3
9. Dryness of skin, hair and vagina	0	1	2	3
10. Painful intercourse..............	0	1	2	3
11. Vaginal pain.......................	0	1	2	3
12. Vaginal itching.................	0	1	2	3
13. Osteoporosis (bone loss)......	No			Yes

Score____

Part X

Section A:

1. Pain in fingers.................	0	1	2	3
2. Bones sore/painful..............	0	1	2	3
3. Eat meat..........................	0	1	2	3
4. Cavities.........................	0	1	2	3
5. Arthritis.........................	0	1	2	3
6. Drink carbonated beverages/soda...	No			Yes
7. Gum disease....................	No			Yes
8. Bone loss..........................	No			Yes
9. Calcium deposits.................	No			Yes
10. Use antacids....................	No			Yes
11. Dentures..........................	No			Yes

12. Bone deformity..................	No			Yes
13. Told you have osteoporosis/ osteomalacia....	No			Yes (5)
14. Recent bone fracture............	No			Yes
15. Are you post menopausal?.......	No			Yes
			Score____	

Section B:

1. Muscle spasms.................	0	1	2	3
2. Tightness in shoulder muscles	0	1	2	3
3. Muscle cramps..................	0	1	2	3
4. Pain in arms, hands...............	0	1	2	3
5. Leg cramps at night...........	0	1	2	3
6. Stiff all over.....................	0	1	2	3
7. Stiff in morning..................	0	1	2	3
8. Unable to sit straight...........	0	1	2	3
9. Pain in neck and/or shoulders	0	1	2	3
10. Back pain..........................	0	1	2	3
			Score____	

Section C:

1. Over flexible joints (double-jointed).........	0	1	2	3
2. Back pain.......................	0	1	2	3
3. Swollen knees/elbows.........	0	1	2	3
4. Athletic injury.....................	0	1	2	3
5. Bursitis..........................	0	1	2	3
6. Tendonitis.......................	0	1	2	3
7. Joint pain.......................	0	1	2	3
8. Slipped disc..............	No			Yes (5)
9. Herniated disc...............	No			Yes (10)
10. Loss in height....................	No			Yes
11. Injure easily.......................	No			Yes
			Score____	

Part XI

1. Head feels heavy..............	0	1	2	3
2. Light headedness/fainting.....	0	1	2	3

3. Loss of balance..............	0	1	2	3
4. Dizziness..........................	0	1	2	3
5. Ringing/buzzing in ears.........	0	1	2	3
6. Trembling hands.................	0	1	2	3
7. Loss of feeling in hands and /or feet (toes)...	0	1	2	3
8. Exhaustion on slightest effort	0	1	2	3
9. Limbs feel too heavy to hold up..............	0	1	2	3
10. Loss of grip strength...........	0	1	2	3
11. Tingling pain sensation.........	0	1	2	3
12. Convulsions.................	No			Yes (10)
13. Incoordination.................	0	1	2	3
14. Nervousness....................	0	1	2	3
15. Accident prone..............	No			Yes
16. Loss of muscle tone...........	No			Yes
17. Need for 10-12 hours sleep...	No			Yes
18. Have had shingles..............	No			Yes

Score____

Part XII

1. Nightmares....................	0	1	2	3
2. Can't fall asleep.................	0	1	2	3
3. Intense dreams.................	0	1	2	3
4. Leg cramps/restless leg at night	0	1	2	3
5. Restless, uneasy sleeper.........	0	1	2	3
6. Awake frequently throughout night	No			Yes
7. Wake up in the middle of night, can't fall back to sleep.................	No			Yes
8. Sleep walk.................	No			Yes

Score____

Example of <u>Answered</u> Questionnaire Key

Now that you have answered the questionnaire, add up the points from each Part and **Enter** in the Questionnaire Key in the far right column. Circle the corresponding number to the left of your total for that part. Ideally, all of your numbers will fall in the *low* range. The higher the score the more at risk you are for developing a condition under the heading of that evaluation or system. This is an actual result from a patient of mine.

Risk Level:	High	Medium	Low
Part I - Digestion			
A. Hypoacidity			1
B. Small Intestine		7	
C. Hyperacidity	9		
D. Colon	13		
Part II - Fat Metabolism			
A. Liver/gallbladder		5	
B. Thyroid			3
Part III - Immune			
A. Hypoadrenal	12		
B. Hypoimmune	15		
C. Hyperimmune			3
Part IV - Cardiovascular			
A. Heart		9	
B. Circulation		9	
C. Hypertension	8		
Part V - Sugar Tolerance			
A. Hypoglycemia			1
B. Hyperglycemia	12		
Part VI Lungs			
A. Lungs			2
Part VII - Urological			
A. Urological			2

Dis-ease is defined as lack of ease or harmony, it is NOT the same as "disease," a medical term for illness treated by medicine. *<u>NEVER</u>* attempt to stop or reduce your medication without the supervision of your medical doctor.

Risk Level: High Medium Low

Part VIII - Male

A. Prostate..3
B. Reproduction...3
C. Genital Infection..............................4

Part IX - Female

A. PMS
B. Amenorrhea
C. Dysmenorrhea
D. Fibrocystic
E. Menopause

Did not apply. Male took the test.

Part X - Musculo-skeletal

A. Bone Integrity....................................3
B. Muscle...5
C. Connective Tissue..............................3

Part XI - Neurological

A. Neurological...3

Part XII - Abnormal Sleep

A. Sleep...5

Now it's your turn. Answer the following questionnaire and see how you do. Remember, this is only a test. Nothing is set is stone. Regardless of your results, you can always improve using natural healing protocols.

When you combine this questionnaire with the hair toxic-metal mineral analysis, the Optimum Wellness Urine and Saliva Test and a SMAC 26 or CBC blood test, you have a significant amount of information. Working with a chiropractic, traditional naturopathic or natural healer, you should be able to detoxify and balance your entire body. Remember, only sick people get sick.

Getting to the cause of your complaint(s) by understanding the *signs* your body reflects as *signals* is paramount to optimum health and longevity.

QUESTIONNAIRE SCORE SHEET

		100 High-75	Mod-50	Low-25	Enter#
XII	Abnormal Sleep patterns	9 7 6	5 4 3	2 1	
XI	Neurological	30 25 20 15	10 5	3 1	
Part X Musculo	C. Connective tissue	12 9 7	5 3	2 1	
	B. Muscle	15 12 9	7 5 3	2 1	
	A. Bone integrity	15 13 11	9 7 5	3 1	
Part IX Female	E. Menopause	19 17 13 11	9 7 3	2 1	
	D. Fibrocystic	30 25 20 15	12 9	5 1	
	C. Dysmenorrhea	30 24 21 18	15 9 6	3 1	
	B. Amenorrhea	15 12 9	6 3	2 1	
	A. PMS	25 20 15 11	8 5	3 1	
Part VIII Male	C. Genital Infection	9 7 5	4 3	2 1	
	B. Reproduction	15 12 9	7 5 3	2 1	
	A. Prostate	15 12 9	7 5 3	2 1	
VII Uro	Urological	21 18 15 9	6 3	2 1	
VI Lung	Lungs	15 13 11 9	6 3	2 1	
Part V Sugar	B. Hyperglycemia	24 18 15 12	9 6	3 1	
	A. Hypoglycemia	21 18 15 12	9 6	3 1	
Part IV Cardio-	C. Hypertension	9 8 7 6	5 4 3	2 1	
	B. Circulation	15 13 11	9 7	4 1	
	A. Heart	15 13 11	9 7	4 1	
Part III Immune	C. Hyperimmune	45 35 25 15	10 5	3 1	
	B. Hypoimmune	30 20 15 12	9 6	3 1	
	A. Hypoadrenal	20 18 14 12	9 6	3 1	
Part II Fat Meta-	B. Thyroid	25 15 12 9	7 5	3 1	
	A. Liver/gallbladders	18 12 9 6	5 4 3	2 1	
Part I Digestion	D. Colon	15 13 11 9	7 5	3 1	
	C. Hyperacidity	15 13 11 9	7 5	3 1	
	B. Small Intestine	15 13 11 9	7 5	3 1	
	A. Hypoacidity	15 13 11 9	7 5	3 1	

Dis-ease is defined as lack of ease or harmony, it is NOT the same as "disease," a medical term for illness treated by medicine. *NEVER* attempt to stop or reduce your medication without the supervision of your medical doctor.

Understanding pH

As I have discussed, keeping the proper pH is critical for not only maintaining optimum health, it is vital for life. Because of this fact, the body will do anything and everything to maintain normal pH levels, including but not limited to, de-mineralizing the bones and teeth and sacrificing other structures and functions.

As Herman Aihara describes in his book, *Acid and Alkaline*, when carbohydrates, proteins and fats are metabolized they produce acids in the body. Protein produces sulfuric and phosphoric acid. Carbohydrates and fats produce acetic and lactic acid. These acids are neutralized by mineral compounds. The family of mineral compounds which neutralize acids are carbonic salts, symbolized as BaCO3. The Ba stands for any one of the four alkaline elements: Sodium (Na), Calcium (Ca), Potassium (K) and Magnesium (Mg). The CO3 stands for carbonate ions.

When the carbonic salts react with the strong metabolic acids, the alkaline minerals making up the carbonic salts leave the salt and combine with the acids to make new salts.

For example:
BaCO3 (carbonic salt) + H2SO4 (sulfuric acid) =
BaSO4 (sulfuric salt) + H2O (water) +
CO2 (carbon dioxide).

These acid salts are then excreted from the body in our urine, saliva, feces and sweat. Thus the acid is neutralized and the pH of the body is raised to a proper alkalinity.

The easiest way to test your pH is from your urine and saliva. The following chart may be used to test both on a daily basis. Catch the urine in mid-stream and hold paper strip to colored chart on back of pH paper holder. When testing saliva, spit on paper. Do NOT place paper in your mouth.

Remember, balance is the key to health. You do not want to be over acidic or alkaline. Adjust diet, attitude, exercise and lifestyle accordingly.

(To purchase pH testing paper see Index E - *Resources* in back of book.)

Our pH fluctuates four times within 24 hours. Depending on what you eat, drink, how you think & what time of the day/night, will determine what your pH will be. The below is merely a guide demonstrating a normal range between acid of 5.8 to slightly alkaline at 7.2. Test your pH for seven days and then log the average. Adjust diet accordingly.

7.2

5.8

4 A.M. 6 8 10 12 P.M. 2 4 6 8 10 12 2 4 A.M.

Today's Date	Time of Last Food	Urine pH 5.8 - 6.8	Saliva pH 6.8 - 7.2	Time Taken	Technician Performed

Food Eaten Last: ______________________

Today's Date	Time of Last Food	Urine pH 5.8 - 6.8	Saliva pH 6.8 - 7.2	Time Taken	Technician Performed

Food Eaten Last: ______________________

Today's Date	Time of Last Food	Urine pH 5.8 - 6.8	Saliva pH 6.8 - 7.2	Time Taken	Technician Performed

Food Eaten Last: ______________________

Today's Date	Time of Last Food	Urine pH 5.8 - 6.8	Saliva pH 6.8 - 7.2	Time Taken	Technician Performed

Food Eaten Last: ______________________

Today's Date	Time of Last Food	Urine pH 5.8 - 6.8	Saliva pH 6.8 - 7.2	Time Taken	Technician Performed

Food Eaten Last: ______________________

Dis-ease is defined as lack of ease or harmony, it is NOT the same as "disease," a medical term for illness treated by medicine. *NEVER* attempt to stop or reduce your medication without the supervision of your medical doctor.

Iridology

As mentioned in Chapter 3 under *eyes*, Iridology is the study of the iris as it relates to health and vitality of humans and animals.

Currently, the most knowledgeable practitioner of this fascinating science is David J. Pesek, Ph.D. of Waynesville, NC. Dr. Pesek is the president of the International Institute of Iridology and the American College of Iridology.

The following is his explanation of Iridology:

The iris is the most complex external structure of the human anatomy. It is connected to every organ and tissue of the body by way of the nervous system. Through the optic nerves, which are attached to the eyes, vision information is sent to the brain. At the same time, in a "looping feedback effect," information is sent to the eyes from the brain about your overall level of health.

Iridology reveals the level of health and the presence of tissue inflammation in the body, where it is located and what stage it has reached: acute, subacute, chronic or degenerative. The iris reveals the level of constitutional strength, inherent weaknesses and the transitions that take place in a person's organs and tissues according to the way they eat, drink, feel, think and live.

The science and practice of iridology is not new. The oldest records uncovered thus far have shown that a form of iris interpretation was used in Central Asia (Mesopotamia) as far back as 1,000 B.C., approximately 3,000 years ago.

In the year 1670, the physician Phillippus Meyens, in his book, *Physiognomia Medica*, described the iris as reflecting the various organs in the body according to specific regions in the irises. The Viennese ophthalmologist, Beer, did not know of these old views on iris analysis. Yet, in his publication of 1813, *Textbook of Eye Diseases*, he wrote, "Everything that affects the organism of an individual cannot remain without effect on the eye and vice versa."

A Hungarian, Dr. Ignaz von Peczely, published a book in 1881 entitled, *Discovery in Natural History and Medical Science, a Guide to the Study and Diagnosis from the Eye.* This book achieved an international fame and he is now considered the Father of Modern Iridology.

In the 20th century, doctors and scientists primarily from the United States (Benard Jensen, D.C., N.D.) and Germany (Josef Deck, Hp. and Josef Angerer, Hp.), have brought Iridology into worldwide recognition. I have studied the work of these pioneers extensively and have lectured internationally on the subject.

The actual fiber structures and various colors we see in the iris tell us about the level of physical health and constitutional strength of our body. These features also relate to personality traits as well as conscious and subconscious thought/emotional patterns.

Incorporating all information available from the pioneers of iridology before me, I have developed a system called Holistic Iridology. For the first time, we can now go way beyond the physical level of iris interpretation and delve into the mental, emotional and spiritual aspects as well.

Each eye gives us different information. The left eye correlates with the left side of our body, that which is feminine, creative, conceptual and intuitive. The right eye correlates to the right side of the body, the analytical, practical, linear and masculine side of us.

By being made aware of their conscious and subconscious behavior patterns and influences of genetic memory, individuals are able to understand the origins of their conditions and afflictions, enabling them to positively transform their lives on all levels. Thus, iridology is an excellent tool of analysis for prevention of illness and dis-ease. In many cases, conditions can be detected 20 years or more prior to symptoms. The potential for a high-risk area in the body can actually be observed in an infant.

As "windows of the soul," our eyes are clearly and literally reflecting the essence of our being. With the help of this fascinating science, we have just scratched the surface of what we will know about the human condition in the future.

Dis-ease is defined as lack of ease or harmony, it is NOT the same as "disease," a medical term for illness treated by medicine. *NEVER* attempt to stop or reduce your medication without the supervision of your medical doctor.

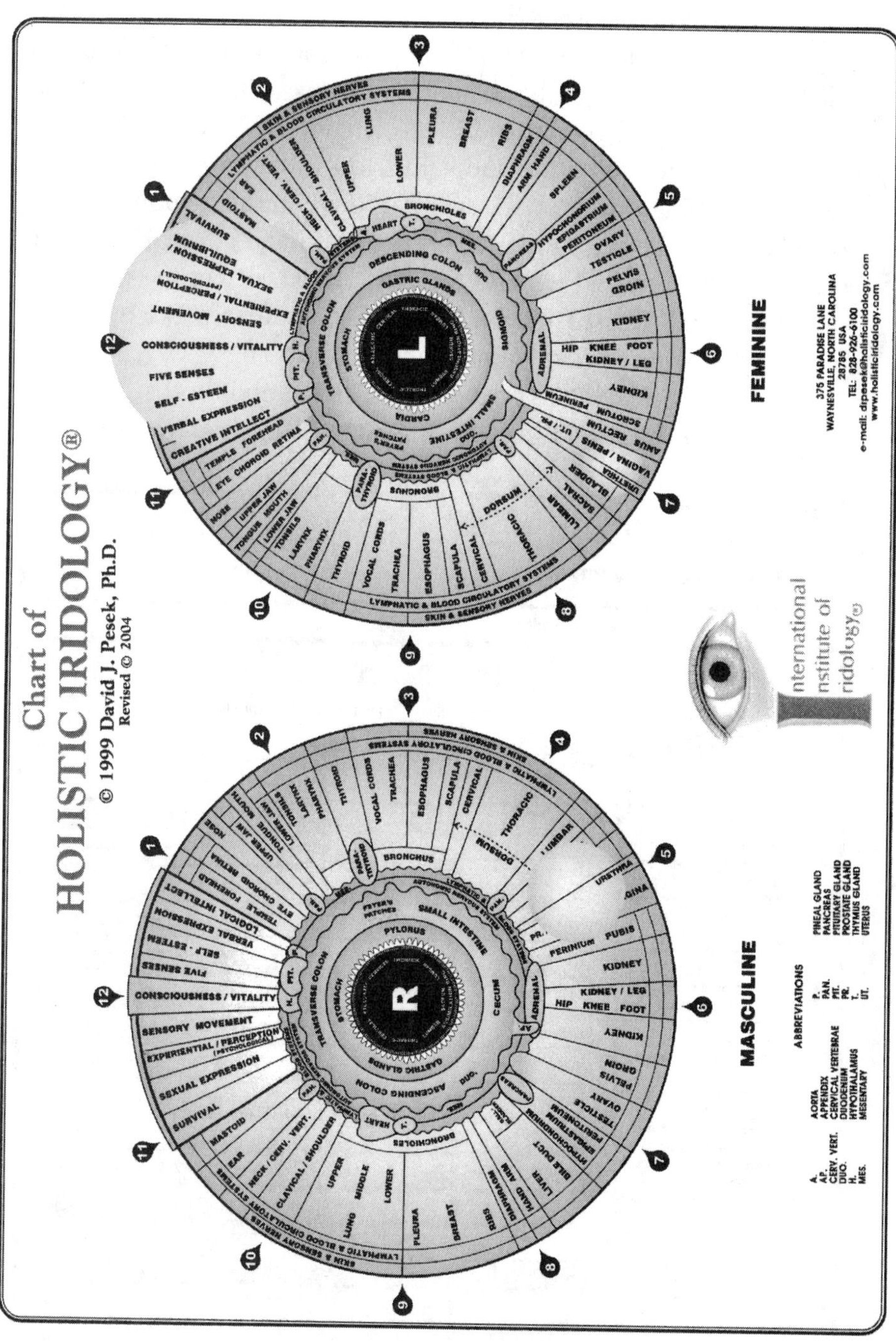

Dis-ease is defined as lack of ease or harmony, it is NOT the same as "disease," a medical term for illness treated by medicine. *NEVER* attempt to stop or reduce your medication without the supervision of your medical doctor.

Optimal Wellness Test

This is an example of one of the most revolutionary diagnostic tests currently available. It is called the *Optimal Wellness Test.* Developed by a brilliant researcher, Melonie Montgomery, it uses urine and saliva to evaluate oxidative stress, cellular respiration, protein and carbohydrate metabolism, pH, blood sugar balance, kidney, liver, digestion and adrenal function, cellular hydration and general toxicity. It can detect the presence of fungus and viruses by evaluating the cellular make-up years before symptoms of involvement appear.

This is truly state-of-the-art medicine and works perfectly with natural healing. (To order this test, see Index *E-Resources*).

Patient Name: OTR
Phone:
Test Date: 1/25/2005 10:12:18 AM
Test ID: 194
Print Date: 01/25/05 10:12 am

	Patient Results								Optimum							
	pH	rH2	r	Cond.	Nitr.	Amm.	Brix	SG	pH	rH2	r	Cond.	Nitr.	Amm.	Brix	SG
Saliva	6.17	19.4	327						6.4	21.5-23.5	210-230					
Urine	6.00	20.3	189	5.3	2.	12.	15.1		6.4	22.5-24.5	30-50	6-7	3	3	1.5-5	

Acidosis
Oxidative Stress
Cellular Respiration
Renal
Hepatic
Digestion
Hydration
Toxicity
Adrenal
Protein Metabolism
Carbohydrate Metabolism
Blood Sugar Balance

Anabolic | Catabolic

Anabolic / Catabolic

Dis-ease is defined as lack of ease or harmony, it is NOT the same as "disease," a medical term for illness treated by medicine.
NEVER attempt to stop or reduce your medication without the supervision of your medical doctor.

This is an example of what a hair toxic metal mineral analysis report looks like. As you can see, this patient had high copper, mercury and aluminum. These metals can cause fatigue, mood swings, weight gain and frequent infections, exactly what this patient was complaining of. (See actual case on next page). To order a hair toxic-metal mineral analysis test see Index E *Resources* in back of book.

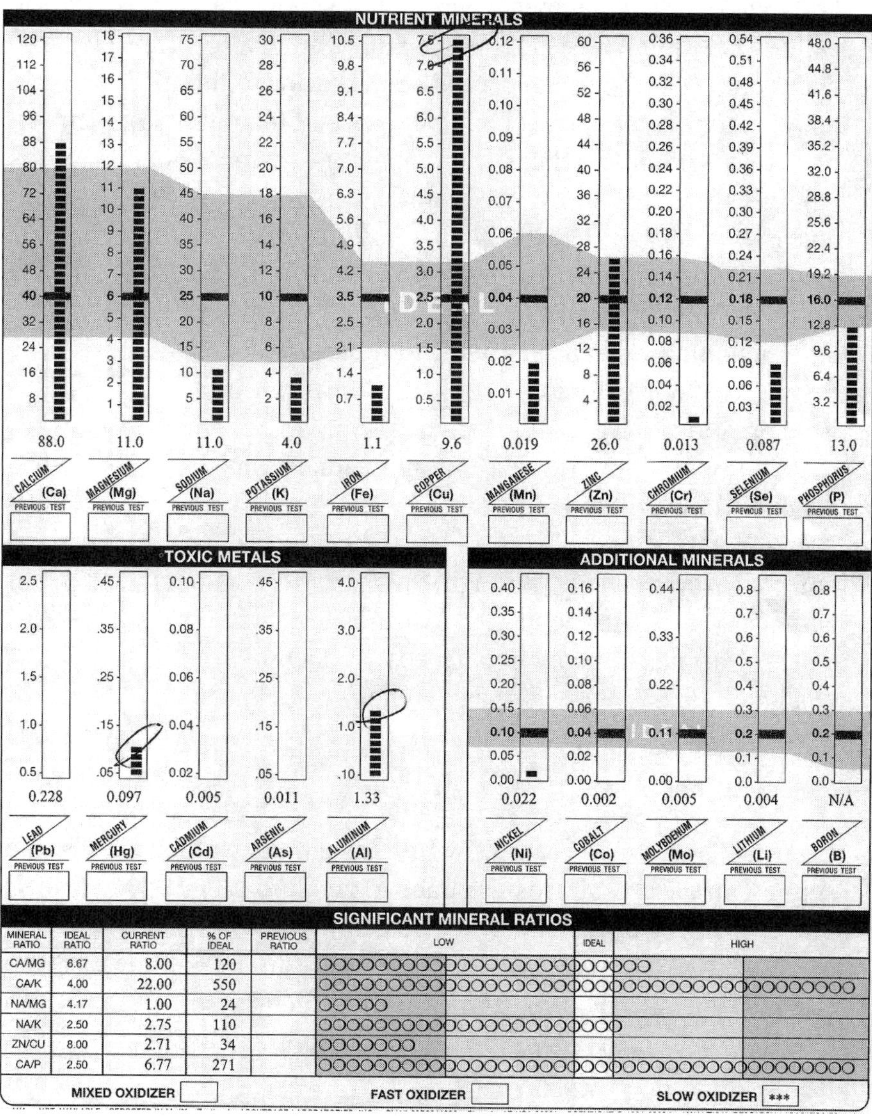

NUTRIENT MINERALS

CALCIUM (Ca)	MAGNESIUM (Mg)	SODIUM (Na)	POTASSIUM (K)	IRON (Fe)	COPPER (Cu)	MANGANESE (Mn)	ZINC (Zn)	CHROMIUM (Cr)	SELENIUM (Se)	PHOSPHORUS (P)
88.0	11.0	11.0	4.0	1.1	9.6	0.019	26.0	0.013	0.087	13.0

TOXIC METALS

LEAD (Pb)	MERCURY (Hg)	CADMIUM (Cd)	ARSENIC (As)	ALUMINUM (Al)
0.228	0.097	0.005	0.011	1.33

ADDITIONAL MINERALS

NICKEL (Ni)	COBALT (Co)	MOLYBDENUM (Mo)	LITHIUM (Li)	BORON (B)
0.022	0.002	0.005	0.004	N/A

SIGNIFICANT MINERAL RATIOS

MINERAL RATIO	IDEAL RATIO	CURRENT RATIO	% OF IDEAL	PREVIOUS RATIO
CA/MG	6.67	8.00	120	
CA/K	4.00	22.00	550	
NA/MG	4.17	1.00	24	
NA/K	2.50	2.75	110	
ZN/CU	8.00	2.71	34	
CA/P	2.50	6.77	271	

MIXED OXIDIZER ☐ FAST OXIDIZER ☐ SLOW OXIDIZER ***

Dis-ease is defined as lack of ease or harmony, it is NOT the same as "disease," a medical term for illness treated by medicine. *NEVER* attempt to stop or reduce your medication without the supervision of your medical doctor.

Hair Toxic Metal Mineral Analysis

Linda was fifty years old with *waist-length hair*, a child of the sixties, a vegan for thirty years. Much to her disappointment, she came to me for Myalgic Encephalomyelitis (ME), commonly called Chronic Fatigue Syndrome (CFS). I guess when you can't get out of bed, even after 12 hours sleep, feel pain throughout your body and can't remember where you put your keys, they have to call it something. CFS does come with fibromyalgia (muscle pain) and brain fog (poor concentration); however, these *signals* are merely *signs* of imbalance, deficiencies and toxicities. Remember, one reason our medical establishment names conditions as "diseases" is to allow their union members to "treat" these "disease" - and no one else. In addition, they can now attach an insurance code to their "disease" for financial reimbursement.

An example of this is arthritis. If one has inflammation in an articulation or joint, the term to describe this condition is only descriptive, not pathological. 'Arth' means joint and 'itis' means inflammation. That's all. Plain and simple.

I not only had Linda fill out the questionnaire, she also had a hair toxic-metal mineral analysis test. Simply called a hair test, it is a laboratory test that measures the mineral and toxic metal content of your body through the hair. If a mineral excess or deficiency exists in the hair, it indicates the same within the body.

Various mineral imbalances frequently lead to metabolic dysfunctions (signs) *before* any symptoms (signals) of a "disease" develop. This falls under the **N** in The H.O.N.S.T.E.C. Syndrome for nutrition. This is called pre-clinical.

Minerals are the "spark plugs" of life. The are involved in almost all enzyme reactions within the body. Without enzyme activity, life ceases to exist. A trace mineral, toxic-metal analysis is preventive as well as useful as a screening tool.

To take a sample of hair, you cut directly up against the scalp. Typically, you only use the first inch or so of the sample closest to the scalp, about the size of a pea in diameter.

Since hair usually takes three to six months to grow an inch, a sample taken this way provides mineral and toxic metal information over this period of time, However, of the thousands of hair tests I have ordered over the last 30 years, because of the length of Linda's hair (down to her waist), I was able to track her pattern for several years, not just a few months. Actually, I submitted ten years or twenty individual hair samples on Linda. The results of were absolutely astounding!

In addition to multiple mineral imbalances and deficiencies, Linda's hair closest to the scalp demonstrated high levels of aluminum at 3.0 parts per million (ppm) and high levels of mercury at 0.9. Mercury and aluminum are major toxic metals, both of which can severely compromise the immune system.

Mercury

Sources of mercury poisoning come from dental filings, fish, fungicides, body powders and talc, cosmetics, latex and solvent-thinned paints, diuretic and other medicines, air pollution, fabric softeners, floor waxes and polishes, air conditioner filters, wood preservative, cinnabar (used in jewelry), batteries, tanning leather, felt, adhesives, laxatives, skin lightening creams, psoriatic ointments, tattooing and sewage sludge used as fertilizer and to grow bacteria to make synthetic vitamin B12.

Signs and signals of mercury toxicity include immune depression, with frequent infections and central nervous system damage, from mental disorders, physical motor challenges to organ and gland dysfunction.

Mercury toxicity can cause insomnia, dizziness, weakness, depression, tremors, seizures, loss of appetite, loss of memory, nervousness, shyness, headache, uncoordination, dermatitis, numbness and tingling of the lips and feet, loss of vision and hearing, emotional instability and kidney damage.

Aluminum

Sources of aluminum poisoning come from food additives, cosmetics, over-the-counter drugs, prescribed drugs, pots and pans, foil, sodium aluminum sulfate in baking powder, cheese and potassium alum in white flour, beverages from aluminum cans, antacids, anti-perspirants, municipal drinking water and drying agents in table salt and other products.

Signs and signals of aluminum toxicity include immune depression, chronic infections, nervous system damage, behavioral problems, dementia, memory loss, loss of coordination, confusion, disorientation as well as intestinal digestive disturbances, colic, etc.

How many of you have any of these signs and signals and yet have never had a hair test to rule out heavy-metal toxicity? Instead, you have gone from doctor to doctor trying to "find" the cause of your problem(s), when it has been sitting on top of your head all along!

Because of the length of Linda's hair and the multiple samples I took, I was able to back track her toxic metal levels from zero, ten years ago, to her current high levels. It was about eight years earlier that she had some dental work done using mercury based amalgam filings. Her hair test showed the results of that mercury contamination. About four years ago, as her mercury levels increased, her so-called "Chronic Fatigue" started.

Although she ate only organic fruits and vegetables, nuts, seeds, sprouts and legumes (part of what I always recommend we eat), because our top soil is depleted of minerals, she demonstrated mineral imbalances. Because of her mercury based amalgams and other unknown mercury contributors, she had mercury poisoning. Cooking with aluminum pots and pans and using anti-perspirant, contributed to her aluminum problems.

Linda needed the complete intensive protocol as found in Chapter 6, along with oral and IV chelation. Once her minerals were balanced and the toxic metals removed, her "Chronic Fatigue" disappeared.

Remember, I had the same condition after having surgery. From Chronic Fatigue, cancer, diabetes, lupus to every other so-called "disease," you haven't tried it all until you have tried natural healing.

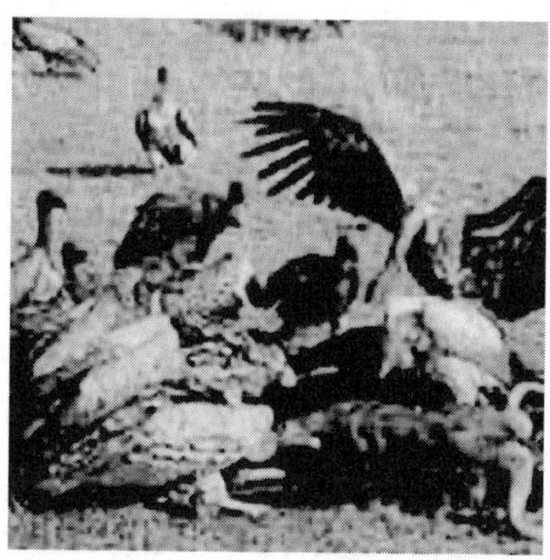

CHAPTER 9 - CURRENT HEALTH STATUS IN AMERICA

"I had a dream. I saw my decaying body torn to shreds by ravenous vultures fighting for every scrap. I struggled to awake from this paralyzing nightmare only to find I was waiting in my doctor's office."

- EC Wyndham

There are two major reasons we don't have a *cure* for cancer. First, the governmental meddling of the National Institutes of Health and second, The National Cancer Institute along with the Food and Drug Administration (FDA) making it difficult, if not impossible, for doctors with breakthrough cancer therapies to bring their healing discoveries to those who need them.

The *experimental* orthodox medical establishment is committed to destroy anyone who dares to challenge the status quo on cancer treatment. Even though we have lost the war on cancer, we continue to use and promote the very methods that *don't* work while banishing those who try non-pharmaceutical modalities to the scrap heap of healing. Through protectionism, patents and the swinging-door policy at the FDA and drugs companies, the "vultures" are picking our bones. Consider the following:

The New England Journal of Medicine reported that women who had their entire breast removed (radical mastectomy) didn't live any longer than those who opted for the less-invasive lumpectomy.

Men who had their prostate gland removed after a diagnosis of cancer lived just as long as those who didn't. Either way the men lived about 14 years after diagnosis.

Chemotherapy helps only 2% of cancer patients, short term.

Infection is the most frequent cause of death in cancer patients; and those infections are likely to have been picked up in a hospital.

Medical Doctors Now Are *Leading* Cause of Death

Writing for the Journal of the American Medical Association (JAMA) volume 284 Number 4, July 26, 2000, Barbara Starfield, M.D., states, "The fact is that the US population does not have anywhere near the best health in the world. Of 13 countries in a recent comparison, the United States ranks an average of 12th out of 16 available health indicators. Countries in order of their average ranking on the health indicators, with the first being the best, are Japan, Sweden, Canada, France, Australia, Spain, Finland, the Netherlands, the United Kingdom, Denmark, Belgium, the United States and Germany."

Our healthcare system also may contribute to poor health through its adverse effects. For example, United States estimates of the combined effect of errors and adverse effects that occur because of iatrogenic (physician caused) damage not associated with recognizable error include:

1. 69,136 deaths/year from unnecessary surgery and procedures
2. 98,000 deaths/year from medical errors in hospitals
3. 108,000 deaths/year from hospital induced malnutrition
4. 203,000 deaths/year from nosocomial (hospital acquired) infections and bed sores.
5. 106,000 deaths/year from non-error, adverse effects of medications
6. 199,000 deaths/year from doctors treating outpatients

The above equals **783,136** deaths per year from iatrogenic causes. These are for deaths only and do not include adverse effects that are associated with disability or discomfort.

The above deaths per year caused by orthodox medical doctors, now constitutes the *leading* cause of death in the United States, after deaths from cancer and heart "disease."

Adverse effects in outpatient care, other than death concluded between 4% and 18% of consecutive patients experience adverse effects in out-patients settings causing:

1. 116 million extra physician visits
2. 77 million extra prescriptions
3. 17 million emergency department visits
4. 8 million hospitalizations
5. 3 million long-term admissions
6. 77 billion dollars in EXTRA COSTS!

Remember, it took ten years to lose 55,000 American soldiers in the Vietnam Conflict. People were rioting in the streets to stop the carnage. Modern medicine kills more than that every 30 days! Why aren't we at least picketing the hospitals or demanding accountability and improvement?

Cancer - According to the International Agency for Research on Cancer of the World Health Organization, the following information was reported:

Females

In 1950 for females - newborn to 85 years old, there were 103,690 deaths or 136.7 individuals per 100,000 population died from cancer.

Increasing every year, in 1998 for females - newborn to 85 years old, there were 259,462 deaths or 187.7 individuals per 100,000 population died from cancer. This is an increase of almost 40%.

Males

In 1950 for males - newborn to 85 years old, there were 106,904 deaths or 142.9 individuals per 100,000 population died from cancer.

Increasing every year, in 1998 for males - newborn to 85 years old, there were 282,057 deaths or 213.6 per 100,000 population died from cancer. This is an increase of almost 50%.

When I first started practicing natural healing 34 years ago, one out of ten people were acquiring cancer. As of 2004, one out of every 2.5 people is getting cancer. The majority of Americans still haven't learned how to "bridge the gap," detoxify the body, avoid contaminant's, rebuild their immune system with whole-food nutrition, and eat all organic foods. We still suffer for our ignorance. However, after reading this book, it is my sincere hope you have learned enough to effectuate a significant change in your life.

California Sun

As reported in the Fall 2001 issue in the *California Sun*, a science, health and environmental newspaper, *"Allopathic Doctors Kill More People than Guns and Traffic Accidents."*

According to the report taken from the *Journal of the American Medical Association* (JAMA), in the year 2000 the drug and pharmaceutical industry did $182 *billion* in sales world-wide. However, there was a little extra in it for those prescribing all those drugs; they made $183 *billion* to treat the adverse reactions. This is not the cost of treating regular illnesses and injuries; this is just what it cost to treat the aftereffects of toxic drug therapy.

Basically, the number of people that medical doctors kill per day from medical malpractice is roughly equal to the amount of people that would die if everyday, three jumbo jets crashed and killed everyone on board. Just imagine the headlines if a chiropractor or naturopath accidentally killed just one patient?

These statistics are cleverly covered up under the heading of *iatrogenic* deaths. Of course the average person on the street has no idea what that means. It literally means physician-induced or caused. According to JAMA as of 2000, one out of every five people (20%) who visit an allopath (orthodox medical doctor) will suffer an *iatrogenic* injury and/or death. I am sure these "reported" percentages have risen yearly ever since.

Again, according to JAMA, sixteen (16%) percent of all people who die in the hospital are determined by autopsy to have died of something other than their admission diagnosis. In other words, the doctor had no idea what was really wrong with the patient and therefore, the patient may have died for want of appropriate care that would have been subsequent to an accurate diagnosis.

Los Angeles Times

In an in-depth article by David Willman as reported in the Los Angeles Times, ten drugs were finally pulled by the FDA after allowing these killers to be on the market for years. It is interesting to note, although parents, doctors, scientists and others vehemently complained about many of these "medicines," it wasn't until most of the drugs reached profitability status before they were banned.

1. Lotronex - (by Glaxo-Wellcome). FDA administrators dismissed one of its medical officer's emphatic warnings and approved Lotronex, a drug for treating irritable bowel syndrome. Lotronex has been linked to five deaths, the removal of a patient's colon and other bowel surgeries. It was pulled off the market November 28, 2000.

2. The diet pill **Redux** (by Wyeth-Ayerst) was approved in April of 1996 despite an advisory committee's vote against it, was then withdrawn in September 1997 after heart-valve damage and pulmonary hypertension was detected in patients put on the drug. The FDA later received reports identifying Redux as a suspect in 123 deaths.

3. The antibiotic **Raxar** (by Glaxo-Wellcome) was approved in November of 1997 in the face of evidence that it may have caused several fatal heart-rhythm disruptions in clinical studies. FDA officials chose to exclude any mention of the deaths from the drug's label. The maker of the pill withdrew it in October of 1999. Raxar was cited as a suspect in the deaths of 13 patients.

4. The blood pressure medication **Posicor** (by Roche Labs) was approved in June 1997 despite findings by FDA specialists that it might fatally disrupt heart rhythm and interact with certain other drugs, posing potentially severe risk. Posicor was withdrawn one year later; reports cited it as a suspect in 100 deaths.

5. The painkiller **Duract** (by Wyeth-Ayerst) was approved in July 1997 after FDA medical officers warned repeatedly of the drug's liver toxicity. Senior officials sided with the manufacturer in softening the label's warning on the liver threat. The drug was withdrawn 11 months later. By late 1998, the FDA had received voluntary reports citing Duract as a suspect in 68 deaths, including 17 that involved liver failure .

6. The diabetes drug **Rezulin** (by Parke-Davis) was approved in January 1997 over a medical officer's detailed opposition and was withdrawn March 2004 after the agency had linked 91 liver failures to the pill. Reports cite Rezulin as a suspect in 391 deaths.

7. The nighttime heartburn drug **Propulsid** (by Janseen Pharmiceuticals) was approved in 1993 despite evidence that it caused heart-rhythm disorders. The officials who approved the drug failed to consult the agency's own cardiac specialists about the signs of danger. The drug was taken out of pharmacies in July 2000 after seven years and scores of confirmed heart-rhythm deaths. Overall, Propulsid has been cited as a suspect in 302 deaths.

8. Pondimin (by Wyeth-Ayerst) was approved in 1973 for weight loss and obesity, but was discovered to cause pulmonary hypertension and heart valve "disease." It took 24 years to remove this killer in 1997!

9. Then there was **Seldane** (by Hoescht-Marion-Roussel) approved in 1985 for seasonal allergies. Unfortunately, this pill caused severe liver damage and other associated effects too numerous to list. It was finally removed in 1997, 12 years later.

10. Remember **Baycol** (by Bayer)? This magic pill was released in 1997 and promoted to lower cholesterol. However, while doing so it caused severe muscle deterioration, kidney and other organ failure. It took four years and billions of profit later before the FDA got around to banning it.

11. Now we have **Vioxx** (by Merck) for arthritis and inflammation. First released in 1999, the FDA discovered it causes heart valve and other associated "diseases," so in 2004, it was removed from the shelf. Why did it take 5 years?

12. What about the over-the-counter pain reliever **Aleve** (by Bayer)? Released in 1976, after really investigating this little pill, the FDA decided the drug wasn't that safe, but it's still here.

Buyer beware, the arthritis drug **Celebrex** is next.

It doesn't make any difference what drug they approve or not. All drugs are toxic and eventually will show the real effects of their use. Only when they have killed or crippled enough people will our "protective" agencies such as the FDA pull them. But for every drug removed, there are 100 or more standing in the wings to be their replacement.

With the constant removal of once FDA approved "safe" drugs like the above, people are left confused and bewildered. The good news is more and more people are running for their lives to natural healing. In light of the within statistics, I think its a good idea.

Some people will have read this book and feel they can stop their medication immediately. You must *not* attempt to do that. The reason is simple: Medications are addictive. Your body becomes dependent on the medication you are taking. You must wean yourself off all drugs very carefully. It is best to go to your drug-prescribing doctor and have them help you, if they can. In some cases, you may not be able to fully get off of your medication and your doctor may not want to participate in your attempt to heal yourself. In that case, you may need to find a medical doctor that will work with you.

References

Schuster, M., McGlynn, E., Brook R.
How good is the quality of health care in the United States? Milbank Q. 1998; 76:517-563

Kohn, L. ed, Corrigan, J. ed, Donaldson, M. ed
To Error is Human; Building a Safer Health System. Washington, DC: National Academy Press; 1999.

References continued

Starfield, B.
Primary Care: Balancing Health Needs, Services and Technology.
New York, NY: Oxford University Press; 1998

Kunst, A.
Cross-National Comparisons of Socioeconomic Differences in Mortality.
Rotterdam, the Netherlands: Erasmus University, 1997.

Leape, L.
Unnecessary Surgery
Annual Revue Public Health
1992; 13:363-383

Phillips, D., Christenfeld, N., Glynn L.
Increase in US medication-error deaths between 1983-1993 Lancet. 1998; 351:643-644

Lazarou, J., Pomeranz, B., Corey, P.
Incidence of adverse drug reactions in hospitalized patients. JAMA. 1998; 279:1200-1205.

Weingart, S.N., Wilson, R.M., Gibberd, R.W., Harrison, B.
Epidemiology and medical error.
BMJ. 2000; 320:774-777

Wilkinson, R.
Unhealthy Societies: The Afflictions of Inequality.
London, England: Routledge; 1996

Guyer, B., Hoyert, D., Martin, J., Ventura, S., MacDorman, M., Strobino, D.
Annual summary of vital statistics-1998.
Pediatrics
1999;104:1229-1246.

References continued

Harold, L.R., Field, T.S., Gurwitz, J.H.
Knowledge, patterns of care and outcomes of care for generalists and specialists.
Journal General Internal Medicine
1999;14:499-511.

Donahoe, M.T.
Comparing generalist and specialty care: discrepancies, deficiencies and excesses.
Arch Intern Med.
1998;158:1596-1607

Anderson, G., Poulier, J-P.
Health Spending, Access and Outcomes: Trends in Industrialized Countries.
New York, NY: The Commonwealth Fund; 1999.

Mold, J., Stein, H.
The cascade effect in the clinical care of patients.
New England Journal of Medicine.
1986;314:512-514.

Shi, L., Starfield, B.
Income inequality, primary care and health indicators.
Journal Family Practice.
1999;48:275-284

World Health Report 2000.
Accessed June 28, 2000

Notes

Dis-ease is defined as lack of ease or harmony, it is NOT the
same as "disease," a medical term for illness treated by medicine.
NEVER attempt to stop or reduce your medication without the supervision of your medical doctor.

Summary

Chapter 1 - It Started With A Rose (page 9)

In Chapter 1 we learned how important it is to have a healthy childhood, both mentally, emotional, physically and spiritually. We learned what happens when one suffers through loss, loneliness, shock, abandonment, fear, insecurity, worry, anger, resentment, hatred and anxiety, all - contributing factors to sickness and dis-ease. Regardless of your age, these emotions are damaging to everyone, but particularly detrimental to *children*.

Although my mother was taken care of for the first six years of her life by her loving parents, after that, she was not given proper nutrition, love or attention to at least 18 years old. (I question how healthy her diet was even *after* that time). Coupled with lack of forgiveness, you have the perfect recipe for a litany of health problems. If we want our children to be healthy and happy, we must teach by example how to live and be healthy and happy. How can you teach your children how to do that which you do not know? My daughter has never, ever heard me swear. Nor has she heard her mother swear. That's not to say she hasn't heard others speak this way, but she has been brought up to a level of sophistication, intelligence and elegance that does not include gutter language. We must realize our children merely reflect their environment. If we want to teach them love, we must love. If we seek grace and style, we must demonstrate that as well.

If you are feeding your children fast and other processed unhealthy "food" you should not be surprised when they become unhealthy. Nothing replaces a lovingly prepared home-cooked meal. The time you spend preparing organic, nutritious food pays unmeasurable dividends when you realize how it prevents cancer, diabetes, obesity and all other degenerative dis-eases. At all costs, we must get back to traditional approaches to natural living.

Chapter 1 was the horrific history that lead my mother to a lifetime of sickness, dis-ease, pain, suffering and torment. As we know, she did not have to die so young. With the help of this book, perhaps you won't either.

Chapter 2 - The H.O.N.S.T.E.C. Syndrome: The Only *Cause* of Dis-ease (23)

In Chapter 2 we covered the seven common denominators in *all* dis-ease. For the very first time, a syndrome has been discovered and accurately applied to illness. From hydration or more appropriately dehydration to chemical contamination, the following applies:

H - Hydration or the lack thereof: We learned that the body is 75% water, the brain 85% water and that how we think affects us at a cellular/molecular level. Even light, sound and language can reconfigure our cellular/molecular structure. When we don't consume enough water our organs, glands, muscles and other living tissues shrivel, shrink and cease to function at optimum output.

Without sufficient water, we will die within days; however, not *all* waters are the same. We learned to make our own charged distilled water using Zeta Crystals®. This formulae not only encourages water absorption, but it puts the zeta or electrical potential back into the cells.

O - Oxygen/Tissue deprivation. In this section, we found out how vital oxygen is. We learned without oxygen, we die within minutes. Our atmospheric oxygen has dropped 50% in 150 years. We read how anaerobic organisms and pathogens thrive in low oxygen, and therefore as we continue to lose oxygen, bacteria, viruses, parasites and even cancer proliferate. With the addition of aerobic exercise, increased hydration and supplementing with stabilized oxygen, called Stable 'O', we can reverse tissue hypoxia or low oxygen states.

N - Nutritional deficiencies and/or excesses. Eating too much food can be more detrimental to our health than not enough food. We eat because the body demands nutrition. We tend to over eat because *what* we are eating is *not* nutritious. In addition to fluids and our thoughts, we learned that we become what we eat, assimilate and don't eliminate. Only organic food and whole food supplements will ensure optimum health and longevity.

Dis-ease is defined as lack of ease or harmony, it is NOT the same as "disease," a medical term for illness treated by medicine. *NEVER* attempt to stop or reduce your medication without the supervision of your medical doctor.

S - Spinal/Structural/Neurological aberrations. We discovered that every organ, gland, muscle, bone and tissue in the body has a nerve supply. If anything compromises the electrical or chemical flow of our nerves, we can have reduced electrical energy or "CHI" going to wherever the nerve goes. If we have a neurological block going to the kidneys, they will be affected and may become dis-eased. As so it is for the liver, stomach, colon, ovaries and every part of the body. We also learned of the benefit of body/spinal work. From chiropractic, shiatsu, acupuncture, Rolfing to massage and yoga, we became aware of how important nerve flow is.

T - Toxic-Waste Accumulation. Everything we eat produces metabolic wastes. As long as we eliminate this waste in a timely fashion, we minimize toxic accumulation associated with it. If our *digestion* and more importantly, our *elimination* is not working at optimum levels, we can easily acquire auto-immune and/or severe auto-intoxication disorders.

The key to adequate elimination is hydration, diet, exercise and eliminating those substances that slow down or even paralyze the peristaltic action of the large intestines and colon. We learned that we can safely take specific herbs that stimulate the rhythmatic movement of the intestines. We also were taught how to safely do a coffee or lemon-water enema to evacuate the colon and purge the liver and gallbladder. Finally, we realized that a "cold" and/or flu is nothing more than the body forced to open its elimination channels to detoxify. In other words, these so-called "infections" are really just a forced detoxification. If we stop contributing toxins through what and how much we eat, and detoxify on a regular basis, "colds" and flu will be a thing of the past.

E - Emotional/Energetic blocks or release. Up until this point, most of what we have discussed concerned the physical side of our health. In this chapter, we learned about the mental, emotional and spiritual side of our beingness. We found out that E-motion is Energy-in-motion and that when thoughts or feelings come to us and do *not* move through us, we block them. This causes vibratory chaos. Wherever this energy settles, we develop a lack of harmonious energetic flow. Lack of harmony equals lack of ease. Lack of E-motion or E-motional blocking is actually one of the most important causes of dis-ease. We learned that we are not human doings, but we are human beings. We also now know life is about choice. That stress is not a problem. The problem is the way we perceive or handle it. Through forgiveness, we are able to "lift the burdens of life." Nothing is more important than peace, love, joy, health and happiness. We are not here for a long time, but we are here for a good time. We learned to not take life or ourselves so seriously. Once we practice the art of "letting go and letting God," we see things from a different light.

Of all the things we *can* control, our external environment is somewhat beyond it. As a so-called "civilized" society, we should be able to address our concerns to our government. However, we learned that our government regulates polluting industries with a blind eye. We now know that petro-chemical companies lobby our elected officials to de-regulate legislation that can restrict their polluting practices. From hydrocarbons to chem-trails, our food, water and air contribute to the chemical contamination of our planet and bodies. Again, unless we detoxify on a regular basis, we risk the severe health consequences of living on and in a polluted planet and environment.

Creation Consciousness: The Source of Energy

This section was concerned with the spiritual part of being a human and the role organized religion plays. We talked about how religious dogmas, doctrines and rituals were created to control the way we think and believe. We covered the timeline translation history of the Bible and how the word "sin" came from the archery word "syn" or to miss the mark (bulls eye).

We learned there are many translations and transliterations of the Bible. We now know Jesus spoke a language called Aramaic, which is ancient Hebrew and that the Bible was original scribed in his own language. From an Aramaic scholar, Dr. George Lamsa, we became aware of the possibility of over 12,000 mis-translations

Dis-ease is defined as lack of ease or harmony, it is NOT the same as "disease," a medical term for illness treated by medicine. *NEVER* attempt to stop or reduce your medication without the supervision of your medical doctor.

in the King James Bible from the original Peshitta or Eastern Biblical manuscripts.

Perhaps for the first time, we read about dualistic separation contributing to fear. From fear of death to the fear of the unknown, we were told about the purpose of life, one being to re-discover our own divinity. However, we are also here to enjoy this life, including developing relationships and procreating as a consequence of intimacy.

Chapter 3 - Top Twelve Conditions with Their Signs, Signals and Symptoms (73)

In this chapter we discussed the signs, signals and symptoms of twelve dis-eases. From cancer, heart dis-ease, strokes, emphysema, diabetes, hepatitis, obesity, multiple sclerosis, Parkinson's, Alzheimer's, systemic lupus erathymatosus to chronic fatigue, all the above conditions share one common denominator: The H.O.N.S.T.E.C. Syndrome.

In the beginning, we covered how hormones play a part in our health or lack of it. From the pituitary to the pancreas, we were told how medics typically treat dis-eases without getting to the cause. As an example, the adrenal glands alone can cause a weak heart, dizziness, fatigue, depression and impaired digestion.

We find out how life is about choice, and there is nothing we truly have to do. We are in control of our out of controlness.

I told the story about a little girl I helped with a brain cancer known as a Glioblastoma Multiforma. I gave the exact protocol I used to get rid of this terrible illness.

Chapter 4 - Curing Dis-eases w/ Food, Herbs, Supplements, Exercise & More (141)

We learned about every known vitamin, mineral, enzyme, amino and essential fatty acid, antioxidant and even stabilized oxygen. We went into the history of herbology and in detail concerning my LifePack System® of organic whole-food nutraceuticals.

Dis-ease is defined as lack of ease or harmony, it is NOT the same as "disease," a medical term for illness treated by medicine. *NEVER* attempt to stop or reduce your medication without the supervision of your medical doctor.

We covered chiropractic, naturopathic, acupuncture, Rolfing, massage, yoga and other natural-healing techniques suppressed by the American Medical Association (AMA).

This was the longest chapter in the book going into detail concerning all the above subjects.

Chapter 5 - Experimental Orthodox Medical Treatment: Drugs and Politics (243)

In this chapter we covered the politics of medicine. We re-affirmed the money incentive, and that conditions are labeled as "diseases" for insurance reimbursement, medical protectionism and profit.

We went over the inconsistencies of the failing germ theory and other "bug" concepts. We covered the history of naturopathy and what happened to Drs. Harry Hoxsey and Allen Hoffman when they went up against the AMA and their "clan."

Perhaps for the first time, you were able to read the classical Hippocratic oath, instead of the bastardized version our current doctors recite.

Special mention was made to read Daniel Haley's book *The Politics of Healing* for an unbelievable insight into this subject matter.

Chapter 6 - The Chappell Protocol for Health & Longevity:A Step by Step *Intensive* Clinical Program (257)

This chapter covered a step-by-step system to open the elimination channels, de and re-polarize the blood and lymphatic circulation, detoxify the entire body and heal, repair and rebuild the immune system. It is the exact protocol I used in my health and longevity clinic to help those with chronic, severe and so-called "terminal" illnesses.

We covered how The H.O.N.S.T.E.C. Syndrome must be concerned when on any healing protocol - and how our attitude, perception and stubbornness determine how well we will fare when our health is challenged.

We exposed who and what a real quack is, learning that it started with medical doctors that used Quack Salber or quick silver (mercury) in the treatment of their "diseases." We now know, the only doctor that could ever be a quack is one that uses toxic drugs.

You learned how to go through a cold-sheet treatment and do an effective enema, using coffee or lemon-water. Finally, I gave you the dose recommendations for my all-inclusive LifePack®.

Chapter 7 - Seven Miracle Elements Scientifically Proven to *Cure* Diabetes (283)

In this chapter we covered the six herbs and one trace mineral that have been scientifically proven to lower glucose. In so doing, with a proper diet and exercise program, you were taught how you can actually *cure* diabetes along with other degenerative conditions.

From cinnamon, bitter melon, napol cactus, American ginseng, fenugreek, gymnema sylvestre and chromium picolinate, you now know what it takes to heal yourself of sugar intolerance problems, including pre, Type I and Type II diabetes.

Chapter 8 - Health Questionnaire and Effective Evaluations: The First Step to Optimum Health (319)

With the enclosed health questionnaire, hair toxic-metal mineral analysis, urine and saliva test and CBC blood panel, you can easily evaluate your current health status. Taking a natural-healing approach, you can start on a prevention program designed for optimum health and longevity.

Chapter 9 - Current Health Status in America (349)

The leading cause of death in the US is from iatrogenic "diseases," not cancer or heart attacks. Over 783,000 people die yearly from medical doctor error. The FDA approves the drugs that are later found to be harmful. For everyone they remove, they are replaced ten-fold. Our country is rated 13th in world health.

No Goal, Save One

by

Eric C Wyndham

At this stage in my life, I have no agenda, no goals, as it were.
I am not interested in furthering my institutional education.
I am still trying to *unlearn* the hoards of misinformation gained
in our state-controlled and certified schools.

I am not striving for a better career. Even though money plays a
part in this existence, it does not rule my life.
I may want much, but my "needs" are simple.
And my wants, thank God, are ever changing.

I am not hormonally driven to seek out and conquer sexual
experience. Although I am not celibate, I reserve intimate
relationships for tender, loving romance, not impersonal sex.
I have also come to recognize meaningful conversation with time
spent together in harmony, as spiritual foreplay to true intimacy.

I no longer seek God for I have seen Her and She is reflected in my eyes. I have discovered the purpose of my life both physically and spiritually. This purpose is to joyfully express life and assuredly claim my own divinity in every breath I take. I realize when one sees me, they see that which has sent me.

I am not trying to get to "Heaven" for as Jesus said, "Heaven is *within* you." I have long ago accepted this and live accordingly.

But if I had a goal, it would be easy. My goal is to out Love everyone! It is not for noble cause I Love, rather for pure selfishness. For as I receive and transmit our Creator's gift of Love, I get to keep the original copy. I get to "feel" the pleasure and privilege of Loving.

Can you imagine?
Love, manifested in form, projecting Love to itself
for its own joy and pleasure? I do...

Dis-ease is defined as lack of ease or harmony, it is NOT the same as "disease," a medical term for illness treated by medicine. *NEVER* attempt to stop or reduce your medication without the supervision of your medical doctor.

Love

by
Eric C Wyndham

Love. That's it. That's all we need.
Writing more would be redundant hyperbole,
a fraudulent attempt to expand the infinite.

You are as I am,
untethered,
the physical expression of the *Essence* in manifest.

Ah, as sweet as a yellow rose!
Thy heart you touch again and again,
'til the last petal is forever dropping.
For you, my precious, tender friend,
I open my soul.
Thank you for the joy of doing so.

Love. Is it too much to pray for?
I think not.
Merely claim it and it becomes you,
the you, you were meant to be.

We danced by the moonlight,
in perfect rhythm to the shooting stars.
A glance, a chance at jubilant romance.

Love. The quintessence of our reason to be.
The glitter in the eyes of you and me.

Notes

Alternative Medicine

Use of herbal products in this country jumped by 380 percent between 1980 and 1997. (Institute of Medicine)

Between 1997 and 2002, about 38 million adults regularly use herbal medicine. (Harvard Medical School)

An extract of the root of a plant called butterbur (Petasites hybridus) significantly reduces the frequency of migraine headaches. (Reuters Health)

"I've long held the view that the distinction shouldn't be between complementary medicine and pharmaceuticals, but between treatments that have scientific support and those that don't," lead investigator - Dr. Richard B. Lipton. (Reuters Health)

A new government survey of 31,000 U.S. adults found that 36 percent of respondents said they generally used some sort of alternative medicine, including yoga, natural products or massage. (Amanda Gardner HealthDay Reporter)

Worldwide estimates of alternative-medicine usage hovers at about 80 percent, however, the United States still lags behind. (Dr. Stephen E. Straus, director of NCCAM)

Women, people with higher education levels, people who had been hospitalized and former smokers tended to use alternative medicine more. Black adults were also more likely than whites or Asians to use alternatives, particularly including megavitamin therapy and prayer. (Amanda Gardner HealthDay Reporter)

Cancer patients are twice as likely to turn to acupuncture and herbal therapy as people suffering from other diseases are, claims a new study of alternative medicine use. (HealthDayNews)

In the year 2000, malignant tumors were responsible for 12 per cent of the nearly 56 million deaths worldwide from all causes. (World Health Organization)

In 2000, 5.3 million men and 4.7 million women developed a malignant tumor and altogether 6.2 million died from the disease. (World Health Organization)

7% of adults have been told by a doctor or health professional that they have a form of cancer. (National Health

Interview Survey)

Of all cancers, 23 per cent are caused by infectious agents, including hepatitis B and C virus (liver cancer), human papillomaviruses (cervical and ano-genital cancers), and Helicobacter pylori (stomach cancer). (World Health Organization)

Cancer could further increase by 50% (15 million new cases yearly) by the year 2020. (World Health Organization)

Lung cancer is the most common cancer worldwide, accounting for 1.2 million *new* cases annually; followed by cancer of the breast with just over 1 million cases; colorectal, 940,000; stomach, 870,000; liver, 560,000; cervical, 470,000; esophageal, 410,000; head and neck, 390,000; bladder, 330,000; malignant non-Hodgkin lymphomas, 290,000; leukemia, 250,000; prostate and testicular, 250,000; pancreatic, 216,000; ovarian, 190,000; kidney, 190,000; endometrial, 188,000; nervous system, 175,000; melanoma, 133,000; thyroid, 123,000; pharynx, 65,000; and Hodgkin disease, 62,000 cases. (World Health Organization)

Children

Children are exposed to serious health risks from environmental hazards. Over 40% of the global burden of disease attributed to environmental factors falls on children below five years of age, who account for only about 10% of the world's population. (World Health Organization)

Each year, at least three million children under the age of five die due to environment-related diseases. (World Health Organization)

Acute respiratory infections annually kill an estimated two million children under the age of five. As much as 60 percent of acute respiratory infections worldwide are related to environmental conditions. (World Health Organization)

Climate

Of all the water available on earth, about 2.5% is fresh and a good part is inaccessible to us. Only a small fraction is available in rivers, lakes and underground. Increased water use as well as increased pollution means that the amount of usable freshwater is decreasing. (World Health Organization)

Colon Cancer

Colon and rectal cancer are rare in developing countries, but are the second most frequent malignancy in affluent societies. (World Health Organization)

A major cause of colon cancer is a diet rich in fat, refined carbohydrates and animal protein, combined with low physical activity. (World Health Organization)

Migrant populations rapidly reach the higher level of risk of the adopted country, another sign that environmental factors play a major role in colon cancer. (World Health Organization)

Diabetes

At least *171 million* people worldwide have diabetes. It's predicted that by the year 2030 there will be *366 million* people affected. (World Health Organization)

About 40% of diabetes sufferers require oral agents for satisfactory blood glucose control and some 40% need insulin injections. (World Health Organization)

In 2002 alone, about 1.3 million adults between 18 and 79 years of age were diagnosed with diabetes. From 1997 through 2002, the number of new cases of diagnosed diabetes increased from 878,000 to 1,291,000 (a 47% increase). (National Center for Chronic Disease Prevention and Health Promotion)

From 1980 through 2002, the number of Americans with diabetes more than doubled (from 5.8 million to 13.3 million). (National Center for Chronic Disease Prevention and Health Promotion)

Approximately one in every 400 children and adolescents has Type 1 diabetes. (American Diabetes Association)

Cardiovascular disease (CVD) affects millions of adults with diabetes and is a major cause of morbidity and mortality among persons with diabetes. In 2002, 5 million persons aged 35 years and older with diabetes reported being diagnosed with a cardiovascular disease condition (i.e., coronary heart disease, stroke, or other heart condition). Among this group of 5 million adults, 3.4 million reported being diagnosed with coronary heart disease (self-reported coronary heart disease, angina, or heart attack) and 1.3 million reported being diagnosed with a stroke. (National Center for Chronic Disease Prevention and Health Promotion)

In 2000, $40.3 billion was spent for inpatient hospital care and $13.8 billion for nursing home care for people with diabetes. (American Diabetes Association)

Diabetes-related hospitalizations totaled 16.9 million days in 2002. Rates of outpatient care were highest for physician office visits, which included 62.6 million visits to treat persons with diabetes. (American Diabetes Association)

Cardiovascular disease is the most costly complication of diabetes, accounting for more than $17.6 billion of the $91.8 billion annual direct medical costs for diabetes in 2002. (American Diabetes Association)

In 2002, diabetes accounted for a loss of nearly 88 million disability days. (American Diabetes Association)

People with diabetes are two to four times more likely to suffer strokes and once having had a stroke, are two to four times as likely to have a recurrence. (American Diabetes Association)

Fast Food

People who eat fast food frequently are more likely to gain weight and develop insulin resistance, and such eating habits may increase the risk of obesity and Type 2 diabetes. (HealthDayNews)

"There have been no large-scale, long-term studies examining the health effects of fast food, which is surprising given that this is the dominant dietary pattern among children and young adults today," said Ludwig. "In the absence of such data, the fast-food industry is allowed to market their products without restriction to young children." (Dr. David Ludwig, director of the obesity program at Children's Hospital Boston)

Individuals who ate fast food more than twice a week gained an extra 10 pounds and had a twofold greater increase in insulin resistance than people who ate less than once a week at one of these establishments. (HealthDayNews)

"Fast food is designed to promote consumption of the maximum number of calories in the minimum amount of time," he explained. "This may confuse the mechanisms we have to regulate our appetite and the intake of food." (Dr. David Ludwig, director of the obesity program at Children's Hospital Boston)

The kind of foods that are served in fast-food restaurants are generally high-energy density, the portion sizes have gone up dramatically and also there are a lot of soft drinks where we know the sugar seems to be more fattening than in solid foods." (Dr. Arne Astrup, head of the department of human nutrition at Royal Veterinary and Agricultural University in Copenhagen, Denmark)

Triggering heart disease more than any other fat is trans fat, which can be found in most fast foods. Most fast-food chain restaurants fry their foods with a leading source of trans fat, otherwise known as the artery clogging partially hydrogenated vegetable oil (PHO). Burger King, Wendy's, Applebee's, and Krispy Kreme are currently using PHO. (Center for Science in the Public Interest September 24, 2004)

Fast food franchises are appearing more and more frequently in hospitals.

Food Additives

As of 2000, there are about 3,794 different additives, of which over 3,640 are used purely as cosmetics, 63 as food preservatives and 91 as processing aids. (The London Food Commission: Food Adulteration and How to Beat it).

The growth in the use of *food additives* has increased enormously in the past 30 years, totaling now over 600,000 tons per year. (Based on information from Industrial Aids Ltd Depth Study of the food additives industry, London 2000, updated by discussions with market researchers, and Key Note Food Flavorings and Ingredients, London 2002)

Dr Benjamin F. Feingold, M.D., Chief Emeritus, Allergy Department, Kaiser Permanente Hospital, San Francisco, and his team, when working under a National Institute of Health grant, discovered in 1964 that low molecular weight compounds, like artificial food dyes, can produce behavioral disorders in susceptible individuals. (Feingold BF: Food additives and child development. Hospital Practice, 21, 11-12, 17-18, 1973) This study is over 30 years ago. We now know artificial dyes *absolutely* produce behavioral disorders in children and adults.

Genetic Engineering

Genetic engineering (GE) makes it possible to insert foreign genes into the DNA of a host, such as a plant or crop. For example, a gene from a fish could be inserted into a strawberry. These new life forms have never occurred before in nature and cross species barriers, unlike traditional plant breeding or traditional bio-technology. (Greenpeace)

Most of the GE ingredients found in our food come from genetically engineered soy that forms the basis of many processed foods. The vast majority of all GE crops are grown in just three countries: the United States, Argentina and Canada. Amazingly, one single company, - Monsanto, is responsible for more than 91 percent of all GE crops in the world. (Greenpeace)

The Food and Drug Administration, Environmental Protection Agency and the U.S. Department of Agriculture all have a responsibility to regulate genetic engineering. But these agencies only impose voluntary safety measures on GE companies, and do not require the labeling of a product as GE. Conversely, FDA guidelines are designed to make it as difficult as possible for food producers that reject genetically engineered ingredients to label their products as "Non-GE." (Greenpeace)

There have been no long-term studies to determine the effects this new technology has on human health or the environment. (Greenpeace)

Once these new organisms are released into our food supply, there is no way of recalling them. In the decade since commercial genetically engineered crop plantings began, we have witnessed the development and spread of superweeds, sometimes resistant to three different types of herbicides. (Greenpeace)

Global Warming and Energy

Scientists project that the planet's average surface temperature will rise between 2.5 and 10.4 degrees Fahrenheit over the next 100 years if our use of fossil fuels persists at the current rate. (Greenpeace)

The United States accounts for 25 percent of the world's annual global warming pollution, but we only make up four percent of the world's population. (Greenpeace)

Bush administration has refused to take part in international agreements to curb global warming, such as the Kyoto Protocol. (Greenpeace)

The Bush administration has received hefty campaign contributions from fossil fuel companies, including oil giant, ExxonMobil. ExxonMobil has spearheaded efforts to undermine the validity of the science behind global warming and has sabotaged attempts to reach global-warming solutions. (Greenpeace)

While a small rise in global temperature doesn't sound threatening, it actually causes earth's weather systems to be thrown off balance, causing extreme and unpredictable weather events. (Greenpeace)

The only safe solution to global warming is to rapidly phase out fossil fuels. Instead of spending billions of dollars on dirty energy development and weather disaster relief, energy companies and our government could be investing in renewable energy technologies and energy efficiency. (Greenpeace)

Heart

Heart disease has been the leading cause of death in the United States since 1910. Approximately 57 million Americans currently live with some form of cardiovascular disease. (Centers for Disease Control and Prevention). Iatrogenic (physician caused) "disease" is now the leading cause of death.

Since the 1940s, most deaths in the United States have resulted from heart disease, cancer, and other lifestyle diseases. (National Center for Health Statistics, National Office of Vital

Statistics, 1947)

11% of adults have been told by a doctor or health professional that they had heart disease. (National Health Interview Survey – NHIS)

Number of non-institutionalized adults with diagnosed heart disease is 23 million. (National Center for Health Statistics)

21% of adults have been told on two or more visits that they had hypertension. (NHIS)

696,947 numbers of deaths in the year 2002 from heart disease. (National Center for Health Statistics)

Heart disease strikes people with diabetes twice as often as people without diabetes. (American Diabetes Association)

Deaths from heart disease in women with diabetes have increased 23 percent over the past 30 years compared to a 27 percent decrease in women without diabetes. (American Diabetes Association)

Deaths from heart disease in men with diabetes have decreased by only 13 percent compared to a 36 percent decrease in men without diabetes. (American Diabetes Association)

200,000 new and recurrent cases of coronary attack per year; 41 percent of people who experience a coronary attack in a given year die from it. (National Heart, Lung, and Blood Institute's Atherosclerotic Risk in Communities (ARIC) study, 1987 – 2000)

Ocean

Overfishing and pollution have littered our oceans with industrial machines and have irreparably damaged its ecosystems, threatening marine life. (Greenpeace)

The Food and Agriculture Organization of the United Nations estimates that nearly 75 percent of the world's fisheries are overfished. (Greenpeace)

Hundreds of thousands of seabirds, sea turtles and marine mammals are entangled and drowned by irresponsible fishing practices every year, or simply discarded as bycatch. (Greenpeace)

Whales are rapidly approaching extinction due to decreasing fish populations, noise pollution and whaling. Despite a 1986 moratorium on whaling, Japan, Norway and Iceland continue to flout international law by killing whales for profit. (Greenpeace)

The U.S. Navy is also guilty of noise pollution, deploying low-frequency sonar with no regard to the damage caused to whales. (Greenpeace)

Respiratory

2% of adults have been told by a doctor or health professional that they had emphysema. (National Health Interview Survey)

11% have been told they have asthma. (National Health Interview Survey)

9% of adults have been told they have hay fever. (National Health Interview Survey)

14% of adults have been told they have sinusitis. (National Health Interview Survey)

4% have been told they have chronic bronchitis. (National Health Interview Survey)

Smoking

100 million people died worldwide from tobacco-associated diseases (cancer, chronic lung disease, cardiovascular disease and stroke). (World Health Organization)

Half of regular smokers are killed by the habit. (World Health Organization)

One quarter of smokers will die prematurely during middle age (35 to 69 years). (World Health Organization)

90 per cent of lung cancers in both men and women are attributable to cigarette smoking. (World Health Organization)

22% of adults in the U.S. currently smoke cigarettes and another 23% were former smokers. (National Health Interview Survey)

Lung cancer strikes 900,000 men and 330,000 women yearly. (World Health Organization)

Lung cancer is the most common cancer worldwide, accounting for 1.2 million new cases annually. (World Health

Organization)

Sun - Ultraviolet radiation: solar radiation and human health

United Nations Environment Programme (UNEP) has estimated that more than 2 million nonmelanoma skin cancers and 200,000 malignant melanomas occur globally each year.

In the event of a 10% decrease in stratospheric ozone, an additional 300,000 nonmelanoma and 4,500 melanoma skin cancers could be expected worldwide. (United Nations Environment Programme (UNEP)

The worldwide incidence of malignant melanoma continues to increase, and is strongly related to frequency of recreational exposure to the sun and to history of sunburn. (World Health Organization)

The acute effects of UV on the eye include the development of photokeratitis and photoconjunctivitis, which are like sunburn of the delicate skin-like tissue on the surface of the eyeball (cornea) and eyelids. While painful, they are reversible, easily prevented by protective eyewear and have not been associated with any long-term damage. (World Health Organization)

Chronic effects include the possible development of pterygium (a white or cream-colored opaque growth attached to the cornea), squamous cell cancer of the conjunctiva (scaly or plate-like malignancy) and cataracts. (World Health Organization)

Some 20 million people worldwide are currently blind as a result of cataracts. Of these, WHO estimates that as many as 20% may be due to UV exposure. Experts believe that each 1% sustained decrease in stratospheric ozone would result in an increase of 0.5% in the number of cataracts caused by solar UV. (World Health Organization)

Direct viewing of the sun and other extremely bright objects can also seriously damage the very sensitive part of the retina called the yellow spot, fovea or macula leutea. When cells of the fovea are destroyed, people can no longer view fine detail. This is a serious visual impairment making it impossible to read, sew, watch TV, recognize faces, drive a vehicle or do any task which requires recognition of fine details. (World Health Organization)

Toxins - Pesticides

There are three million cases of severe pesticide poisoning and 20,000 deaths globally in 1996. (World Health Organization)

Based on industry reports to the EPA, there are more than 30 cities in 25 states that contain the 112 chemical facilities that threaten one million or more workers and local residents in the event of a toxic release due to a terrorist attack or accidental release. (Greenpeace)

A survey by the Ministry of Agriculture, Food and Fisheries found that 89% to 99% of all fresh fruit, cereals, and vegetables are sprayed with pesticides! That means that pesticides used in animal feed also contaminate most meat and milk. (World Health Organization)

Association for Public Analysts randomly tested 305 fruits: 31 of the samples contained pesticide residues above the safety levels, and another 72 samples showed lower pesticide residues. (Greenpeace)

Health problems are on the rise, including a dramatic increase in cancer rates for American children. The EPA reports that one in six children are now born with elevated levels of mercury in their blood. Mercury is a dangerous neurotoxin emitted from coal-fired power plants. (Greenpeace)

Trans Fats

Trans fat is made when manufacturers add hydrogen to vegetable oil - a process called hydrogenation. Hydrogenation increases the shelf life and flavor stability of foods containing these fats. About 40% of products in supermarkets contain them.

According to the National Heart, Lung, and Blood Institute of the National Institutes of Health, more than 12.5 million Americans have Coronary Heart Disease (CHD), and more than 500,000 die each year. That makes CHD one of the leading causes of death in the United States. Scientific evidence shows that consumption of saturated fat, trans fat, and dietary cholesterol raises low-density lipoprotein (LDL), or "bad" cholesterol, levels, which increases the risk of coronary heart disease (CHD).

Tommy Thompson, the Secretary of Health and Human Services, said at a news conference on the Guidelines on January 12, 2005 that the FDA may recommend that daily intake of trans fat be less than 2 grams, perhaps less than 1 gram.

"By our most conservative estimate, replacement of partially hydrogenated fat in the U.S. diet with natural unhydrogenated vegetable oils would prevent approximately 30,000 premature coronary deaths per year, and epidemiologic evidence suggests this number is closer to 100,000 premature deaths annually." (Conclusion of the top nutritionists at Harvard University)

If the 100,000 figure is correct, then an average of 274 people are dying each day from consuming trans fatty acids.

On May 18, 2004, CSPI filed a petition with the U.S. Food and Drug Administration (FDA) to ban partially hydrogenated oils from our food supply. The Center for Science in the Public Interest (CSPI), which is based in Washington, D.C., is the premier nutrition advocacy organization in the world. Its Nutrition Action Healthletter has more than 800,000 subscribers. CSPI's efforts resulted in the enactment of the law in 1990 that requires Nutrition Facts labels on packaged products sold in the United States.

Further studies found that unlike saturated fat, trans fat also decreases the "good" (HDL) cholesterol in blood. That may well further increase the risk of heart disease. For that reason, some leading researchers think trans fat is even more harmful than saturated fat. In July 2002, the National Academies' Institute of Medicine concluded that the only safe level of trans fat in the diet is zero. (CSPI)

Researchers at the Harvard School of Public Health suggest replacing dietary trans fats with polyunsaturated fats such as vegetable oils, salmon, etc., can reduce diabetes risk by as much as 40%.

Celebrities that have died prematurely

Name	Age	Year	Cause
Frank Sinatra	82	1998	Heart attack
Dean Martin	68	1995	Liver cancer
Sammy Davis, Jr.	64	1989	Throat cancer
Peter Lawford	62	1984	Heart attack
Johnny Carson	79	2005	Emphysema
John Wayne	72	1979	Cancer
George Harrison	58	2001	Cancer
Dave Thomas	69	2002	Liver Cancer
(Founder of Wendy's)			
Robert Urich	55	2002	Cancer
Johnny Unitas	69	2002	Heart attack
Robert Palmer	54	2003	Heart attack
Joey Ramone	49	2001	Lymphoma
Johnny Ramone	55	2004	Prostate cancer
(Founder & Co-founder of the band The Ramones)			
Laura Branigan	47	2004	Brain aneurysm
Charlie Bell	44	2005	Colon cancer
(CEO of McDonald's)			
Gene Kelly	83	1996	Stroke
Terry Melcher	62	2004	Cancer
Johnny Cash	71	2003	Diabetes
Humphrey Bogart	58	1957	Cancer
Alan Ladd	50	1964	Liver failure
Clark Gable	59	1960	Heart attack
WC Fields	66	1960	Liver failure
John Candy	43	1994	Heart attack
Jack Benny	80	1974	Cancer (stomach)
James Cagney	86	1986	Diabetes/Heart
Reggie White	43	2004	Heart attack

Most of these people, we grew up watching on television or listening to on the radio. They had access to the best medicine money could buy and yet, they died from dis-eases widely known as preventable.

I spent over ten years as one of the lot doctors in the largest film studios in Hollywood, California. I consulted actors, producers and directors on health and nutrition and provided chiropractic care. Some of these people learned a few things from my "lectures," most of them did not. They had other things on their mind. However, remember, we become what we think about.

Life is about priorities. Celebrities, as with most of us, do not put their health at the top of their "to do" list. It's just the way it is.

I am a dedicated, dependable teacher. I have to be. When Mother Nature is concerned, there is no room for negotiation. You can't smoke three packs a day and take a little vitamin C thinking you will prevent cancer, emphysema or some other degenerative dis-ease. It will never happen. If you violate the natural order, the healthy "code of conduct," you *will* experience the consequences. There is no escaping it.

Everyday is a gift. We are truly here today and gone tomorrow. We each have the *right* to live the life we desire, albeit in harmony with the planet and all of its inhabitants. For those wanting health and vitality, it is available. I hope this book provides you with the foundation for achieving your healthy dreams. As you have heard, I promise you will improve your health tremendously, if you only try to do what you have learned.

Index C - Suggested Readings & References

Again, *"You learn more about a person from their library than from their diploma(s)."* The following books are highly recommended for those individuals seeking more information relative to true natural healing. The authors are innovators, creators, inventors and pioneers in their chosen field of medicine, health, research and/or spirituality.

Arthritis and Common Sense, Good Health and Common Sense
by Dale Alexander ©1954
Witkower Press
Hartford, Connecticut

Foundations of Health, Handbook of Herbal Healing, The Herbal Prescriber, Echinacea: The Immune Herb
by Christopher Hobbs
Botanica Press
Santa Cruz, CA 95060

Chronic Fatigue Syndrome and the Yeast Connection
by William G. Crook, M.D., © 1992
Professional Books
Jackson, Tennessee

The Yeast Connection: A Medical Breakthrough
by William G. Crook, M.D., © 1986
Vintage Books
New York, New York

Helping Yourself with Foot Reflexology
by Mildred Carter © 1969
Parker Publishing Company, Inc.
West Nyack, N.Y.

Hand Reflexology: Key to Perfect Health
by Mildred Carter, © 1975
Parker Publishing Company, Inc.
West Nyack, N.Y.

"New" Trition
by Dr. George Meinig, © 1987
Bion Publishing
Ojai, CA

Root Canal Cover Up
by Dr. George Meinig, © 1993
Bion Publishing
Ojai, CA

Light, Radiation, & You
by Dr. John Ott, © 1982
Devin-Adair, Publishers
Greenwich, Connecticut

Diet Does It, Eat and Grow Beautiful, Dictionary of Foods
by Gayelord Hauser, © 1943
Coward-McCann, Inc
New York, New York

The Cancer Cure That Worked! (The story of Royal Rife)
by Barry Lynes, © 1987
Marcus Books
Queensville, Ontario Canada

The Life and Trials of Gaston Naessens:
The Galileo of the Microscope
by Christopher Bird, © 1990
Les Presses de l'Universite de la Personne Inc
St. Lambert, Quebec Canada

A Cancer Therapy: Results of Fifty Cases
by Max Gerson, M.D., © 1958
Totality Books
Del Mar, California

Bach Flower Remedies
by Dr. Philip M. Chancellor, © 1971
Keats Publishing, Inc.
New Canaan, Connecticut

Getting Well Again, The Healing Journey
by O. Carl Simonton, M.D., © 1978
Bantam Books
New York, New York

Nutrition for Women, Progesterone in Orthomolecular Medicine
by Ray Peat, Ph.D., © 1981
Blake College Publishing
Santa Barbara, CA

Arthritis and Folk Medicine
by D.C. Jarvis, M.D.,© 1960
Fawcett Publications
Greenwich, Connecticut

Banish Constipation & Colitis, Medicinal Value of Natural Foods, Cure That Cold
by Dr. W.H. Graves, © 1936, 1950 & 1954
Graves Publishing Company
Santa Barbara, CA

The Choice Is Clear
by Dr. Allen E. Banik, © 1971
Acres USA
Raytown, Missouri

Politics in Healing
by Daniel Haley, © 2000
Potomac Valley Press
Washington, DC
1-800-898-0639

MUST READ!

DMSO: A Short Course on Description use Functions
by Robert D. Gutting, © 1981
Tecbook Publications
Topeka, Kansas

Diagnostic Usefulness of Trace Elements in Human Hair
by Jeffrey Bland, Ph.D., © 1981
Northwest Diagnostic Services
Bellevue, Washington

The Metabolic Types
by Dr. William D. Kelly, © 1980
VM Nutri Inc
Lake Geneva, WI

Medicines for the New Age
by Edgar Cayce, © 1975
Virginia Beach, Virginia

The Oxygen Answer for Health and Healing
by Tonita d'Raye, © 1999
Awieca Publishing Company
Keizer, Oregon

Assess Your True Risk of Breast Cancer
by Patricia T. Kelly, Ph.D., © 2000
Henry Holt and Company
New York, New York

Water: The Shocking Truth
by Drs. Patricia and Paul Bragg
Health Science
Santa Barbara, CA

The Stress of Life
by Hans Selye, M.D., © 1956
McGraw-Hill
New York, New York

Get Off The Menopause Roller Coaster
by Dr. Shari Lieberman
Avery Publishing
New York, New York

Chelation Extends Life
by James J. Julian, M.D., © 1981
Wellness Press
Hollywood, CA

Vitamin E for Ailing and Healthy Hearts
by Wilfrid E. Shute, M.D., © 1969
Pyramid House
New York, New York

God's Healing Leaves
by Robert McClintock, N.D., © 1998
Remnant Publications
Rice, WA

Vaccines: Are They Really Safe and Effective?
by Neil Z. Miller, © 1992
New Atlantean Press
Santa Fe, New Mexico

MUST READ!

Hemp Foods & Oils for Health
by Gero Leson and Petra Pless, © 1999
Hemptech
Sebastopol, CA

Alive and Well
by Philip E. Binzel, M.D., © 1994
American Media
Westlake, CA

Olive Leaf Extract
by Dr. Morton Walker, © 1997
Kensington Publishing
New York, New York

Glutathione GSH, The Ultimate GSH
by Jimmy Gutman, M.D., © 1998
Gutman & Schettini
Montreal, Canada

Quantum Medicine
by Paul Yanick Jr., Ph.D., N.D., © 2000
WriterService Publications
Portland, OR

Health in the 21st Century
by Francisco Contrereas, M.D., © 1997
InterPacific Press
Chula Vista, CA

Miracle Healing from China: QIGONG
by Charles T. McGee, M.D., © 1994
MEDIPRESS
Coeur d'Alene, ID

The Complete Book of Essential Oils & Aromatherapy
by Valerie Ann Worwood, © 1991
New World Library
Navato, CA

Siberian Ginseng: An Introduction to Concept of Adaptogenic Medicine
by Bruce Halstead, M.D., © 1984
Oriental Healing Arts Institute
Long Beach, CA

The DMSO Handbook
by Bruce Halstead, M.D., © 1981
Golden Quill Publishers
Colton, CA

Fossil Stony Coral Minerals and Their Nutritional Application
by Bruce Halstead, M.D., © 1999
Health Digest Publishing Company
Cannon Beach, OR

The Canary and Chronic Fatigue
by Majid Ali, M.D., © 1994
Life Span Press
Denville, New Jersey

Confessions of a Medical Heretic
by Robert S. Mendelsohn, M.D., © 1979
Beaverbooks
Pickering, Ontario Canada

Indium: The Missing Trace Mineral
by Dr. Robert Lyons, © 2000
Lyons Publishing
Budapest, Hungary

The Miracle of Fasting
by Paul C. Bragg, N.D., Ph.D., ©
Health Science
Hot Springs, CA

Back to Eden
by Jethro Kloss, © 1939
Back to Eden Publishing Company
Loma Linda, CA

1. Childhood Diseases, 2. Three Day Cleansing Program and Mucusless Diet, 3. The Cold Sheet Treatment, 4. The Incurables, 5. Dr. John Christopher: School of Natural Healing
by Dr. John Christopher, © 1976
BiWorld Publishers
Provo, Utah

1. Let's Have Healthy Children, 2. Let's Cook It Right, 3. Let's Get Well, 4. Let's Eat Right to Keep Fit, 5. Vitality Through Planned Nutrition
by Adelle Davis, © 1951
Harcourt, Brace and Company
New York, New York

1. How to Get Well, 2. Every Women's Book, 3. Airola Diet Cookbook, 4. Miracle of Garlic, 5. Are You Confused?, 6. How to Keep Slim, 7. Healthy and Young with Juice Fasting, 8. Cancer: Causes, Prevention and Treatment, 9. Rejuvenation 10. Secrets from Around the World, 11. Swedish Beauty Secrets, 12. Stop Hair Loss, 13. There Is a Cure for Arthritis, 14. Health Secrets from Europe, 15. Sex and Nutrition, 16. Hypoglycemia.
by Paavo Airola, N.D., Ph.D., © 1974
Health Plus Publishers
Phoenix, Arizona

Trace Elements, Hair Analysis and Nutrition
by Richard Passwater, Ph.D. and Elmer M. Cranton, M.D. © 1983
Keats Publishing
New Canaan, Connecticut

Perfect Health
by Deepak Chopra, M.D., © 1991
Harmony Books
New York, New York

World Without Cancer
by G. Edward Griffin, © 1974 - 2001
America Media
Westlake Village, CA 91359
www.realityzone.com
1-800-595-6596
All books of G. Edward Griffin.
Mr. Griffin is one of my favorite writers
and the most courageous man I have ever met.

MUST READ!

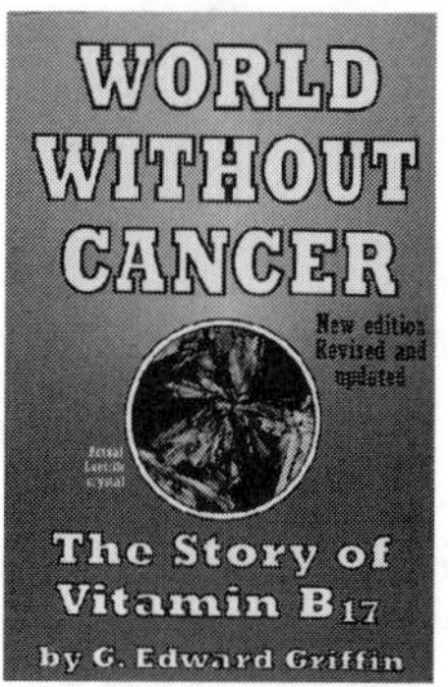

Reflections on a Philosophy
by Forrest C. Shaklee, Sr., © 1973
Benjamin Company
New York, New York

1. Seeds and Sprouts for Life, 2. You Can Feel Wonderful: Enjoy It Now, 3. Joy of Living and How to Attain It, 4. Vital Foods for Total Health, 5. You Can Master Disease, 6. Beauty & Charm at a Glance
by Bernard Jensen, D.C.
Bernard Jensen Publishing
Solana Beach, CA

Notes

"The birth of a man is the birth of his sorrow. The longer he lives, the more stupid he becomes, because his anxiety to avoid unavoidable death becomes more and more acute. What bitterness! He lives for what is always out of reach! His thirst for survival in the future makes him incapable of living in the present."

- Chang-Tzu

"Man did not weave the web of life, he is merely a strand in it. Whatever he does to the web, he does to himself." **- Chief Seattle**

"We shall overcome because a lie can not live forever."

- Martin Luther King, Jr.

"The most serious potential danger associated with experimental orthodox medicine is that a patient may avoid or delay receipt of safe, natural healing care in a timely fashion leading to irreversible damage caused by toxic drugs, mutilating surgeries and medieval carcinogenic radiation." ***- James Chappell, D.C., N.D., Ph.D.***

"Health is a frame of mind, a matter of attitude, of eating proper foods and knowing what elements are available to us to facilitate healing." ***- Kurt Donsbach, D.C.***

"The laws of God and Nature are immutable: They can not long be broken without retribution. Life in its fullness is Mother Nature obeyed." **- Weston Price, D.D.S.**

"There is no room in the Hall of Fame for the founder of a cure that involves eating certain foods and giving up others. Dis-ease is so easily prevented and so easily cured, it warrants no 'heroes'."

- Giraud Campbell, D.O.

"Germs, bacteria, virus and alike, are scavengers and can live only on wasting-away cells, mucous and toxic conditions. They can never exist in a healthy and clean cell structure or body."

- John Christopher, N.D., M.H.

Dis-ease is defined as lack of ease or harmony, it is NOT the
same as "disease," a medical term for illness treated by medicine.
NEVER attempt to stop or reduce your medication without the supervision of your medical doctor.

"The key to health is simple: If we do not eat the kind of food, prepared properly, which will nourish the body constructively, we not only die prematurely, we suffer along the way."

- Norman Walker, D.Sc.

"It is never too late to begin creating the bodies we want instead of the ones we mistakenly assume we are stuck with."

- Deepak Chopra, M.D.

"There is only one thing more powerful than all the armies of the world, that is an idea whose time has come." **- Victor Hugo**

"Science without religion is lame, religion without science is blind." **- Albert Einstein**

"Our scientific power has outrun our spiritual power. We have guided missiles and misguided men." **- Martin Luther King, Jr.**

"I do not feel obliged to believe that the same God who has endowed us with sense, reason, and intellect has intended us to forgo their use." **- Galileo Galilei**

"The whole history of science has been the gradual realization that events do not happen in an arbitrary manner, but that they reflect a certain underlying order, which may or may not be divinely inspired." **- Stephen W. Hawking**

"When I despair, I remember that all through history the ways of truth and love have always won. There have been tyrants, and murderers, and for a time they can seem invincible, but in the end they always fall. Think of it...always." **- Mahatma Gandhi**

"To confine our attention to terrestrial matters would be to limit the human spirit." **- Stephen W. Hawking**

"I believe there is no source of deception in the investigation of nature which can compare with a fixed belief that certain kinds of phenomena are impossible." **- William James**

"No theory of reality compatible with quantum theory can require spatially separate events to be independent." ` **- J.S. Bell**

"The visible world is the invisible organization of energy."
- Heinz Pagels

"There is no reality in the absence of observation."
- The Copenhagen Interpretation of Quantum Mechanics

"If quantum mechanics hasn't profoundly shocked you, you haven't understood it yet." **- Niels Bohr**

"Man can learn nothing except by going from the known to the unknown." **- Claude Bernard**

"The warrior steps forth to accept the unknown and challenge disbelief, for if it lies in mind it Is, by God!" **- Ramtha**

"Sometimes I've believed as many as six impossible things before breakfast." **- Lewis Carroll**

"Your theory is crazy, but it's not crazy enough to be true."
- Niels Bohr

"To know that we know what we know, and to know that we do not know what we do not know, that is true knowledge." **- Copernicus**

"Few people are capable of expressing with equanimity opinions which differ from the prejudices of their social environment. Most people are even incapable of forming such opinions."
- Albert Einstein

"Whoever talks about Planck's constant and does not feel at least a little giddy obviously doesn't appreciate what he is talking about." **- Niels Bohr**

"The opposite of a fact is falsehood, but the opposite of one profound truth may very well be another profound truth."
- Niels Bohr

"The sense of being which in calm hours arises, we know not how, in the soul, is not diverse from things, from space, from light, from time, from man, but one with them and proceeds obviously from the same source. Here is the fountain of action and of thought. We lie in the lap of immense intelligence." **- Ralph Waldo Emerson**

"The power of Thought, the magic of the Mind!" **- Lord Byron**

"How wonderful that we have met with a paradox. Now we have some hope of making progress." **- Niels Bohr**

"The most beautiful thing we can experience is the mystical. It is the source of all true art and science." **- Albert Einstein**

"Do you remember how electrical currents and 'unseen waves' were laughed at? The knowledge about man is still in its infancy."
- Albert Einstein

"It gives me a deep comforting sense that 'things seen are temporal and things unseen are eternal." **- Helen Keller**

"You cannot see anything that you do not first contemplate as a reality."
- Ramtha

"The greatest discovery of my generation is that a human being can alter his life by altering his attitudes." **- William James**

"We feel and know that we are eternal." **- Edmund Spenser**

"As far as we can discern, the sole purpose of existence is to kindle a light in the darkness of being." **- Carl Jung**

"Time is not a line, but a series of now points." **- Taisen Deshimaru**

"Consciousness is a being, the nature of which is to be conscious of the nothingness of itself." **- Jean-Paul Sartre**

"The spirit down here in man and the spirit up there in the sun, in reality are only one spirit, and there is no other one."
- The Upanishads

"The dissenter is every human being at those moments of his life when he resigns momentarily from the herd and thinks for himself."
- Archibald MacLeish

"The mystery of life is not a problem to be solved but a reality to be experienced." **- Aart Van Der Leeuw**

"Go confidently in the direction of your dreams! Live the life you've imagined. As you simplify your life, the law of the universe will be simpler." **- Henry David Thoreau**

"Cease from practice based on intellectual understanding, pursuing words, and following after speech, and learn the backward step that turns your light inward to illuminate yourself. Body and mind of themselves will drop away, and your original face will be manifest." **- Dogen**

"Although each of us obviously inhabits a separate physical body, the laboratory data from a hundred years of parapsychology research strongly indicate that there is no separation in consciousness." **- Russell Targ**

"Who looks outside, dreams; who looks inside, awakes."
- Carl Gustav Jung

"I can see, and that is why I can be happy, in what you call the dark, but which to me is golden. I can see a God-made world, not a man-made world." **- Helen Keller**

"The gift of fantasy has meant more to me than my talent for absorbing knowledge." **- Albert Einstein**

"Life is short. Eat dessert first." **- James Murray**

"Man will occasionally stumble over the truth, but usually manages to pick himself up, walk over or around it and carry on."
- Winston Churchill

"The truth dazzles gradually, or else the world would be blind."
- Emily Dickinson

"Everything you see has its roots in the unseen world. The forms may change, yet the essence remains the same. Every wonderful sight will vanish; every sweet word will fade, but do not be disheartened. The source they come from is eternal, growing, branching out, giving new life and new joy. Why do you weep? The source is within you And this whole world is springing up from it."
- Jelauddin Rumi

"A full-spectrum approach to human consciousness and behavior means that men and women have available to them a spectrum of knowing. A spectrum that includes at the very least, the eye of flesh, the eye of mind, and the eye of spirit." **- Ken Wilber**

"All speech, action, and behavior are fluctuations of consciousness. All life emerges from and is sustained in, consciousness. The whole universe is the expression of consciousness. The reality of the universe is one unbounded ocean of consciousness in motion. **- Maharishi Mahesh Yogi**

"Consciousness is the basis of all life and the field of all possibilities. Its nature is to expand and unfold its full potential. The impulse to evolve is thus inherent in the very nature of life."
- Maharishi Mahesh Yogi

"Knowledge is structured in consciousness. The process of education takes place in the field of consciousness; the prerequisite to complete education is therefore the full development of consciousness; enlightenment. Knowledge is not the basis of enlightenment, enlightenment is the basis of knowledge."
- Maharishi Mahesh Yogi

"We are the physical manifestation of the essence of our collective consciousness. We are the I AM. To see us is to see that which sent us." **- James Chappell**

"All that we are is the result of what we have thought. The mind is everything. What we think, we become."
- Maharishi Mahesh Yogi

"All truths are easy to understand once they are discovered; the point is to discover them." **- Galileo Galilei**

"Perhaps in time the so-called Dark Ages will be thought of as including our own." **- George C. Lichtenberg**

"That which the dream shows is the shadow of such wisdom as exists in man, even if during his waking state he may know nothing about it. We do not know it because we are fooling away our time with outward and perishing things, and are asleep in regard to that which is real within ourself." **- Philipus Aureolus Paracelsus**

"When a man undertakes to create something, he establishes a new heaven, as it were, and from it the work that he desires to create flows into him... For such is the immensity of man that he is greater than heaven and earth." **- Philipus Aureolus Paracelsus**

"The universe on a very basic level could be a vast web of particles which remain in contact with one another over distance, and in no time." **- R. Nadeau and M. Kafatos**

"The state of least excitation of consciousness is the field of all possibilities." **- Maharishi Mahesh Yogi**

"If I could take all your words away and give you but a sparse few, they would be: 'I now know, I am absolute, I am complete, I am God, I am.' If there were no other words but these, you would no longer be limited to this plane." **- Ramtha**

"Two things are infinite: the universe and human stupidity and I'm not sure about the universe." **- Albert Einstein**

"Perhaps there is a pattern set up in the heavens for one who desires to see it, and having seen it, to find one in himself." **- Plato**

"Know thyself." **- Socrates**

"Reality is not only stranger than we suppose but stranger than we can suppose." **- J. B. S. Haldane**

"Quit thy childhood, my friend, and wake up!"
- Jean-Jacques Rousseau

"I want to know how God created this world. I am not interested in this or that phenomenon, in the spectrum of this or that element. I want to know His thoughts; the rest are details. " **- Albert Einstein**

"Suddenly, from behind the rim of the moon, in long, slow-motion moments of immense majesty, there emerges a sparkling blue and white jewel, a light, delicate, sky-blue sphere laced with slowly swirling veils of white, rising gradually like a small pearl in a thick sea of black mystery. It takes more than a moment to fully realize this is Earth, home. My view of our planet was a glimpse of divinity." **- Edgar Mitchell, Apollo 14 astronaut and founder, Institute of Noetic Sciences**

"All matter originates and exists only by virtue of a force. We must assume behind this force the existence of a conscious and intelligent Mind. This Mind is the matrix of all matter."
- Max Planck, Nobel Prize-winning Father of Quantum Theory

"I used to be a truth seeker until I realized I AM that which I AM seeking." **- James Chappell**

"Mind and intelligence are woven into the fabric of our universe in a way that altogether surpasses our understanding."
- Freeman Dyson

"A man of genius makes no mistakes. His errors are volitional and are the portals of discovery." **- James Joyce**

"Time has ceased to exist, now that I have found my Bliss."
- EC Wyndham

"I have yet to meet a single person from our culture, no matter what his or her educational background, IQ, and specific training, who had powerful transpersonal experiences and continues to subscribe to the materialistic monism of Western science." **- Albert Einstein**

"A hundred times every day I remind myself that my inner and outer life depend upon the labors of other men, living and dead, and that I must exert myself in order to give in the measure as I have received and am still receiving." **- Albert Einstein**

"The significant problems we face cannot be solved at the same level of thinking we were at when we created them."

- Albert Einstein

"Darkness cannot drive out darkness; only light can do that. Hate cannot drive out hate; only love can do that. Hate multiplies hate, violence multiplies violence, and toughness multiplies toughness, in a descending spiral of destruction. The chain reaction of evil must be broken or we shall be plunged into the dark abyss of annihilation." **- Martin Luther King Jr.**

"In the century now dawning, spirituality, visionary consciousness, and the ability to build and mend human relationships will be more important for the fate and safety of this nation than our capacity to forcefully subdue an enemy. Creating the world we want is a much more subtle but more powerful mode of operation than destroying the one we don't want." **- Marianne Williamson**

"He who joyfully marches in rank and file has already earned my contempt. He has been given a large brain by mistake, since for him the spinal cord would suffice." **- Albert Einstein**

"Nothing exists except atoms and empty space; everything else is opinion." **- Democritus of Abdera**

"To put the world in order, we must first put the nation in order; to put the nation in order, we must put the family in order; to put the family in order, we must cultivate our personal life; and to cultivate our personal life, we must first set our hearts right." **- Confucius**

"The truth is incontrovertible. Malice may attack it, ignorance may deride it, but in the end, there it is." **- Winston Churchill**

"Words ought to be a little wild, for they are the assaults of thoughts on the unthinking." **- John Maynard Keynes**

"We shall not cease from exploration. And the end of all our exploring will be to arrive where we started and know the place for the first time." **- T. S. Eliot**

"All great truths begin as blasphemies." **- George Bernard Shaw**

"What lies behind us and what lies before us are small matters to what lies within us." **- Ralph Waldo Emerson**

"What we are looking for is what is looking." **- St. Francis of Assisi**

"The purpose of life is two-fold: On the physical level, we are here to merely express and enjoy it; as creation, to create. On the spiritual level, we are here to re-discover our own divinity and help others re-discover theirs since we tend to forget this truth as we pass through the portal." **- James Chappell**

"First, a new theory is attacked as absurd; then it is admitted to be true, but obvious and insignificant; finally it is seen to be so important that its adversaries claim that they themselves discovered it." **- William James**

The Greatest Quotes of Benjamin Disraeli:

1. "The secret of success is constancy of purpose."
2. "There are three kinds of lies: lies, damned lies and statistics."
3. "My idea of an agreeable person, said Hugo Bohun, is the person who agrees with me."
4. "To be conscious that you are ignorant is a great step to knowledge."
5. "It is easier to be critical than be correct."
6. "The magic of first love is our ignorance that it can never end."
7. "Patience is a necessary ingredient of genius."
8. "Nature is more powerful than education; time will develop everything."
9. "The disappointment of manhood succeeds to the delusions of youth; let us hope that the heritage of old age is not despair."
10. "Man is not the creature of circumstances. Circumstances are the creatures of men."
11. "Experience is the child of Thought and Thought is the child of Action. We can not learn men from books."
12. " Gladstone is a sophisticated rhetorician, inebriated with the exuberance of his own verbosity and gifted with a egotistical imagination that can at all times command an interminable and inconsistent series of arguments to malign an opponent and to glorify himself."
13. "Everything comes if a man will only wait."
14. "Nurture your mind with great thoughts. To believe in the heroic makes heroes."
15. "The health of the people is really the foundation upon which all their happiness and all their powers as a state depend."

"They that can give up essential liberty to obtain a little temporary safety deserve neither liberty nor safety." -**Benjamin Franklin**

"Never try to teach a hog to sing. It frustrates you and aggravates the hog. In other words, don't throw your pearls before swine."
– Unknown

"Don't follow any advice, no matter how good, until you feel as deeply in your spirit as you think in your mind that the counsel is wise." . **-- David Seabury**

"The world is a dangerous place to live; not because of the people who are evil, but because of the people who don't do anything about it." **-- Albert Einstein**

"There is a sufficiency in the world for man's need but not for man's greed." **~Mohandas K. Gandhi**

"It wasn't the Exxon Valdez captain's driving that caused the Alaskan oil spill. It was yours." ***- Greenpeace advertisement, New York Times, 25 February 1990***

"Your grandchildren will likely find it incredible - or even sinful - that you burned up a gallon of gasoline to fetch a pack of cigarettes!" **- Dr. Paul MacCready, Jr.**

"I have no doubt that we will be successful in harnessing the sun's energy.... If sunbeams were weapons of war, we would have had solar energy centuries ago." **- Sir George Porter**

"When we heal the earth, we heal ourselves." **- David Orr**

"There are some remedies worse than the disease."
- Pubilius Syrus

"Most diseases are the result of medication which has been prescribed to relieve and take away a beneficial and warning symptom on the part of Nature." **- Elbert Hubbard**

"Our own physical body possesses a wisdom which we who inhabit the body lack. We give it orders which make no sense." **- Henry Miller**

"A man too busy to take care of his health is like a mechanic too busy to take care of his tools." **- Spanish Proverb**

"I am dying with the help of too many physicians." **- Alexander the Great**

"America's health care system is second only to Japan, Canada, Sweden, Great Britain ... well, all of Europe. But you can thank your lucky stars we don't live in Paraguay!" **- Homer Simpson**

"Life expectancy would grow by leaps and bounds if green vegetables smelled as good as bacon." - **Doug Larson**

"Health is a state of complete physical, mental and social well-being, and not merely the absence of disease or infirmity." **- World Health Organization, 1948**

"The power of love to change bodies is legendary, built into folklore, common sense, and everyday experience. Love moves the flesh, it pushes matter around. Throughout history, "tender loving care" has uniformly been recognized as a valuable element in healing." **- Larry Dossey**

"In order to change we must be sick and tired of being sick and tired." **- Author Unknown**

Notes

Index E - Resources

As of the date of this printing, the following companies and their prices are still available and good for the products listed.

Other than *QCI Products, LLC* (a company I founded and serve as President), I can *not* publicly endorse any other company. However, I would never *knowingly* recommend a product or company that is <u>not</u> EcoPure, EcoSafe, organic or wild harvested.

Relative to herbal companies, their organic herbs must also be *non*-genetically engineered, *non*-fumigated and *non*-irradiated. I believe the following listed companies are reputable and honorable. When contacting any of the companies below, make sure you ask them if they still use products that fit the above strict recommendations. If not, please let me know.

You can also go on the Internet and seek your own sources, however, please proceed with caution. You *never* know what you are getting.

A Herbal Promise, LLC
Lake Tahoe, NV
1-888-880-2182 or 1-775-831-9320
www.herbalpromise.us

1. Individual Herbs and Compounds

Al Low & Associates, Inc
San Marcos, TX
1-800-807-4779
www.4Rhealthproducts.com

1. Nopal Cactus
2. Aloe Immune (excellent immune modulator)

Arizona Sauna of California, LLC
San Diego, CA
1-619-685-3463
www.azsaunaca.com

1. FAR InFrared Portable Sauna
Est. Cost: $595.00

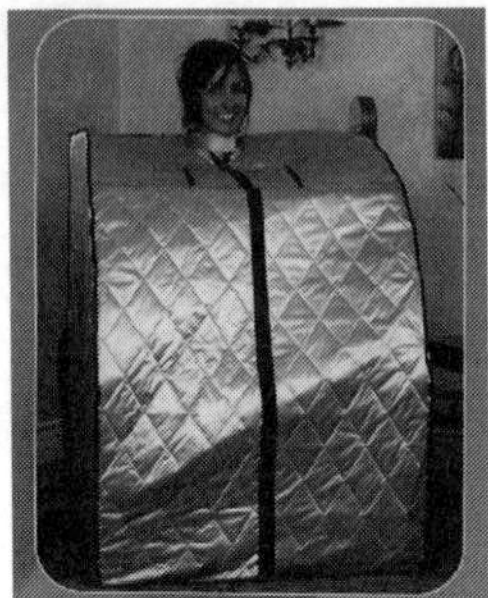

There are over 82,000 lower extremity amputations per year because of diabetes and lack of proper circulation. In addition to the seven elements scientifically proven to lower and stabilize glucose, I highly recommend the Arizona (FAR Infrared) Sauna of California. It is the only *effective* portable unit on the market.

Humans at normal body temperature radiate most strongly in the infrared at a wavelength of about 10 microns (a micron equals one millionth of a meter). The long wave infrared occurs just below "infra" to red light as the next lowest energy band. This level of light is not visible to the human eye, but we can feel this type of light as heat. The earth radiates rays in the 7 to 14 micron range with its peak output at 10 microns.

The *Arizona Sauna of California* has a 95% radiant efficient and a majority of output from 7 to 12 microns during use. It only takes five minutes to pre-heat the unit with operating costs of approximately 10 cents per hour. Only the *Arizona Sauna of California* has a conductive heating of 1030 Watts plus FIR radiation equivalent to 1780 watts thermal energy.

The net result of using this device is that it stimulates the blood and lymphatic circulation, thereby releasing an average volume of perspiration of 500cc per 10 minutes of use. As long as you drink plenty of charged distilled water before, during or after your treatment, you will easily re-hydrate.

The best feature about this sauna is its portability. It takes less than two minutes to set up and weighs only 14 pounds. It is truly state-of-the-art and very affordable. I own and use this unit every day. If you have any health challenge you need to increase your circulation. This FIR Infrared will do it.

Banyon Trading Company
Albuquerque, NM
1-800-953-6424 www.banyantrading.com

1. Gymnema sylvestre
2. Traditional Ayurvedic Herbs & Products

Dis-ease is defined as lack of ease or harmony, it is NOT the same as "disease," a medical term for illness treated by medicine. *NEVER* attempt to stop or reduce your medication without the supervision of your medical doctor.

Coral, LLC
Incline Village, NV
1-800-678-9884
www.coralcalcium.com

1. CoralWhite® (toothtreatment)
Est. Cost: $12.95/tube
2. Fossilized Stony Coral Products: labeled & bulk.

Ecuadorian Rain Forest
West Patterson, NJ
1-973-237-9833
www.intotherainforest.com

1. Bitter melon

EM Labs, LLC
Los Angeles, CA
1-310-364-4558

1. Urine/Saliva Test - Est. Cost $275.00
2. Oxy-Charge® (Ozone) Water Purification System. Est. Cost: $2,500.00 Plus S/H

Farm Sanctuary
Lorri & Gene Bauston
P.O. Box 150
Watkins Glen, NY 14891
www.farmsanctuary.org
1-607-583-2225 (East)
1-530-865-4617 (West)

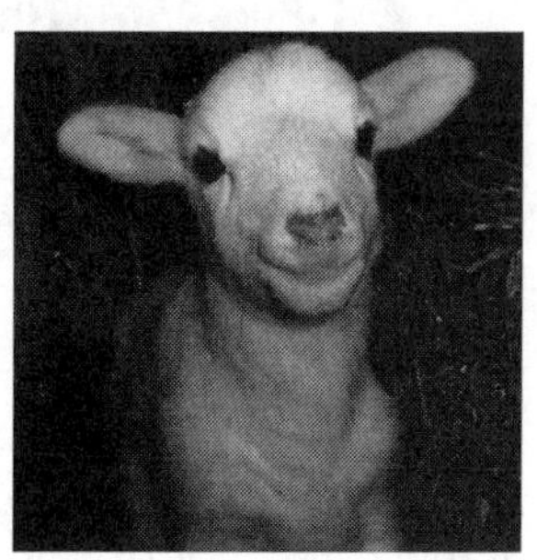

Herba Labs
Courtenay, BC Canada
1-800-209-1723
Att: Ray Neuls

IN CANADA!

1. Above Sea Coral Minerals

Dis-ease is defined as lack of ease or harmony, it is NOT the same as "disease," a medical term for illness treated by medicine. *NEVER* attempt to stop or reduce your medication without the supervision of your medical doctor.

Integrity Health Marketing
19918 Stagg Street
Winnetka, CA 91306
800-850-0355
Att: Cathy Catsoulas

They supply a complete line of nutraceuticals, botanicals and other health products to doctors and retailers. If you want, they can get it!

International Association of Infant Massage
1891 Goodyear Avenue, Suite 622
Ventura, CA 93003
1-805-644-8524

International Institute of Iridology
American College of Iridology
David J. Pesek, Ph.D.
375 Paradise Lane
Waynesville, NC 28785
drpesek@myexcel.com
1-866-456-6100

Life Dynamics
Tustin, CA 92780
1-714-730-0021

Acai

Acai has been used by the people of Brazil for over 500 years. It is one of their most nutritious foods known and now science has confirmed it may be the most nutritious and powerful healing food in the world.

Acai is a dark blueish-purple berry found on the Acai palm tree deep in the Amazon rainforest. For the first time, we now have it in the United States. Even Oprah Winfrey suggests Acai as the #1 "super food" for obtaining optimum health.

It is a well documented fact the French have one of the lowest incidences of heart "disease" of any Westernized society despite smoking and a diet high in saturated animal fats and cholesterol. However, they do love their red wine! (In that respect, they are a lot like the Italiano's). What we now know is red wine is high in an antioxidant, a phytochemical called anthocyanin. Acai is up to 3,000 (30 times) higher in this specific cholesterol controlling substance.

In addition, the United States Department of Agriculture and the American Heart Association suggest we consume at least five servings of fresh fruits and vegetables per day. At that amount, we would be consuming 2,500 ORAC-rated antioxidants. ORAC simply means Oxygen Radical Absorption Capacity. This is a way science rates how many free radicals a substance can neutralize. By adhering to the above 2,500 ORAC recommendations, you can lower your chance of a heart attack by 28%.

Our goal should be to consume the highest ORAC-rated foods possible. For every ounce of Noni juice, you get an ORAC rating of 500. One ounce of Mangosteen is rated at about 550 and Wolfberry juice is rated at 875. However, just two capsules of Acai or Acai PLUS, will give you an ORAC rating of 3,871! This lowers your heart attack risk by 47%. If you then eat five servings of fresh fruits and vegetables daily, you lower your risk by 75%!

With its essential and amino acids, macro and trace minerals, electrolytes, antioxidants, fiber and vitamin C and E, Acai is truly a "super food." It is also part of my LifePack System®.

Ministry Minerals
Brookings, OR
1-888-818-5580
Att: Eva Melody

1. Above Sea Coral Minerals

Pure-Rest®/Earth Pure Products
Ojai, CA 93024 1-805-646-2012
The All Organic Green Sleep Pure-Rest® System

Toxins are a major contributing factor to illness, as I covered under the H.O.N.S.T.E.C. Syndrome. Indoor pollution is one pathway for toxemia. Since we spend most of our time indoors, it is imperative we reduce and/or eliminate as many electro-magnetic, petro-chemical and zeno (synthetic) estrogen based products and materials as possibile.

Because we spend 1/3 of our life in bed, it is critical we create a clean, toxin-free environment. Neuro-excito-toxins not only contribute to restless sleeping patterns and insomina, they cause illness and dis-ease.

I personally use and only recommend the *Atlantis Green Sleep Organic Pure-Rest® System.* The mattress is made of non-treated organic rubber covered in organic wool. It comes in two pieces: one is firm and the other medium density. The box has adjustable wooden slats. This bed does NOT conduct electro- magnetic frequencies (EMF'S) nor has it been sprayed with fire retardant or any other toxic chemical.

Conventional beds conduct EMF's because of the wire coils. They are also made with synthetic fibers treated with different chemicals, fire retardant being one. Pure-Rest® offers a wide assortment of linens, towels, pillows, baby clothes and bedding. The baby mattress is a must for a newborn, if you care about their health.

To purchase a *Green Sleep Pure-Rest® System from Earth Pure Products*, call the number above.

QCI Products, LLC (Membership Only)
P.O. Box 1221
Placentia, CA 92871
1-800-492-1849
www.qciproducts.com

1. Dr. Chappell's LifePack System®

Est. Cost: $199.95/mth
2. Zeta Crystals® Est. Cost: $4.95/mth
3. Glucose Meter & Testing Strips
Est. Cost: $25.00 Meter
$60.00/testing strips (box of 100)
4. pH Testing Paper
Est. Cost: $9.50/roll

Sabinsa
Payson, Utah
1-801-465-8400
www.sabinsa.com

1. Gymnema sylvestre
2. Bitter melon

San Francisco Herbs
Fremont, CA
www.herbspicetea.com
1-800-227-2830

1. Individual Herbs

Talmage Solar Engineering Inc.
/Solar Market/Blue Link Solar Systems
Arundel, Maine 04046
www.bluelinksolar.net.
1-877-785-0088

1. Solar units for homes and business

The Oasis of Hope Hospital
Tijuana, Mexico
1-888-500-4673

Note: This is a complete hospital. It is the only one I am currently recommending for all advanced health challenges. I have been sending patients here for over 30 years.

A Final Word…

When we appreciate, we are appreciated. When we respect, we are respected. A peaceful heart gives one a peaceful mind. And when we Love, we are loved. If your life is *not* what you want it to be, look at who you are, how you think and how you spend your time.

What books, magazines or newspapers do you read? If you still watch television, what do you watch? What music do you listen to? Who do you choose to have as friends? What do you talk about? Do you listen to "talk" radio, if so, who are your favorites and more important, why? Do you belong to any groups, clubs, organizations, religious sects, political parties or associations with rules, regulations, dogmas, rituals or doctrines? Do you practice any new or old traditions? Do you pray or meditate daily? Do you know not to project when praying, but to be quiet, still and listen? Take the time and evaluate your life.

What do you think about? As you know, we become what we think about all day long. If you don't like what you have become, change your thoughts. Change your life. If you are in a dysfunctional relationship or marriage, either fix it or end it. If you hate your job, find another. What are you doing and why?

Some faithful believe God wants them to suffer. If so, why? I thought He was our loving father? Or perhaps She is our loving Mother? There is nothing more powerful than God, yet nothing more loving, for God IS Love. Our ignorance keeps us bound to pain, suffering, anger, resentment, jealousy, sickness and ultimately, a premature death. Even the Christian Bible says in Hosea 4 verse 6, "My people are destroyed (suffer) for their lack of knowledge."

Perhaps knowledge is the key to a happy, healthy life?

Can we ever know too much or Love too much? I don't think so. Knowledge negates fear, fear of the unknown. Without fear, wouldn't your life drastically change? Love also comes from knowing. Once we know who we are, where we came from and where we are going, it is easy to Love ourselves, then Love others. Our goal should be to out Love everyone. In so doing, we become

Love and help others learn how to give and receive it.

When we truly Love life, we Love all of it. The plants, flowers, trees, mountains, rivers, lakes, oceans, deserts, forests and all the life in the sky, water and on land. When we truly Love, we see the invisible thread that connects all life. We become respectful of everything and everyone. After all, how could you hurt or kill someone or thing you Love? That's right, you can't nor can the Great Mystery.

If we want to end war, we could in an instant. However, not if we don't see the connecting thread. Without the thread, we divide humans into male/female, black, white, brown and others, then by political and religious sects, by rich or poor, by city, state, country and continent. Instead of seeing the connecting thread, we divide, divide and divide some more. What if all you saw was energy-in-motion with no discernible form? How could one discriminate then? What if you couldn't tell where your hand ends and the sky starts? What if all you saw were dots on a page, this page? I know we can, for I do.

I hope this book helps you to *unlearn* everything that has kept you from realizing the truth: Love is all there is and we are that!

Dr. James Chappell
October 19, 2005

Of all the songs and poems I have read in my life, nothing has come closer to how I feel about my mother passing then the following song written by the incomparable Beth Nielsen Chapman. Although her words are piercingly soothing, her voice is soulfully angelic. The below song came from her CD entitled, *Sand and Water.* It was written when Beth experienced the loss of her husband and yet it was as if she wrote it for me after losing my mother. May it bless you as it has me a thousand-fold...

No One Knows But You

©1997 Beth Nielsen Chapman

I can almost feel you smiling
From beyond those silver skies
As you watch me finding my way
Here without you in my life

No one knows but you
How I feel inside
No one knows
No one knows but you

I've come so close to believing
All the echoes in the wind
Brushing my hair off my shoulders
I feel you there once again

No one knows but you
How I feel inside
No one knows
No one knows but you

And if there is some magic
Some way around these stars
Some road that I can travel
To get to where you are
I'll cry this empty canyon
An ocean full of tears
And I won't stop believing
That your love is always near

No one knows but you
How I feel inside
No one knows
No one knows but you

[Sweet dreams Mama 'Lucia.' May you finally rest in peace.]